TOPICS IN CLINICAL CHIROPRACTIC Series

Robert D. Mootz, Editor

Chiropractic Technologies

TOPICS IN CLINICAL CHIROPRACTIC Series
Robert D. Mootz, Editor

Chiropractic Care of Special Populations
Robert D. Mootz and Linda J. Bowers

Chiropractic Technologies
Robert D. Mootz and Daniel T. Hansen

Sports Chiropractic
Robert D. Mootz and Kevin A. McCarthy

Best Practices in Clinical Chiropractic
Robert D. Mootz and Howard T. Vernon

TOPICS IN CLINICAL CHIROPRACTIC Series
Robert D. Mootz, Editor

Chiropractic Technologies

Robert D. Mootz, DC
Editor
Topics in Clinical Chiropractic
Associate Medical Director for Chiropractic
State of Washington Department of Labor and Industries
Olympia, Washington

Daniel T. Hansen, DC
Associate Editor
Topics in Clinical Chiropractic
Chiropractic Provider
Assistant Medical Director for Quality and Outcomes Management
Texas Back Institute
Plano, Texas

AN ASPEN PUBLICATION®
Aspen Publishers, Inc.
Gaithersburg, Maryland
1999

The author has made every effort to ensure the accuracy of the information herein. However, appropriate information sources should be consulted, especially for new or unfamiliar procedures. It is the responsibility of every practitioner to evaluate the appropriateness of a particular opinion in the context of actual clinical situations and with due consideration to new developments. The author, editors, and the publisher cannot be held responsible for any typographical or other errors found in this book.

Library of Congress Cataloging-in-Publication Data

Chiropractic technologies/
[edited by] Robert D. Mootz, Daniel T. Hansen.
p. cm.—(Topics in clinical chiropractic series)
Consists of updated articles from Topics in clinical chiropractic.
Includes bibliographical references and index.
ISBN 0-8342-1373-7 (pbk. : alk. paper)
1. Chiropractic Miscellanea.   I. Mootz, Robert D.
II. Hansen, Daniel T.   III. Series. [DNLM: 1. Chiropractic—methods.
WB 905   C545   1999]
RZ242.C456   1999
615.5'34—dc21
DNLM/DLC
for Library of Congress
99-31808
CIP

Copyright © 1999 by Aspen Publishers, Inc.
All rights reserved.

Aspen Publishers, Inc., grants permission for photocopying for limited personal or internal use. This consent does not extend to other kinds of copying, such as copying for general distribution, for advertising or promotional purposes, for creating new collective works, or for resale. For information, address Aspen Publishers, Inc., Permissions Department, 200 Orchard Ridge Drive, Suite 200, Gaithersburg, Maryland 20878.

Orders: (800) 638-8437
Customer Service: (800) 234-1660

About Aspen Publishers • For more than 35 years, Aspen has been a leading professional publisher in a variety of disciplines. Aspen's vast information resources are available in both print and electronic formats. We are committed to providing the highest quality information available in the most appropriate format for our customers. Visit Aspen's Internet site for more information resources, directories, articles, and a searchable version of Aspen's full catalog, including the most recent publications: http://www.aspenpublishers.com
Aspen Publishers, Inc. • The hallmark of quality in publishing
Member of the worldwide Wolters Kluwer group.

Editorial Services: Stephanie Neuben
Library of Congress Catalog Card Number: 99-31808
ISBN: 0-8342-1373-7
Series ISBN: 0-8342-1710-4

Printed in the United States of America

1 2 3 4 5

For Karen, Gayle, Eric, Aren, and Stefan.

Table of Contents

Contributors	ix
Series Preface	xi
Preface	xiii
Understanding and Appropriate Use of Clinical Algorithms	xv
PART I—OVERVIEW	**1**
1—Formal Processes in Health Care Technology Assessment: A Primer for the Chiropractic Profession *Daniel T. Hansen and Robert D. Mootz*	3
2—Public and Occupational Health Regulations in Chiropractic Practice *David Wickes, Grant Iannelli, and John Livingston*	18
3—Decision Analysis: Are Calculations and Clinicians Really on a Collision Course? *Gary D. Schultz*	28
4—Technology Assessment of the Chiropractic Subluxation *Paul J. Osterbauer*	37
APPENDIX I–A—Resource List for Technology Assessment in Health Care	45
APPENDIX I–B—Directory of State and National Public Health Offices	50
APPENDIX I–C—Public Health Resources on the Internet	53
PART II—DIAGNOSTIC TECHNOLOGIES	**57**
5—Improving the Clinician's Use of Orthopedic Testing: An Application to Low Back Pain *Kevin A. McCarthy*	59
6—Clinical Considerations in the Mechanical Assessment of the Cervical Spine *Austin D. McMillin*	70
7—Is Radiography Appropriate for Detecting Subluxations? *Gary D. Schultz and John M. Bassano*	88

8—Diagnostic Imaging of the Cervical Spine following Whiplash-Induced Injury 96
John S. Miller and M. Maggie Craw

9—Imaging Modalities for the Lumbar Spine 106
Sandra M. O'Connor, William S.W. Hsu, and Constance Columbus

10—Advanced Diagnostic Imaging of Adults with Neck or Low Back Pain: A Seed Algorithm 119
Michael Perillo, Mark Hannan, and David Lemberg

11—Diagnostic Ultrasound of the Adult Spine: State of the Technology 126
Gary D. Schultz

12—Optimizing Clinical Use of Radiography and Minimizing Radiation Exposure in Chiropractic Practice 131
Robert D. Mootz, Lisa E. Hoffman, and Daniel T. Hansen

13—Quality Assurance in Chiropractic Radiology 142
John A.M. Taylor and Douglas M. Lawson

PART III—THERAPEUTIC TECHNOLOGIES 147

14—The Use of Expert Panel Results: The RAND Panel for Appropriateness of Manipulation and Mobilization of the Cervical Spine 149
Ian D. Coulter, Paul G. Shekelle, Robert D. Mootz, and Daniel T. Hansen

15—Assessment of Chiropractic Techniques and Procedures 157
Robert Cooperstein and Michael S. Schneider

16—Quantitative Functional Capacity Evaluation: The Missing Link To Outcomes Assessment 165
Steven G. Yeomans and Craig Liebenson

17—Opening Access to Spine Care in the Evolving Market: Integration and Communication 182
John J. Triano, Ralph F. Rashbaum, and Daniel T. Hansen

Index 193

Contributors

John M. Bassano, DC
Los Angeles College of Chiropractic
Whittier, California

Constance Columbus, DC
Department of Radiology
Canadian Memorial Chiropractic
 College
Toronto, Ontario

Robert Cooperstein, DC
Palmer College of Chiropractic–West
San Jose, California

Ian D. Coulter, PhD
RAND
Santa Monica, California
Los Angeles College of Chiropractic
Whittier, California
School of Dentistry, University of
 California Los Angeles
Los Angeles, California

M. Maggie Craw, DC
Private Practice of Radiology
Sacramento, California

Mark Hannan, DC
Private Practice
Merrick, New York

Daniel T. Hansen, DC
Texas Back Institute
Plano, Texas

Lisa E. Hoffman, DC
Western States Chiropractic College
Portland, Oregon

William S.W. Hsu, DC, DACBR
Canadian Memorial Chiropractic
 College
Toronto, Ontario

Grant Iannelli, DC
National College of Chiropractic
Lombard, Illinois

Douglas M. Lawson, DC
College of Chiropractics of Alberta
Private Practice
Calgary, Alberta, Canada

David Lemberg, DC
Private Practice
New York, New York

Craig Liebenson, DC
Private Practice
Santa Monica, California

John Livingston, DC
National College of Chiropractic
Lombard, Illinois

Kevin A. McCarthy, DC
Palmer College of Chiropractic—West
San Jose, California

Austin D. McMillin, DC
Private Practice
Tacoma, Washington

John S. Miller, DC
Private Practice of Radiology and
 Chiropractic
Seattle, Washington

Robert D. Mootz, DC
State of Washington Department of
 Labor and Industries
Olympia, Washington

Sandra M. O'Connor, DC
Canadian Memorial Chiropractic
 College
Toronto, Ontario

Paul J. Osterbauer, DC, MPH
Northwestern College of Chiropractic
Bloomington, Minnesota

Michael Perillo, DC, MPH
Private Practice
Rockville Centre, New York

Ralph F. Rashbaum, MD
Texas Back Institute
Plano, Texas

Michael S. Schneider, DC
Private Practice
Pittsburgh, Pennsylvania

Gary D. Schultz, DC
Los Angeles College of Chiropractic
Whittier, California

Paul G. Shekelle, MD, PhD
West Los Angeles Veteran's Adminis-
 tration Medical Center
RAND
Santa Monica, California

John A.M. Taylor, DC
Western States Chiropractic College
Portland, Oregon

John J. Triano, DC, PhD
Texas Back Institute
Plano, Texas

David Wickes, DC
National College of Chiropractic
Lombard, Illinois

Steven G. Yeomans, DC
Private Practice
Ripon, Wisconsin

Series Preface

This book includes contributions to the first six volumes of *Topics in Clinical Chiropractic* (TICC) that relate the use of "technologies" in chiropractic. Technology in the contemporary health care world includes both the high and low varieties, so basic clinical practices, use of devices, procedural techniques and decision-making are included. This text is part of an initial four-volume series that collects and updates many of the most relevant works from the journal's archives. Where necessary, articles and care pathways have been updated from their initial publication to reflect current practices. The original idea for a scholarly chiropractic journal focusing on clinically relevant topics came from Martha Sasser, an Aspen Publishers, Inc., acquisitions editor at the time. Her first choice for editor was Reed Phillips who was in his ascendancy to president of Los Angeles College of Chiropractic.

Much to the profession's loss, Reed was unable to fit the project on his rather full plate. Martha arranged to meet with me to discuss a "book manuscript review project" during a routine promotional visit to Palmer College of Chiropractic–West where I was professor. Little did I know, but by the time our lunch meeting rolled around, Martha had already met with the President and Dean to secure their support and my release time to take on the editorship of Aspen's new journal, TICC. With great trepidation, I agreed, provided that Aspen would support an expanded associate editor structure that allowed me to spread editorial tasks among eminently more qualified individuals in the publishing world.

Regrettably, most of the people I knew who were experienced with journal editing were also much smarter than I and turned down involvement, leaving me to turn to a cast of good friends and co-workers who knew no more than I did about operating a peer-reviewed scientific journal. And what good fortune that was. Linda Bowers, Dan Hansen, Kevin McCarthy, and Tom Souza all agreed to work on the project under the experienced tutelage of Martha who, before the ink was dry on the contracts, left Aspen for other publishing opportunities.

That left the five of us to make the project into our own, building the editorial board from scratch, developing issue topics, and twisting the arms of chiropractic practitioners, researchers, and academicians to submit their wares to our new upstart of a journal. Luckily, Martha's replacement was Jane Garwood, a bright and supportive Aspen insider who worked diligently and patiently with the five of us to get TICC off and running and assure that resources were there to make it a first class publication. Jane, too, was promoted, followed by Steve Zollo. When Tom Souza left to to write a couple of the profession's most respected textbooks, I was very lucky to have Howie Vernon join our Associate Editor staff.

My thanks go out to Martha Sasser for both her original idea and her persistence in getting it off the ground. I thank Reed Phillips for giving the "second-in-line" the opportunity to make a lasting contribution to chiropractic scholarship. I must especially thank my friends and colleagues, TICC's associate editors, Linda Bowers, Dan Hansen, Kevin McCarthy, Tom Souza, and Howie Vernon for their willingness to give up the incredible amount of time and energy it takes to maintain the quality and consistency that are the journal's hallmarks.

Steve Zollo was responsible for first approaching me to put together this series of essential reading books based on TICC's contributions, but it has been Amy Martin who brought the project through to fruition. Mary Anne Langdon and Stephanie Neuben, whose competence in creating the finished product, has assured its success. In addition, TICC's long-time production editor, Sandy Lunsford, has been an absolute joy to work with. Through three new children she has continued to put up with our publishing naiveté, our missed deadlines, forgotten permission requests, and our stressful last minute revisions. She has been supportive of us, patient, understanding, and resourceful when things just would not come together as planned. She continues to be the behind-the-scenes glue that holds the project together. For our lasting endearment to Sandy: *"Deadlines mean always having to say you're sorry!"*

My thanks also go to all of the authors who submit their work to the journal, particularly the contributors to this book. The quality of their work, and their willingness to share their knowledge is greatly appreciated. A special thanks to the college faculty members that have found value in our publication to make it required reading within their curriculum. And on behalf of the editors and contributors, we would also like to thank our readership—*our customers*—for the valuable feedback toward the improvements we've made and toward the recognition that what we've provided to our profession is meaningful and has made a difference.

I hope you will find the entire series of value for enhancing your educational opportunities, your practice, your community of health care, and mostly to the patients you serve.

—*Robert D. Mootz*
Editor

Preface

The world of health care has changed dramatically in the past decade. Gone forever are the days of the doctor-patient dynamic being the sole constituency for dealing with clinical decision-making. The payers of insurance premiums (mostly employers), the plan administrators (third party administrators, insurance companies, managed care organizations and the like), and government regulators all have a say in the clinical decision-making process today. Unless one chooses to opt out of any kind of third party reimbursement, incorporating communication and partnering strategies between providers, their organizations, and these other constituencies becomes a normal course of business.

Modern health care delivery now requires communication along a common lexicon consistent with customer-focused and community-based health policy. This language is not and should not be reduced to "bureaucratic doublespeak"—it is the language of the industry. Furthermore, contemporary health delivery is now operated according to recognized business and quality management principles. Disciplines desiring to be separate and distinct will face difficult times integrating into this health economy through rejection of accountability by ignoring communication and quality care demands.

In the best of situations, this new multifactorial dynamic can help keep everyone's eye on the laudable objective of optimizing patient outcomes in the most cost-efficient way available. In the worst cases, which sadly make up a large part of modern health care, arbitrary guidelines, uninformed administrative policies, and cutthroat economic competition drive the "individual" need out of individualized care, not to mention the economic jeopardy foisted upon many competent providers.

However, the turmoil and frustration have led to some useful innovations including outcomes management, technology assessment, evidence-based care pathways, and continuous quality improvement processes. As with all good ideas, these approaches have frequently evolved to little more than the latest buzzwords used to justify someone's existing view of the world. Arbitrary cutoffs by payers for all low back pain cases are based on "evidence-based" national guidelines, ignoring that only uncomplicated, acute episodes make up the bulk of the evidence. On the other side, and just as inept, are so-called "evidence-based" guidelines that only interpret the "evidence" to support giving carte blanche for unaccountability to the provider. Somewhere in the middle are reasonable processes and conclusions for providing necessary and effective care that meets patient and community needs. Our goal with this collection is to provide some insight to practitioners on how to best reach that evidence-based middle ground.

As is the case with keeping up with new scientific literature, information overload has seized the world of evidence-based practice. It too is fraught with varying hierarchies of quality, methodology, and underlying agendas. Wrestling with this information, deciding where to invest one's time and energy, and prioritizing which diagnostic tests and care interventions to use requires more skill and insight than ever before. Adding to the equation are proponents of costly new medical devices requiring investments from providers that may never be recouped through payer reimbursement. The end result is a head-turning state of affairs. The sequence from procedure innovation to scientific study to social acceptance to health policy has been formalized and is now well-entrenched in health care communities.

Throughout TICC's tenure, we have tried to solicit submissions and devote entire issues to systematically addressing the various levels of critical appraisal and accountability being established in health care delivery today. This book collects articles that help the practitioner understand what is under the hood of all of the social changes demanding accountability on providers, and reviews the state of available information for a number of technology-specific diagnostic and therapeutic tools DCs regularly grapple with.

We hope that this collection will serve as a useful resource for the things you can offer whether it is in the educational arena, in private or group practice, in newer integrated practice models, in networking within your community of health care, or in health services or health policy pursuits.

Some critics of the movement toward accountability have reduced the efforts of those that have facilitated the chiropractic profession's improved social acceptance as "misguided" and "not representative" of the discipline as a whole. Some have referenced articles or publications using those same key health policy buzzwords as "bureacratic doublespeak." However, some of these critics have turned to the pages of TICC to assist them in shaping their own community-based solutions.

To those responsive and responsible providers, we congratulate you and wish you success. To those who are honorably serving their patients and their community of health care, we hope the material contained in this series of books will help you with communication and ability to network with your "customers." To the students and doctors-in-training, we encourage you to consider this material as your education helps shape your mastery as a Doctor of Chiropractic.

Robert D. Mootz
Daniel T. Hansen

Understanding and Appropriate Use of Clinical Algorithms

Robert D. Mootz and Daniel T. Hansen

Among the most popular features of *Topics in Clinical Chiropractic* (TICC) are the clinical algorithms found in the appendixes of each issue of the journal. When used properly, a well-done clinical algorithm can be an important learning tool in clinical training and can help inform clinical decision making. The editors of TICC decided from the beginning to utilize this tool whenever possible as an adjunct to the presentation of the various clinical topics. Our original 1994 article[1] reviewed the nature and use of clinical algorithms. We update that piece here to allow better appreciation for the intended use and application of these graphic guidelines. In addition to informing the doctors and patients who use them, care pathways for chiropractic procedures can also provide guidance to non-DC providers when a chiropractic referral may be prudent.

RELEVANCE OF ALGORITHMS

The health care system continues to experience turbulent changes in delivery and accountability never before seen in the industry. Where other elements of manufacturing and service industries have been "assuring quality" and "lower costs" for products and services, the health care profession has lagged in its response to this change of culture. Health care providers cannot work a day now without some sort of contact with the new paradigm of health delivery and some element of managed care being applied to their practices. Preauthorization for procedures, benefit limitations, additional or standardized reporting requirements, and utilization reviews are all examples of managed care methodologies that providers must regularly cope with.

These changes are the result of a strong public mandate for the purchase of health care that is patient centered, evidence based and protocol driven. Patient outcome has become the tangible focus of care and coverage decisions. In practice, this means that the selection of diagnostic tests or a sequence of care is increasingly driven by accepted, evidence-based protocols. From a provider's perspective, one of the most useful forms that such guidelines can take are as *algorithms* or *care pathways*.

Because well-done algorithms are clear, concise, and graphically represented, they are an excellent basis for communicating and representing typical considerations in delivering optimal clinical care. They help convey the sequential and linked nature of many care decisions. Well-done algorithms can facilitate thinking through tiers of decisions and can systematically identify emergent and ambiguous clinical considerations. When viewed by other providers and health care administrators, they can offer a sense of predictability and a systematic organization to case management that provides assurance that the approach a chiropractor is using is reasonable and well founded.

Many common conditions have management sequences shown to be clinically efficient. Less variation in the use of

---

Algorithms offered in this book are presented with the intention of clarifying the relationships among various conditions. They are not intended for use as diagnostic guides for individual patients. Each patient's case has its own unique characteristics and must be addressed by someone well trained and competent to render a diagnosis and care. These guidelines are not presented as definitive but rather as examples of typical kinds of thought processes the practicing chiropractor might want to consider. Parameters such as these are designed to assist the DC by providing a framework for the evaluation of the patient in situations characterized by the algorithms. These guidelines are not intended to replace the physician's clinical judgment or to establish a protocol for diagnosis and/or treatment of patients with any particular set of symptoms.

resources can contribute to quicker and more optimal outcomes and, ultimately, to a reduction in health costs.[2] Algorithmic care pathways can be used to communicate expected ranges of care for a majority of patients presenting with those common problems. Physician discretion is then applied to those patients who may exhibit exceptions based on age, sex, comorbidities, or other health complications. Ideally, the algorithm should include insight as to when additional variables or confounding issues can come into play. In the era of highly competitive care, the better we can do in terms of outcomes and cost, compared with others, the more likely it is that we will be considered the provider of choice.

For doctors, this provides benefit, in that those issues that have been demonstrated to impact quality and efficiency (eg, when to order tests, how long to pursue a course of care, and how to sequence second opinions or additional diagnostics) are accessible from an algorithm in a readily identifiable fashion. Such "expert" evidence-based guidance may also benefit the doctor by providing protection from malpractice exposure. On the flip side, poorly written algorithms or inappropriate interpretation by payers may contribute to confusion and inept oversight in managed care settings. An understanding by doctors of algorithm processes and quality can promote the benefits and reduce possibilities of negative consequences from inappropriate use.

Health care disciplines have been developing and publishing algorithms for more than 30 years. In today's environment of accountability, there has been a virtual explosion of these kinds of guidelines, particularly in managed care settings.[1] Development of care pathways is a part of *continuous quality improvement* (CQI) programs. As we move into the twenty-first century, health care "best practice" algorithms are being embedded into sophisticated, network-based or internet-based information systems for ready access and data retrieval by health planners, providers, and even patients themselves. Those who purchase, use, and refer for health services are better informed than ever before. The need for well-done, provider-developed, evidence-based algorithms cannot be understated.

The chiropractic profession is responding to this charge and has developed and published several pertinent algorithms in the management of common presenting patient complaints. Chiropractic colleges and privately owned chiropractic managed care organizations (MCOs) are developing and implementing clinical algorithms for teaching and management purposes.[3]

With the recent surge in algorithm development and publication, there appears to be greater variation in algorithm formats. It has become necessary for some standards to be developed and implemented in the design, development, and production of algorithms. The standards adopted by the editorial board of TICC are included here.

HISTORY OF ALGORITHM USE IN HEALTH CARE

Graphic algorithms have been widely incorporated in health care literature since the mid-1960s. Algorithms have also been seen in the popular press in self-help books focused on common, uncomplicated health management, such as back pain and headache. Technical algorithms are currently being used in many diverse health delivery systems, such as hospitals and health maintenance organizations (HMOs), and among cohesive physician groups, such as IPAs and EPOs. Governmental and academic institutions, as well as both public and private sector payers, are increasingly turning to such graphical presentations to efficiently summarize key clinical thresholds and decision points.

The Hartford Foundation was the primary funding organization in a nationwide demonstration project that incorporated quality improvement principles used in major industries into health delivery systems. From this effort came projects aimed at identifying wasteful health practices and designing solutions for improvement and systems to implement the improvement processes.[4] The National Demonstration Project on Health Care Quality Improvement developed logical sequences for creating clinical algorithms using "quality improvement teams."[5] The effort sought to develop systems and procedures that assure reliability and validity of the algorithms.

The approach taken in the demonstration project was first validated at the Harvard Community Health Plan in Boston. The process incorporated systematically developed algorithms, review and feedback by providers expected to incorporate them, and measurement and follow-up on patient outcomes and quality markers.[5] Since then, the methods for constructing and implementing clinical algorithms have been distributed widely through course work and published literature. Currently, these methods are widely incorporated as essential steps for quality improvement in health care in both the private and public sectors.[6] There are examples of state level requirements that any health care that is purchased be protocol driven, to the extent possible, and based on published evidence and the consensus of recognized experts and community-based practitioners.[7]

ALGORITHM TERMINOLOGY

It is important to distinguish between some of the terms mentioned in this chapter. Whereas for the most part, there are conceptual similarities, there may indeed be subtle or specific differences.

Algorithms are a series of specifically shaped boxes connected by lines, usually with arrow tips. They can serve as pathways for clinical decision making in a step-wise fashion, identifying the more important or critical steps in the beginning and allowing for transitions into other management sequences or terminal steps. Clinical algorithms have their origins from *decision charts*, which analyze the various clinical decisions that can be made for a problem or patient complaint.

Care pathways are essentially the decision-making and process flow components that appear in algorithms. Algorithms represent one way to graphically illustrate a care pathway in a sophisticated, standardized, graphical manner. Whereas a care pathway may be represented by an algorithm, it may also be characterized in narrative fashion, by step-by-step lists or in a nonstandardized flow chart fashion.

Clinical guidelines are systematically developed statements to assist practitioner and patient decisions about appropriate health care for specific clinical circumstances. These can be in the form of rules or algorithms that reflect the best or most appropriate way to care for certain clinical conditions. Ideally, the use of the term *guideline* implies that some form of formalized review or consensus process has been applied to the content. Examples include recent publications from the Agency for Health Care Policy and Research and the Canadian Chiropractic Association.[8,9]

Practice parameters relate to the inventory of health practice in general. The recommendations found in parameters of care documents relate to the acceptance of procedures, devices, and other attributes of medical or chiropractic practice, according to the available science and opinions of recognized experts. They do not make any distinction for the management of condition-specific issues commonly found in practice.[10]

"Seed" algorithms, guidelines, or *pathways* are ideally well-thought-out first efforts at characterizing the components of clinical decision making in an informal fashion by an individual or a small group of authors. Any time the word *seed* appears as a modifier, it can be implied that minimal or no formalized processes of consensus or review were applied in their development. Peer review, local input, and revisions may or may not be inherent in seed efforts but formalized testing, implementation, and consensus methodologies are unlikely to have been incorporated.

Standards of care are legal standards, established by the trier of the fact in malpractice cases, describing the conduct that society finds acceptable. If a doctor's conduct falls below the applicable standard of care, liability may result. Standards of care are identified by evidentiary rules of discovery and expert testimony, and may vary from region to region and from case to case. The legal test of a standard of care is typically based on the trier of fact's assessment as to whether or not a "reasonable" doctor in a "similar" situation would have acted in a "similar" fashion.[11]

Clinical algorithms or clinical guidelines are not the same as standards of care. However, under common law in most states, a practice parameter or practice guideline may be introduced as evidence of a standard of care in a medical negligence case, as long as it is relevant to the clinical issues involved and is demonstrated to be reliable. Even if a practice parameter or practice guideline is introduced as evidence, it is not considered a predetermined standard of care that a court is required to apply.

WHAT ARE ALGORITHMS?

Algorithms are simply a series of "if, then" statements with dichotomous choices and action steps. For example, a paragraph of complex prose could describe how to compute capital gains tax where there are statements that "*if* you did this, that, and the other thing" with your real estate, "*then* you pay this amount." Alternatively, a series of boxes and lines could be used where the "if" questions are asked and the "then" action steps are clearly presented graphically. Obviously, there can be many different applications of algorithmic sequences, and specific situations can involve additional information that is not addressed in a given algorithm. In the chiropractic literature, we have seen numerous applications of graphical algorithms for assessment of technology;[12] development of standardized terminology;[13] diagnostic decision making;[14-16] and therapeutic management of specific clinical circumstances.[17-19]

Health educators have expressed interest in using clinical algorithms in the teaching and learning environment. Students can use algorithms in learning situations for quick graphic reference to logical clinical decision making. Additionally, applications of clinical algorithms as tools for collaborative and interactive teaching have already shown promise.[20] Generation of seed algorithms has been included as a learning tool for practicing chiropractors in some postgraduate orthopedic programs as a part of their course of study.

Seed clinical parameters for the management of industrial low back injuries have been presented as a part of a prospective clinical trial comparing chiropractic management with medical care.[21] These care pathways are not of the classic algorithm "boxology" but are chronological "if, then" statements identifying anticipated courses of care and expected outcomes. Investigators can then go back and compare the thresholds of care for the individual cases against their projected algorithmic steps.

Despite recent gains in popularity, algorithms and care pathways are still not prevalent in clinical practice at this time. However, with the advance of information systems technology, combined with the development of contemporary clinical pathways, a practitioner may gain access to computerized condition-specific databases with probabilities of successful management.[22] In the future, widespread availability of authoritative software seems likely to allow for the input of clinical characteristics or diagnoses to obtain a series of algorithms or care pathway options that can help the doctor to synthesize the latest clinical research, contemporary outcomes data, and expert opinion into the immediate needs of a given patient.

These computer-based tools will also help the doctor in matters of patient education and informed consent. During the course of treatment, the doctor could be able to track an individual patient through the various decision boxes and action steps, allowing the physician to generate an informative report for the patient in easy-to-understand language. In the meantime, algorithms such as those published thus far can serve to assist competent clinicians as decision-making tools.

It is emphasized that these algorithms are clinical *tools* and are not intended to replace clinical judgment. High-quality clinical guidelines are designed to assist clinicians by providing a framework for the evaluation and treatment of the more common patient problems confronting the physician. It is again emphasized that they are not intended either to replace the clinician's clinical judgment or to establish protocol for all patients with a particular condition. Some patients do not fit the clinical conditions contemplated by such guidelines, and a guideline will rarely establish the only appropriate approach to the problem.

ARE THEY REALLY BEING USED?

Group practices, MCOs, and hospitals have already begun to implement clinical algorithms and expect tighter compliance throughout their system of physicians and support staff. The Harvard Community Health Plan HMO in Boston has shown significant advances in quality of patient care and reduction of health care costs as a result of community-based physician development and refinement of care pathways and algorithms. Additionally, they have documented patient and physician satisfaction with these sequences.[8] Algorithms are also being used in MCOs and utilization management firms to estimate care and to preauthorize expensive diagnostic tests or resource-intensive care. Often, these algorithms are part of a complicated database program and are usually proprietary. Some HMOs have developed algorithms and provided for wide dissemination, expecting system-wide implementation. Applications of algorithms such as these are not "future shock"—this is the present state of the system.

The dynamic nature of algorithms and guidelines embodies the need for modification and attenuation to individual and regional needs. Variations in clinical approach between specialties and disciplines may also account for the compulsion to write, modify, and test a given algorithm or care pathway in different clinical settings. It becomes incumbent, therefore, that modern proactive clinicians be capable of constructing, modifying, critiquing, and implementing clinical care pathways and algorithms.

CONSTRUCTING A "SEED" ALGORITHM

To construct an algorithm, there is a sequence that should be followed. "How" the algorithm is developed is considered to be the "process," but "who" develops it determines how mature and implementable the "structure" is. Applying some purposeful meaning to placing certain clinical information or decision steps into variously shaped and numbered boxes connected by lines and arrows is part of the process of developing an algorithm. This aspect of algorithm development has been termed *medical cartography*,[4] but for the purposes of this book, we can simply refer to it as *boxology*. A mild warning is offered, in that application of adequate critical study toward identifying efficient decision options relative to a given clinical problem is more important than merely arranging boxes and arrows on a page. The development process involves reviewing the pertinent literature and discussing the clinical problem with experienced advisors.

Various authors have developed "seed" algorithms[15,18] as appendixes for a clinical review article. Such algorithms are typically the products of the author (or of an editorial architect) and likely have not had revision through quality improvement teams or consensus panels. The "seeds" are included in their articles merely as suggestions to practitioners, based on clinical experience, and they are ripe for professional discourse.

Conversely, in preparation for a clinical trial on the effectiveness of chiropractic manipulation for headache patients, Nelson and Boline[14] created algorithms using the quality improvement "team approach." Initial "seed" headache algorithms were refined, using consensus methodology with a community-based physician panel, then readied for implementation. These two components, the *seed algorithm* versus the *algorithm by consensus*, represent two distinct but complementary approaches in the *structure* or "design" of algorithm development.

This discussion offers a systematic review of an approach for the development of a "seed" algorithm. A common patient problem or one that is a source of clinical uncertainty and/or variations in practice is appropriate for algorithm development. Clinical algorithms can sometimes emphasize diagnostic pathways as distinct from treatment pathways, or they can be a combination of both. Often, space and page size available for the algorithm will influence how much text or information can be included. The shape of the boxes gives the reader an idea of the various logic sequences or steps in the care pathway, but the detail of the text gives meaning to the logic. An algorithm is "user friendly" when the decision logic is makes clinical sense and the content of the text is useful to the physician and patient.

Development of an algorithm requires a scholarly review of relevant literature. For some of the more common conditions that patients present with, there is a knowledge base in the literature ranging from reliability and validity studies for diagnostic technologies to case studies, cohort trials, and, in some cases, randomized clinical trials. Synthesis of information from these studies should identify which methods and procedures have been shown to be effective and which might be ineffective or even controversial. Often, the scientific and more rigorous clinical literature provides only a small piece of the puzzle. A good place to start is to find a series of qualitative literature reviews or, where possible, metanalyses (or literature syntheses) that have systematically searched for and critically appraised the scientific and clinical investigation that has been done.[23,24] The product of this literature review will eventually be made available to consultants or consensus panelists later in the sequence of algorithm development (see Figure 1).

1. Define the problem	• Users • Patient population • Resources
2. Differential diagnosis	• List all causes • Review pathophysiology
3. Sequencing of boxes	• Clinical State Box • Most urgent • Most common • Rare causes in annotation
4. Specify therapy	• Management (freq/duration) • Modalities and doses • Monitor treatment
5. Specify end- or transition points	• Functional status • Modify treatment plan • Referral • Discharge
6. Annotations	• Clarify rationale • Explain controversy • Expand information in box • Review less essential details omitted from algorithm

Fig 1. How to write a clinical algorithm.

Consideration should also be given to identifying who the end-users of this algorithm will be. Practicing doctors, clinical staff, and quality assurance managers may all find utility in a given clinical algorithm. If an algorithm is geared toward a specific end-user, it may be best to include it in the algorithm's title (eg, "Efficient Hypertension Screening for the Nurse Practitioner"). Who the guideline is designed for can make a difference. Additionally, it is important to identify the patient population for which the guide is intended. Again, this may best be dealt with in the title or in the beginning statement (eg, "Hypertension Screening in the Elderly"). A clinical flow chart designed for the management of hypertension in a geriatric population cannot necessarily be generalized to the adolescent or to "twenty-something" populations. Additionally, the designer of the algorithm should be sensitive to the resources reasonably available to the end-user and the patient population.

In studying diagnostic sequences, all etiologies of the patient's presenting complaint should be identified, including pathophysiologic conditions that might be less readily apparent to the end-user. These diagnostic steps should be sequenced in a fashion designed to flush out and manage emergent and urgent conditions earlier in the algorithm. Often, the first diagnostic step is a triage-type decision and usually results in the patient exiting the algorithm. The next priority is to identify and manage the more common conditions through a series of alternating diagnostic and treatment steps. For all the common causes of the clinical condition and its treatment, details of the management should be provided. This includes treatment modalities, doses, frequency, and duration. Intermediate steps for monitoring treatment response (outcomes) should be included when indicated.

Endpoints of therapeutic cycles or phases should be noted by a discrete statement or by action steps (eg, discharge from further care, send to emergency room, etc.). Other endpoints of an algorithm may include referral for a particular diagnostic procedure, referral to a specialist, or referral to another algorithm. Typically, the algorithm will end by identifying some of the rare conditions or by determining that the patient does not fit the algorithm. Experience has shown that it is often easiest to begin by simply listing the various management considerations (etiologies, urgent situations, endpoints, etc.) and trying out various graphic sequences to identify the best way to present the first draft of the algorithm.

Once there is an appreciation for clinical decision making concerning the patient complaint and for the diagnostic or therapeutic options, it is time to start designing boxes and decision steps for the algorithm. How the boxes are shaped, sequenced, connected, and identified is now standardized through an international oversight committee.[6] Figure 2 describes the functions given to the various box shapes.

The *clinical state box* should describe the clinical problem to be addressed. Clinical state boxes that occur in the body of the algorithm are used to clarify the status of the patient or diagnosis along the path of the algorithm (ie, describe a subset of patients with a particular clinical entity).

The *decision box* contains statements that are phrased as questions and punctuated with question marks. If two assessments are to be determined, specify whether both ("and") or one ("or") must be positive for a "yes" response. Multiple questions can be asked in one box, with criteria specified for a "yes" response to the entire box (ie, are two of three present, are all present, are any present?). An example would be a multiple-choice decision box that asks whether the patient has a fever greater than 102° F, history of cancer, sudden weight loss, *or* diabetes. If any of these findings are present, it begs a "yes" response and the appropriate action step. If none are present, it receives a "no" response and the appropriate action.

The *action box* contains a single phrase, indicating a therapeutic or diagnostic action within a box. This box prompts the end-user or patient to "do" something. For clarity's sake, multiple actions that do not need to be sequenced in time may be listed in one box. When multiple actions are presented in one box, each action should be listed on a separate line (preceded with an optional number, dash, or bullet). Typically, the action phrase is not punctuated by a period.

The *link box* can be either a five-sided box or an oval shape. It is a transition step to another box sequence or page of the algorithm. The message in the box may simply read "Go to Page___" or "Go to Box___."

Figure 3 lists the standards for sequencing, connecting, and numbering the algorithm boxes. Lines and arrows should connect boxes closely, such that no lines are unduly long or angled. Boxes are numbered according to the listed guidelines. Numbers should appear outside the upper righthand corner of the box and should be large enough to be easily read. Numbering provides ease in communication between users of the algorithm and is very convenient during consensus exercises. Algorithms should ideally be on one page but can be on multiple pages, according to the recommended guidelines.

Table 1 provides guidance on titling and use of annotations. The *title* of the algorithm is located at the top right of the page. The title should be crafted carefully because it sets the tone of the algorithm. A title of "Chiropractic Management of Pediatric Headaches" is short and succinct, and it identifies the clinical topic, the patient population, and the intended users. Identification of the author(s) and publication dates is appropriate. It is also advised that there be some designation of the explicit process used in the development of the algorithm; this can be designated as a footnote. *Annotations* are like expanded footnotes that are found at the end of the algorithm, often on a separate page. They are used to clarify rationale or to explain a controversy, with citations to references in the literature used to support the

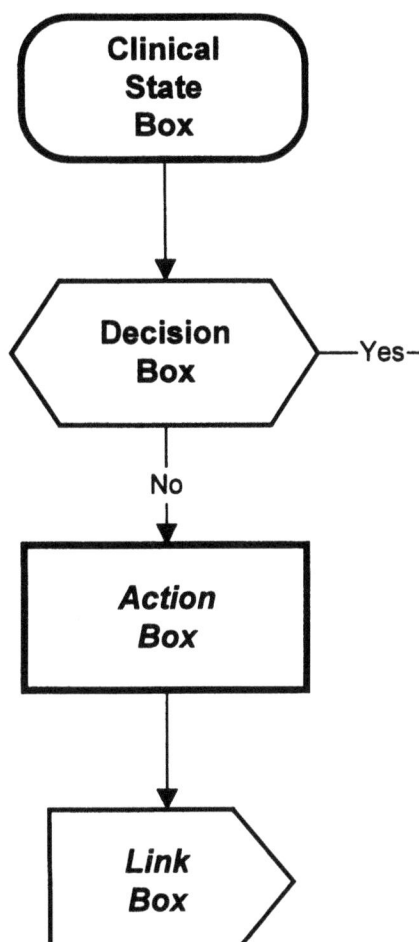

Clinical State Box
Rounded rectangle. This box defines the clinical state or problem. It has only one exit path and may or may not have an entry path. This box always appears at the beginning of an algorithm.

Decision Box
Hexagon in shape. This box requires a branching decision, whose response will lead to one of two alternative paths. It always has one entry path and two exit paths. The text is phrased in the form of a question leading to a "yes" or "no" response.

Action Box
Rectangle. This box indicates instruction for a specific action, usually therapeutic or diagnostic. Oftentimes it serves as an end-point and may suggest transfer to another place on the algorithm.

Link Box
Five-sided (can be oval). This box can be used in place of an arrow, to link boxes for graphic clarity (at page breaks or between separated nodes to maintain path continuity).

Annotations:
(A) Make annotations here...

Fig 2. Algorithm box shapes and functions.

recommendation(s) of the algorithm. They can expand on a statement in an algorithm box (ie, how to perform a procedure, possible side effects, or recommended therapy and when to monitor). Alternatively, they can explain clinical details not essential to the clinical algorithm (ie, a relatively rare etiology).

With this overview of algorithm construction and the established standards for content and clarity, the care pathway can be developed as a "seed" algorithm. Once a seed algorithm is developed, multiple attempts should be made to run through various types of patient presentations to see how well the algorithm can be applied. It is a good idea to ask

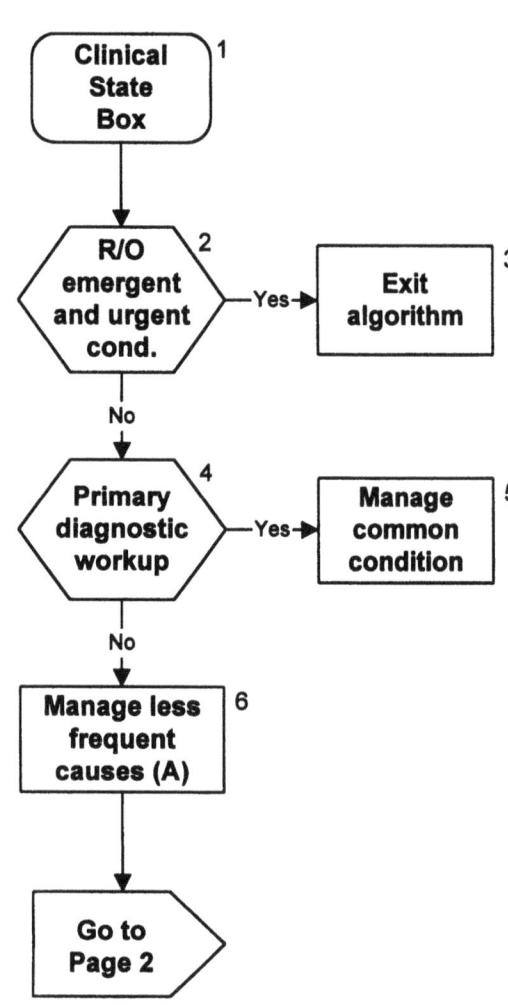

Sequencing Boxes
Present the diagnostic steps in order to rule out emergent and urgent conditions or conditions where the algorithm doesn't apply; alternate diagnostic and therapeutic steps in sequence to then rule out common to frequent to rare causes of the patient complaint.

Connecting Boxes - Arrows
Lines and arrows flow from top to bottom, and in general flow from left to right (exception: where side branch rejoins main stem).
Arrows should never intersect - link boxes can be used to avoid crossing paths.
Arrows originating from decision boxes should be labelled "yes" or "no".
No other text should be used over the arrow. Whenever possible, "yes" arrows should point right, and "no" arrows down.

Numbering Boxes
Clinical state boxes, decision boxes, and action boxes should be numbered sequentially, left to right and top to bottom. Link boxes should not be numbered.

Paging
Whenever possible, consolidation should be sought so an algorithm can be presented on one page.
When page breaks are needed, they should be inserted where clinically logical.
A single box should never be isolated on a page.
For complex algorithms, the first page could best serve as a directory to clinical subsets of patients, identified as clinical state boxes.

(A) *Annotation* regarding rare causes, controversies or clarification of clinical issues.

R/O, rule out; cond., conditions

Fig 3. Algorithm box sequencing, connecting and numbering standards.

---

other potential end-users to try it out, offer their input, and make any further refinements that may be needed. The next step is to seek broader dissemination for testing. In-house algorithms may be tried for a period of time, then evaluated; or seed algorithms can be submitted for peer review and publication. Once it is published as a seed, it can be explicitly reviewed in a number of ways to refine, edit, and improve its content, flow, logic, appearance, and applicability to the intended users. Just getting this far is often a challenge to many clinicians and educators but is usually characterized as a fun and rewarding scholarly accomplishment.

Algorithms can be generated using computer graphic programs such as *Harvard Graphics, Corel Draw, ABC Flowcharter,* or *Visio* (preferred by editors of TICC). It is advisable to utilize a program that features "click and drag" and ample templates of box shapes and line/arrow configura-

Table 1. Algorithm title and annotations

Title
- ❏ Title should define clinical topics and intended users.
- ❏ Authors should be listed under the title, including degree and institutional affiliation.
- ❏ Date of publication and revisions (if applicable) should be specified.
- ❏ A footnote to the title should state the explicit process by which algorithm logic was decided (ie, group consensus after literature review, individual recommendation based on clinical experience, and so forth).

Annotations
- ❏ Annotations are an intrinsic part of the algorithm, and they are used to clarify the rationale of the decisions and cite the supporting literature, or expand on less essential details of the clinical information contained in the box.
- ❏ Annotations following a single phrase should be cited by a capital letter (A) at the end of the phrase.
- ❏ When multiple statements are contained in a single box, annotation(s) should appear at the end of the phrase(s) to which applicable.
- ❏ If an annotation is applicable to the entire box with multiple statements, the annotation should be cited by a capital letter (A) centered on a separate line at the bottom of the box.
- ❏ Annotations should be written in text format, appearing on the bottom of the algorithm page or on a separate page.

---

tions. It is also helpful to have diversity in text formatting and merge capabilities with other supportable software. The value of these desired features will become very apparent once the algorithm is edited or reworked.

FORMAL PROCESSES FOR IMPROVING, CRITIQUING, AND TESTING ALGORITHMS

For a detailed description of the formal processes employed in refining algorithms through consensus methods, critiquing algorithmic guidelines, and testing these pathways and guidelines for reliability and validity, refer to the full text of the article offered in TICC Volume 4, Number 1, 1994.[1] This article has been used extensively as a basis of training in college teaching situations, as well as in practice environments.

The article also offers an explanation of how these development and improvement tools find their way into practice applications in a socially meaningful way. This response by delivery and reimbursement systems has been due to the changes in social tolerances for variations in practice and quality of care. Unfortunately, not all applications of clinical or system-based algorithms are done correctly, or their implementation has occurred without critical input from the respective end-users. Practitioners must be wary of clinical algorithms and guideline systems that do not employ those formal development and implementation processes.

CONCLUSIONS

As mentioned previously, algorithms and care pathways are intended to clarify relationships among clinical conditions and possible decisions—not as diagnostic or treatment guides for individual patients. They just synthesize graphically or in an organized narrative fashion a reasonable hierarchy of clinical decision making. This is especially important to understand when attempting to apply or test a seed algorithm. The thought processes illustrated in guidelines and algorithms are not definitive, but rather examples of typical and supportable thought processes that a clinician might want to consider when addressing a similar clinical situation. They neither replace a clinician's judgment nor establish a protocol, standard for diagnosis, and/or treatment of patients with any particular set of symptoms.

As sometimes happens with medical, chiropractic, and clinical information, a flawed care pathway may be used, or inappropriate interpretation or application of an algorithm may occur, as the result of a well-intentioned attempt by an overseer to standardize an adjudication processes or to contain costs. The best defense against such misuse is to have a good working knowledge of the basis of a guideline, the process by which it was developed, and the unique circumstances of any given case. Overall, the utility of condition-specific synthesis of literature and expert opinion through the vehicle of clinical algorithms has been demonstrated to improve quality of care for patients and to improve efficiency of application of clinical resources.[1,24]

Algorithms are dynamic tools and are subject to continuous revision, based on new knowledge, new technology, and, most importantly, new experience gained through implementation, evaluation, and revision.[25] Critical debate and scholarly discourse in the letters to editors sections of journals—in which both seed and refined algorithms have been published—are fertile grounds for important new input for the ongoing revision of clinical guidelines and algorithms.

Development of a useful clinical algorithm is best accomplished by following these steps (refer to Algorithm 1):

1. Review quality clinical and scientific literature on a given clinical situation. This may most easily be accomplished by searching for any published qualitative literature reviews or metanalyses on the topic.
2. Using this review and an algorithm architect's clinical experience, draft a list of key clinical issues, decisions, and options to address in constructing the algorithm.

3. Next, use the tools described in the "boxology" section of this paper to construct a seed algorithm. Attempt to identify a direct strategic endpoint to work toward in the lower portion of the page, identifying key yes or no decisions that can branch off to other clinical options horizontally.
4. Follow through the algorithm using a variety of different clinical situations to see whether it flows adequately.
5. Ask peers to also review and critique it, offering their suggestions and revisions. Incorporate them and repeat steps 4 and 5 until the flow is smooth and limitations have been dealt with.
6. A seed algorithm should now be ready for publication and dissemination. Peer scrutiny is an important step in development and refinement of workable algorithms. TICC requests authors of clinical protocol articles to develop seed algorithms for publications as an appendix.[15-19] Seed algorithms and care pathways are quite common in medical literature[24] because they can be useful references for practicing clinicians.
7. Next, algorithms should be subjected to expert consensus, implementation, testing, and further revision. After testing and refinement, algorithms should again be disseminated through publication, with a full report of the methodology and revisions that resulted from the process. These kinds of algorithms are likely to be the most reliable and useful form of this clinical aid. It should be pointed out that as new technologies are developed and validated, and other new knowledge arises, all clinical algorithms are likely to need revisiting for further upgrading.

Seed algorithms and care pathways can be useful clinical aids for chiropractors in documenting clinical thought processes. This profession has often been misunderstood by other providers, policy makers, and payers. Much of this lack of understanding of chiropractic procedures can be attributed to inadequate information from chiropractors themselves in documenting and refining their methodologies and clinical decision-making practices. There are no clinicians better prepared to describe and refine chiropractic protocols than DCs.

When well designed, not only can these tools be useful clinical adjuncts to practicing chiropractic physicians, but an abundance of such protocols available for peer review, scrutiny, and refinement can help position chiropractic as a responsible and viable health care resource. Perhaps the biggest complaints about chiropractic from policy makers and purchasers center around the disunity, unpredictability, and practice variation that often characterize chiropractic care. An evidence-based process of algorithm development can be axiomatic in both providing clinicians with important clinical insight and improving the credibility of and comfort with chiropractic services. Rather than limiting the decision-making capabilities of individual physicians, condition-specific algorithms can actually stimulate more appropriate patient referrals to chiropractors from other providers, as well as help to assure quality and consistency for the most important constituent—the patient.

REFERENCES

1. Hansen DT, Mootz RD. Understanding, developing and utilizing clinical algorithms. *Top Clin Chiro*. 1994;1(4):44–57.
2. Gottlieb LK, Margolis CA, Schoenbaum SC. Clinical practice guidelines at an HMO: Development and implementation in a quality improvement model. *Quality Rev Bull*. 16(2):80–86, 1990.
3. Hansen DT. Development and use of clinical algorithms in chiropractic. *J Manipulative Physiol Ther*. 1991;14(8):478–482.
4. Berwick DM, Godfrey AB, Roessner J. *Curing Health Care: New Strategies for Quality Improvement*. San Francisco, CA: Jossey-Bass, Publishers; 1990:23–28.
5. Berwick D, Gottlieb L. *Clinical Quality Improvement: Designing Care*. Brookline, MA: National Demonstration Project on Quality Improvement in Health Care; 1990.
6. Margolis CZ. Proposal for clinical algorithm standards. Society for Medical Decision Making Committee on Standardization of Clinical Algorithms. *Medical Decision Making*. 1992;12(2):149–154.
7. Cheadle A, Franklin G, Wolfhagen C, et al: Factors influencing the duration of work-related disability: A population-based study of Washington state Workers' Compensation. *Am J Publ Health*. 1994;84(2):190–196.
8. Vibbert S, Reichard J, eds. *The 1993–4 Medical Outcomes and Guidelines Source Book*. Washington, DC: Faulkner & Gray; 1993:169–318.
9. Henderson D, Chapman-Smith D, Mior S, Vernon H. Clinical guidelines for chiropractic practice in Canada. *J Can Chiro Assoc Suppl*. 1994;38(1):1–203.
10. Haldeman S, Chapman-Smith D, Petersen DM. *Guidelines for Chiropractic Quality Assurance and Practice Parameters*. Gaithersburg, MD: Aspen Publishers; 1993.
11. Adler RH, Giersch EP, Ennis ML, Heermans H. *Survival Guide: Chiropractic Practice Guidelines*. Seattle, WA: self-published; 1993.
12. Kaminski M, Boal R, Gillete RG, Peterson DH, Villnave TJ. A model for the evaluation of chiropractic methods. *J Manipulative Physiol Ther*. 1987;10:61–64.
13. Gatterman MI, Hansen DT. Development of chiropractic nomenclature through consensus. *J Manipulative Physiol Ther*. 1994;17(5):351–359.
14. Nelson C, Boline P. A consensus on the assessment and treatment of headache. *J Chiro Technique*. 1991;3(4):151–168.
15. Souza TA. Back to basics: Differentiating mechanical pain from visceral pain. *Top Clin Chiro*. 1994;1(1):67–69.

16. Henninger R. Back to basics: Evaluation of soft tissue pain. *Top Clin Chiro.* 1994;1(2):77.
17. Cook RD, Mootz RD. Determining appropriateness of exercise and rehabilitation for chiropractic patients. *Top Clin Chiro.* 1994;1(1):75–77.
18. Mullen D, Bowers LJ. Myofascial pain syndromes: A look at the lower extremity. *Top Clin Chiro.* 1994;1(2):81.
19. Souza TA. Conservative management of orthopedic conditions of the lower leg, foot, and ankle. *Top Clin Chiro.* 1994;1(2):82–83.
20. Hansen DT. Construction of "seed" algorithms in chiropractic postgraduate interactive learning opportunities. In: Hansen DT. ed. *Proceedings of 1993 Conference on Research and Education, Consortium for Chiropractic Research.* San Jose, CA: 1993;182–183.
21. Mootz RD, Waldorf VT. Chiropractic care parameters for common industrial low back conditions. *J Chiro Technique.* 1993;5(3):119–125.
22. Office of Quality Assurance and Medical Review. *Directory of Practice Parameters: Titles, Sources and Updates.* Chicago, IL: American Medical Association; 1993.
23. Goertz C, Mootz R. A review of chiropractic management strategies in the care of hypertensive patients. *J Neuromusculoskel System.* 1993;1(3):91–108.
24. Hadorn DC, McCormack K, Diokno A. An annotated algorithm approach to clinical guideline development. *JAMA.* 1992;267(24):3311–3314.
25. Hansen DT. Prospect for the future of chiropractic guidelines. In: Lawrence D, ed. *Advances in Chiropractic.* Vol. 1. St. Louis, MO: Mosby-Year Book; 1994:372–409.

Algorithm 1

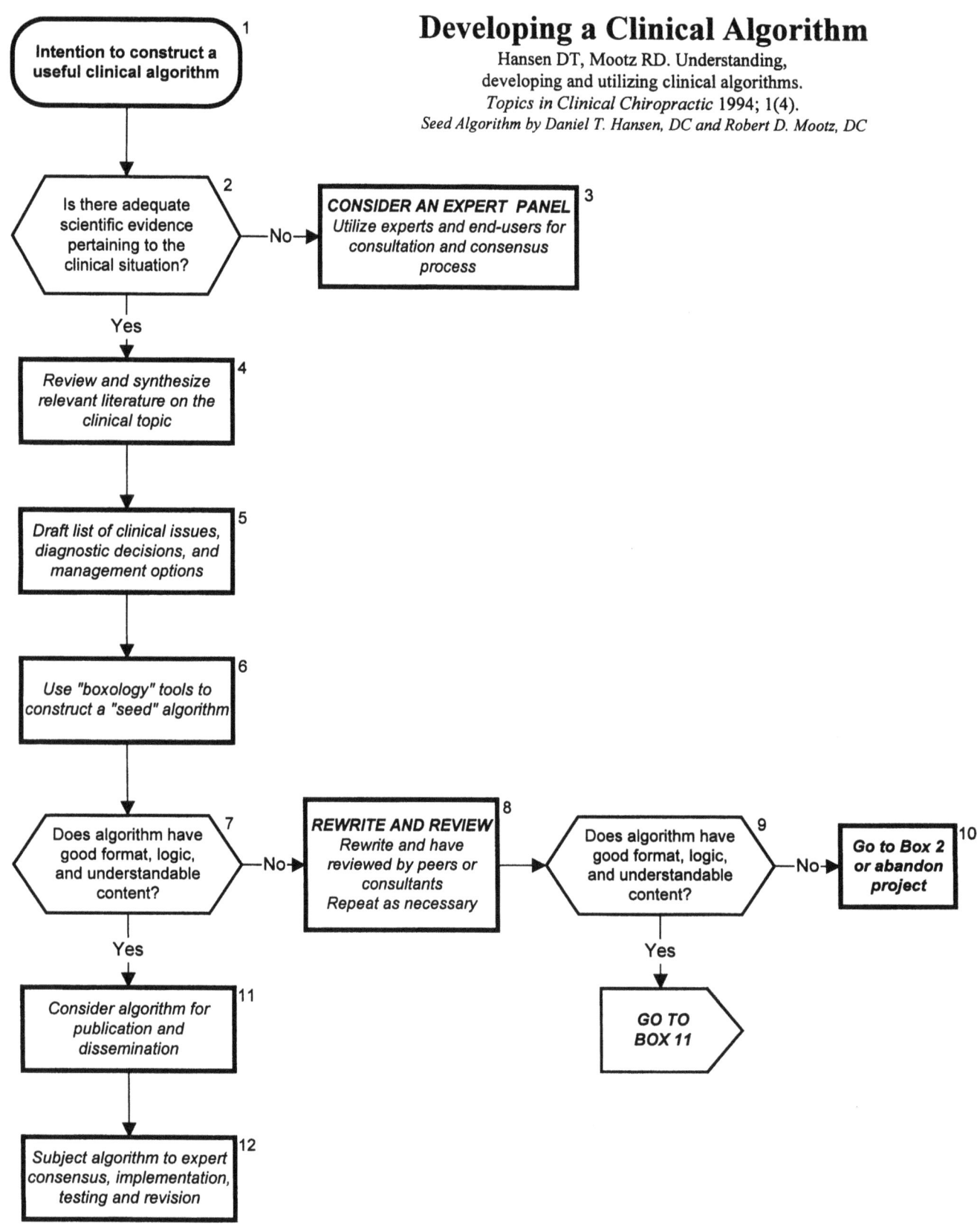

Developing a Clinical Algorithm
Hansen DT, Mootz RD. Understanding, developing and utilizing clinical algorithms.
Topics in Clinical Chiropractic 1994; 1(4).
Seed Algorithm by Daniel T. Hansen, DC and Robert D. Mootz, DC

Part I

Overview

1

Formal Processes in Health Care Technology Assessment: A Primer for the Chiropractic Profession

Daniel T. Hansen and Robert D. Mootz

Imagine that you are the chief executive officer of a Fortune 500 company. Your company employs more than 8,000 people nationwide, and you are accountable for their livelihoods and their health benefits. You are also accountable to the stockholders and the company's board of directors. New competitors have emerged offshore that can pay lower wages and provide minimal health benefits. They are thus able to deliver a rival, quality product for far less. This past year your organization responded by lowering prices, maximizing efficiency, and reducing overhead costs. Still, sales are down, and three of the last four quarters have been in the red. You have reduced and stabilized your fixed expenses and optimized inventory and raw materials expenditures. One cost has not remained fixed, however. Health care expenditures went up 74% in the current year, and you have just received word that just to maintain the same level of benefits for your employees in the coming year, costs are going to increase another 124%. A significant portion of your total health care dollars go to medical pension benefits for retired workers who are no longer a productive part of the company. Your employee demographics have remained relatively constant for the past 5 years, and the rate of inflation has not exceeded 4% for 4 years running. What are you going to do?

A CONTEMPORARY DILEMMA

If you were to react like most health care purchasers and other consumers, you might start trying to contain and stabilize the escalating costs. What are your options? Letting employees go? Moving offshore? Or, what about seeking new "suppliers" for health care services? Have you ever changed your automobile policy when suddenly faced with a large rate increase? Have you ever stopped buying office supplies from the local stationery store when a new discount store opened up?

In the past, when individuals paid most of their own health care costs out of pocket, cost containment was very much in the hands of the patient. Today, many patients do not even see bills for services or, when they do, they sigh with relief that most of the cost is dealt with by third parties. In an age of instant information and rapidly increasing technology, patient demand for access to the latest and greatest test procedures, the best specialists, and multiple clinical opinions and options has been high. This demand remained high until employers start to offer employees a range of health plans, with a variety of cost sharing options. Although free choice and unrestricted access plans are still available, patients and purchasers alike are opting for programs that have small or no copayment requirements and that restrict access to a group of preselected providers in exchange for lower premiums.

Similar scenarios are confronting American businesses, employees, and consumers on a daily basis. Many of the fundamental, underlying problems that have contributed to escalating and unpredictable health care costs are only beginning to be addressed. Health care purchasers and policy makers are asking tougher questions of providers and the health care system at large. Are there any health care services being paid for that are unnecessary or redundant? Are any ineffective? Are there procedures or techniques that help people heal more quickly, or for less money, than others? If a test or procedure is paid for, will it ensure a better outcome than cheaper alternatives or natural progression alone? If a cheaper alternative is found, are the quality and outcome of the service comparable?

The health care demands on contemporary society require careful, systematic assessment of complex problems along with thorough, reasoned, and coordinated responses from a

Adapted from *Top Clin Chiro* 1996; 3(1): 71–83
© 1996 Aspen Publishers, Inc.

variety of key constituents in private and public sectors. Over the past decade, there has been an explosion in approaches to find solutions to spiraling health care costs. In the public sector, fledgling attempts at health care reform, reimbursement policy, and cost containment have been floated with varying degrees of success. Intrinsic to the public domain are the shifting sands of political reality. The private sector has seen responses ranging from changes in insurance plans and products to radical redesign of health care delivery in the form of managed care and managed competition. The health care industry itself has responded through promotion of physician design practice guidelines and innovative new business collaborations between medical specialties, corporate users, and the insurance industry itself.

A couple of constants exist within all attempts to find solutions. Any potential solution must address cost control and predictability; quality and appropriateness of care; and integration of the needs of patients, purchasers, and physicians into workable delivery and reimbursement systems. The issues are emotionally and politically charged, and everyone from consumer groups, labor unions, physician trade associations, the insurance industry, and tax payer groups can find special interest organizations that support their perspectives.

There is a clear need for strategies to appraise and incorporate systematically the needs of all stakeholders in the identification and development of solutions. One of the current buzzwords in health services research is technology assessment (TA). This evolving field of critical appraisal of complex issues is making significant strides forward in problem solving for the health care community. Table 1 lists many of the major questions being asked of the health care system. As practitioners, DCs are often in a position of advocating for the needs of an individual patient and for fair practice rights. Both are legitimate needs of a functional health care system. However, providers are increasingly finding themselves polarized in adversarial and competitive relationships with other providers, health purchasers, and overseers of the system. A number of recently developed and evolving TA strategies can serve as tools to help the chiropractic community navigate the ever-changing morass of the modern health care system.

This article identifies a number of important issues confronting individual DCs, regional community-based physician groups, chiropractic licensing and oversight bodies, and professional trade associations. In addition, it presents TA tools and strategies that can assist DCs in addressing, evaluating, and constructively contributing to the health care information gap.

PROVIDER-CENTERED ISSUES THAT CONTRIBUTE TO HEALTH CARE DILEMMAS

There are more than enough problems to spread around the health care system. Poorly conceived policies and sluggish bureaucracies in the public sector, inadequate access to primary care services, overemphasis of expensive technologies, and cumbersome and financially driven insurance companies illustrate but a few.

With increased development and application of health care technology, health care costs have risen. Innovations that extend the capabilities of existing technologies are generally more expensive to operate than those they replace. For example, computed tomography (CT) scans are replacing radiographs, and magnetic resonance imaging (MRI) is replacing CT scans, both at substantially increased costs. General consensus exists that technological innovation is cost increasing, although theoretically it can be cost decreasing or cost saving if a less expensive technology is substituted for a more expensive one, or if the new procedure replaces a variety of procedures. Simple survival is no longer the only important outcome; rather, quality of life and associated costs have become important issues for both consumers and providers.[1]

Vendors of technology (devices, procedures, and so forth) have tended to push their products into the chiropractic marketplace without much testing for efficacy, reliability, validity, and so on. The result has been "waves" of popularity for devices that claim that they "objectify" the need for chiropractic care (eg, Moire photography, thermography, surface electrode electromyography, special radiographic studies, and spinal ultrasound). The claims for their objectivity are often accompanied by promises of increased revenues and reimbursement by insurance companies. These "constructs" of their application are typically doctor centered, in that the applications and outcomes have clear benefit only to the practitioner. They typically do not address the patient's perspective; that is, they do not respond to the question of whether the device or procedure will help the patient get better faster, be more functional, or have an improved quality of life.

Table 1. Questions confronting the health care system

- Which tests and treatments currently being paid for are unnecessary or redundant?
- Which procedures are ineffective?
- Which procedures, services, and techniques promote improved health status more quickly and at a lower cost?
- If a test or procedure is purchased now will it ensure a better outcome than a cheaper alternative or natural progression alone?
- What are the important elements related to quality of health care?
- Which doctors, clinics, and interventions do patients want to meet community needs?

Many popular systems of patient management are also doctor, rather than patient, focused. Business and clinic management strategies that have been popular in chiropractic practices over the past three decades offer patient treatment plans (frequency and duration) that are concerned more with practice volume than individual patient goals. That is, regardless of presenting complaint, age, or severity of spinal problem, all patients receive the same level of care, requiring frequent visits over a long period of time.[2] From the patient or payer's perspective, these management strategies are seen as being "cookbook" treatment plans from the book of doctor excess. Paying customers are asking legitimate questions such as: Is this kind of care really effective? What evidence is it based on? Is it merely based on theory or treatment philosophy? Does this kind of care improve quality of life? Is this kind of care better (superior, faster, or less expensive clinical and social outcomes) than the care received from the traditional allopathic approaches or from those of other alternative health care disciplines?

These questions are tough, modern-day ones. They are being asked of all players in health care, including traditional allopathic generalists and specialists, hospital systems, rehabilitation centers, long-term care centers, dentists, and most allied health care providers. Related health education and administrative support systems are now taking responsibility for educating health professionals about the current expectations for implementation and application of TA issues in day-to-day practice. In the chiropractic profession, chiropractic colleges, state licensing boards, and professional associations hold this responsibility. Notably, in the days of doctor-centered attitudes, licensing boards were seen as doctor/philosophy protectors rather than consumer protectors. Today there is strong evidence suggesting a new consumer-centered trend among many boards and commissions.

The chiropractic profession is no longer an insignificant commodity of health care. The profession is reaching over 11%[3] of the American public, and an even greater percentage is being treated for back-related disorders.[4] Thus, more social entities are taking notice of chiropractic. Added to the already well-established oversight organizations, agencies, and institutions (chiropractic organization, licensing boards, educational agencies, and institutions), chiropractors and chiropractic practice are now being overseen by public and private sector health purchasing authorities, managed care organizations (MCOs), and patient advocacy groups. The increased attention is a byproduct of greater public acceptance and demand. Although this increased attention yields greater practice opportunities for chiropractors, with this change comes greater scrutiny of all aspects of the profession including belief systems, education and clinical exposure, delivery settings, and quality of recordkeeping.

Chiropractic institutions produce practitioners who contribute to communities throughout the world, in rural, urban, and underserved regions. These colleges have been generating a constant flow of practicing doctors, but very few doctors who are properly trained experts in the administrative, quality assurance, policy setting, and health services research capacities that are currently in high demand. Thus much of the analysis and policy setting related to chiropractic services is occurring without input from chiropractors who understand the greater epidemiologic and health services administration issues confronting society.[5]

The assessment of technology involves more than just an appreciation of the reliability and validity of a particular device or procedure. Comparative costs, quality of life outcomes, and resource capabilities of a discipline or specialty must also form a part of global TA in health care delivery.

To overcome hurdles (such as skepticism and sniping from the medical profession), chiropractic will be pushed hard by insurers, employers, workers' compensation programs, and managed care plans to demonstrate successful clinical outcomes using cost-effective care methods. US health care is being rapidly restructured by a combination of public policy initiatives and market reforms. To gain acceptance, the chiropractic profession must align with, not avoid, these critical environmental shifts.[6]

DESCRIPTION OF TA

Technology assessment can be defined as a form of policy research that evaluates technology for the purpose of providing decision makers with information on different policy options. These options may include the allocation of resources to research and development, development of regulations or legislation, and the establishment of standards or guidelines for health planning and health practice.[1] *Technology* refers to any medical procedure or intervention (whether or not it is considered high or low tech); it includes everything from the latest medical device to the basic clinical examination or treatment.

Managed care companies have identified the area of technology utilization as a focal point for the establishment of mechanisms to enhance effectiveness and efficiency. Through the 1970s, payers generally reimbursed for whatever use of a technology (ie, drug, device, procedure) a recognized provider billed for. However, during the 1980s managed care companies began to make explicit determinations about the safety and effectiveness of technologies for which payment was to be made. Payers began to establish formal processes for the rigorous evaluation of the various applications of technologies. This process of TA is now widely recognized as an essential tool for improving the quality of health care delivered and maximizing the efficiency of the health care system.[7]

Cost-effectiveness analysis will also become an important outcome in health care decision making. Managed care companies are adapting their processes and products to permit explicit application of cost-effectiveness analysis to coverage and medical necessity determinations. This evolution is only natural given the fact that only a few major managed care companies have established formal, quality-driven TA processes.[7]

TAs can be used in a variety of ways. Some serve as tools to ensure appropriate use of resources and enhance the delivery of high-quality care. TA can also be misused or applied in a way that fails to incorporate the legitimate needs of the patient. How TA functions depends on the organization performing the assessment and its particular goals or needs. TAs are designed to help elucidate what "works" in health practices. At its best, assessment produces information regarding the impact of a particular technology on safety, efficacy, effectiveness, cost-effectiveness and cost-benefit, and quality of care. It may also address the broader social, legal, and ethical consequences of technology. TA may be used for various purposes including the following:

- To improve well-being and the quality of care delivered, consistent with the effective use of resources;
- To assist in choosing among alternative treatments or the delivery of those treatments (services);
- To provide a foundation for practice guideline development;
- To contribute to decisions regarding allocation of resources; and
- To provide information for making decisions regarding coverage and reimbursement of health care services.

The increasing interest in TA reflects an understanding that the exponential growth of health and medical technology and the spiraling cost of health care are related phenomena. In evaluating health care technologies, decision makers must balance the costs and benefits for both the consumer and the provider. The allocation of resources to constant and continuous care of the critically ill newborn illustrates a relevant example of the tradeoff between costs and quality of life in a highly expensive health technology. Treatment for angina, including coronary artery bypass graft surgery, serves as another example for which contemporary society requires cost and outcomes comparisons for a moderate-cost technology that is available to a large number of persons in the United States and elsewhere.[1] By comparison, chiropractic services being offered to the public could be considered as minor-cost technologies in the management of back pain accessible to a large number of persons globally, particularly in industrialized nations. While some technologies reduce costs, others add expenses. Increased costs must be balanced against meaningful patient outcomes such as mortality, lowered morbidity, and improved quality of life.[8]

TA in health care has become an integral part of broad government oversight in recent years. Historically, there have been committees and commissions in federal and state agencies that formally appraise assessment of health care technologies and public health programs. The activity of these groups has been focused largely on high-cost facilities or technologies that would have significant impact on regional community economies. By design, government TA programs incorporate public input and due process. Extension of the public sector involvement in TA has included community-based decision making through the Health System Agency (HSA) model of the 1970s and 1980s. HSA councils included physicians, health administrators, allied professionals, and consumer representatives. Although they were well-conceived, community-based efforts, HSAs may have been ahead of their time and thus subject to political annihilation.

However, purchasers in the private sector, as well as a number of state and federal agencies, have continued to pay significant attention to assessment of health technologies, particularly through private or university-based research centers and health care "think tanks." Recently chiropractors experienced first-hand the impact that the public sector technology and guidelines process can have when the Agency for Health Care Policy and Research published treatment guidelines for acute back pain in adults.[9] Table 2 lists some of the major TA entities and presents descriptions of their activities, processes, and products.

Initiatives from these kinds of organizations and implementation of their reports and assessments have had an effect. Changes are occurring throughout the health care industry as a result. For example, guidelines and technology reports have affected resource allocation within community health systems, hospitals, specialty and private primary care practices by bringing about the development of practice policies and precertification criteria for many popular but expensive clinical procedures. Such an impact is not only expected but also increasingly evident throughout many publicly funded reimbursement systems including workers' compensation programs, Medicare, and Medicaid. Many employee benefits health plans that use managed care formats, especially those of large employers, are contractually requiring approval of procedures and devices from formal TA exercises.

The social and non-technical aspects of TA include such things as human resource and legal issues. It is believed that significant cost savings can be realized by using nurses in advanced practice roles such as nurse practitioners (NPs), clinical nurse specialists (CNSs), and certified nurse midwives (CNMs) to deliver primary care and other basic health services. It can be argued that nurses can provide the majority of primary care and other basic services currently provided by physicians (MDs) and they can do so at substantially lower costs without any sacrifice in quality of care. Thus, the wide-scale use of nurses in advanced practice roles can help to make health care reform an affordable possibility.[10]

Table 2. Organizations involved in TA

Office of Medical Applications of Research (OMAR) of the National Institutes of Health (NIH). This organization has a number of activities related to medical applications of research, technology transfer, and TA. OMAR operates the NIH Consensus Development Program, which evaluates the use of biomedical technologies in a public forum, publishes a consensus statement relevant to the public at large that provides guidelines for practitioners on the use of the technology, and disseminates this information.

NIH Technology Assessment Conferences and Workshops. These conferences and workshops are convened to evaluate available scientific information related to a biomedical technology when topic selection criteria for a consensus development conference are not met. The assessment statements are intended to advance understanding of the technology or issue in question and to be useful to health professionals and the public.

Office of Health Technology Assessment (OHTA). This organization is currently functioning under the Agency for Health Care Policy and Research (AHCPR) and performs TAs for the Health Care Financing Administration (HCFA). OHTA assessments focus on the safety and effectiveness of a particular technology and include recommendations to HCFA regarding coverage and reimbursement.

Council on Health Care Technology. This organization was established in 1986 at the Institute of Medicine (IOM) to promote the development and application of TA in health and medicine. The council was charged by Congress to identify needs in the assessment of health care technology and expanded its role to identifying priority clinical conditions as well as medical technologies and practices. The council has been particularly interested in outcome measures that coincide with patient well-being, quality of health care, and quality of life.

Clinical Efficacy and Assessment Project (CEAP). CEAP was established by the American College of Physicians to evaluate medical technology. This program selects technologies for evaluation based on their degree of interest to internists, potential for widespread use, and anticipated benefits and risks. It has reviewed topics that include diagnostic tests, surgical indications, and others. CEAP has also worked jointly with the Blue Cross and Blue Shield Medical Necessity Project, which prioritizes projects on the basis of requests from member plans.

Diagnostic and Therapeutic Technology Assessment (DATTA). The American Medical Association (AMA) sponsors multiple activities related to TA that are typically published in the *Journal of the American Medical Association*. In 1982, the AMA formed the DATTA program, which is a physician consensus panel that evaluates medical technologies using different methodologies.

Note: This listing does not describe the activities of technology manufacturers and distributors in testing and achieving approval for new medical technologies and devices from the Food and Drug Administration. Both have major roles in TA, regulation, and approval for specific clinical purposes.

This list is based on a compendium of organizations involved in TAs as listed in 1988 edition of The Medical Technology Assessment Directory published by the Council on Health Care Technology.

Source: Ferrara EP, Servis KW. *State Task Force on Clinical Guidelines and Medical Technology Assessment.* Albany, NY: New York State Department of Health; 1994.

ATTEMPTS AT TA RESOURCE DEVELOPMENT IN CHIROPRACTIC

Prior to 1990

Historically, chiropractors have not been involved in all of the various government organizations that oversee TA in health care. It was not until the mid-1980s that any chiropractors were selected to serve in any substantive capacity on committees of state and federal agencies. Prior to 1990, the only broad, profession-wide effort by chiropractors to assess methods or procedures was the 1974 Houston Conference that led to the development of the subsequent Medicare radiographic manifestations of subluxation that would be weakly implemented in the years to come. That conference led to a vast administrative perception that radiographic examination was essential for the establishment of a chiropractic diagnosis or clinical assessment. The mandatory radiographic verification of the presence of subluxation became "policy" and ultimately found its way into the administrative management of all Medicare and federally funded employee health programs (employee benefits and workers' compensation). It is the only example in federal health care reimbursement where a procedure or technology is mandated for administrative reimbursement, regardless of the clinical need for the procedure. Unfortunately, this issue has been allowed to stand the test of time. Even now, 20 years later, in the face of mounting evidence to the contrary,[11,12] most Medicare regional operations still require the compulsory radiographic findings. As of this writing, however, there is movement afoot to remove this administrative barrier.

Prior to 1990, the only ecumenical effort to assess chiropractic therapeutic procedures by applying explicit methods was spearheaded by the American Chiropractic Association

(ACA) Council on Technique. That early effort forged the beginning of a sequence of events that generated widely accepted terminology[13,14] and led to the development of a formal sequence to assess chiropractic techniques eventually advanced by Kaminski and colleagues.[15,16] Unfortunately, the Kaminski sequence of assessment of chiropractic techniques looked only at the formal assessment of a few technique procedures.[17] There is no evidence in the literature that it was used for any other technique or procedure.

Also, prior to 1990, the chiropractic profession addressed technologies and methods as being approved or disapproved through association policy statements[18] and actions taken by state licensing authorities. Typically, the actions of the associations or administrative boards are published either in the minutes (proceedings) or formally as policies, but without detail of the methodology used in the determination. Because the chiropractic profession lacks the universal scope of practice enjoyed by other health disciplines, administrative decisions are typically made as to whether certain diagnostic or therapeutic procedures are consistent with the locally legislated scope of practice. Inventory of statutory interpretations in states and provinces throughout North America shows not only great diversity[19] but also magnifies the potential impact of inconsistencies in costs and completeness of health care received for the ever increasing mobile population and multistate nature of reimbursement. In addition to scope of practice issues, licensing boards in many jurisdictions extend themselves to make policy relative to assessment of technologies. The competency of the licensing boards and individual board members of chiropractic licensing authorities in their understanding, performance, or implementation of formal technology assessments has not been studied, and, given the political nature of such appointments, it is rare to see DCs with extensive TA or research experience hold such positions. It is also unknown to what extent these decisions have had a bearing on the reimbursement system, quality of care, or patient outcomes.

Prior to 1990, chiropractic saw the emergence of its first generation of practice guidelines, erroneously referred to as "standards of care." The Washington State committee's early effort for the workers' compensation system acknowledged lack of process capability especially in the performance of formal TAs and left that chapter unfinished.[20] It was that recognized void of TA capacity in the discipline that ultimately was the impetus for the convening of the formal, profession-wide "consensus conferences" that began in 1990.

Seattle, 1990

The Consortium for Chiropractic Research (CCR), ACA Council on Technique, and the Washington Chiropractic Association cosponsored the first consensus conference on the validation of chiropractic methods in Seattle, early in 1990. This watershed conference was attended by some of the most influential chiropractic leaders from academia, research, technique methods, licensing boards, and state and national associations. Participants heard presentations on current trends in guideline development and assessment of technologies from noted experts from within and outside the chiropractic profession. Proceedings of this conference were published in the chiropractic literature.[21] The meaningful outcome of this conference was that the chiropractic profession appeared willing to commit to use of explicit science and/or formal consensus in all efforts to establish validity in chiropractic diagnostic and therapeutic procedures. It was not the intent of the 1990 conference to validate any procedure or device. The CCR subsequently developed and adopted attributes to be used in the development of chiropractic guidelines based on similar criteria from the Agency for Health Care Policy and Research (AHCPR) and the Institute of Medicine (part of the National Institutes of Health).[22,23]

Intramural chiropractic consensus exercises, 1991 to present

Following the Seattle conference, the CCR embarked on assembling a number of expert panels during their annual Conference on Research and Education (CORE) programs. The panels included formal reviews of the literature and testimony of respected experts. The panels were also designed to accept public testimony through gallery interaction. The literature reviews and summaries of many of the panels have been published in refereed literature and are available as proceedings.[24,25] The information and consensus statements from the panels are available in the literature for consideration in the development of clinical guidelines and practice policies.

Extramural TA and consensus exercises

Studies[5,26,27] performed at RAND on the appropriateness of spinal manipulation for back pain and neck complaints represent the best examples to date of formal TA efforts by the chiropractic profession. The appropriateness processes used by RAND have been recognized throughout the health care industry for their reliability, validity, and generalizability. Many health conditions and technologies have been studied in this fashion. Pertinent to chiropractic, RAND continues to study practice issues such as patient and practitioner satisfaction and compliance.[28–30]

AHCPR ratings for procedures used by chiropractors (eg, manipulation, physiologic therapeutics, exercise, examination, and radiographs) for adults with acute low back pain are found in its Clinical Practice Guideline 14.[9] These ratings reflect the consensus of a panel of experts composed of world-wide authorities from all neuromusculoskeletal disciplines as well as representatives from the consumer segment, which makes these recommendations even more significant. As of this writing, the AHCPR consensus panel on cervical spine complaints and headaches is underway with chiropractic representation on the consensus panel. The AHCPR guideline efforts are preceded by another AHCPR process of patient outcomes research teams (PORTs) where there is systematic review of the literature, including quantitative and qualitative analysis of data studies (meta-analysis), prospective comparative study of health measures (eg, chiropractic management versus physical therapy), and design of implementation and outcome measurement strategies. Chiropractors have been serving as technical advisors to the PORT project on low back pain since 1989.

Although chiropractic trade organizations have not actively pursued TA, they have endorsed the results of TA exercises performed by RAND and AHCPR.[31] The International Chiropractors Association (ICA) prepared its own response to the AHCPR by adding its interpretation of Guideline 14.[32] The editors of the ICA response demonstrated cautious optimism with the outcome of the AHCPR panel and offered an interpretation on chiropractic use of radiographs but de-emphasized references and expert resources, consultants, and reviewers.

Evaluation of manpower resources

Recently, an extensive analysis of chiropractic resources in the United States was undertaken and reported through the National Board of Chiropractic Examiners (NBCE).[33] The data were collected using survey methodology of practicing doctors representative of population distributions across the United States. The study resulted in a "job analysis" report providing insight into resources available within the chiropractic profession that may be available to meet community needs. The report also serves as an inventory of self-reported practice attitudes and habits. Future questions arising from communities or from health planning concerns might look to the chiropractic profession to meet local or regional needs for primary care.[34] Such consideration could assure access or provide care within integrated systems to reduce direct and indirect costs in injury care models. The NBCE report also provides statistical analysis of diagnostic and therapeutic methods employed by chiropractors. The same process was employed by the NBCE using data sets from Canada and Australia-Asia leading to the publication of those respective geographic reports.

DETAILS AND EXAMPLES OF TA/GUIDELINE PROCESSES

Current examples of medical TA can be found in government-based organizations and efforts undertaken by various health care purchasers and policy makers. Assessments of technology are an important administrative segment of most health care purchasers, especially MCOs. Recently, quality standards developed by the National Commission on Quality Assurance have included language mandating that MCOs have a process in place to assess health care technologies using formal appraisal methods.[35]

There are four basic components of a scientific, defensible process for both clinical and coverage decision making. These components are

1. Outcomes data are preferably derived from controlled clinical trials that support the safety and effectiveness of a specific indication.
2. There is evidence of acceptance by the practicing medical community of specific applications of a technology.
3. There is a rigorous, evaluative process that synthesizes and analyzes outcomes data and expert opinion.
4. There is consistency in the use of terminology, as it is translated from the technology assessment process to coverage policy.

The process must be designed to assure scientific and methodologic defensibility. Also, it must be designed to facilitate and substantiate the medical and coverage decision-making processes. Last, the process must be designed to enable and expedite the implementation of the managed care philosophy (ie, outcomes-based decision making) within a particular health plan.[7]

Ferrara and associates[8] state that various methodologies exist for technology assessment. These methodologies are not mutually exclusive. Many organizations have attempted to combine the strengths of several techniques to improve their results.

The method most familiar to the scientific and health care community is the *randomized controlled clinical trial* (RCT). An RCT is rigorous and challenging to conduct and involves considerable time and expense because it depends on well-designed research protocols and large numbers of patients assigned in a randomized fashion.

Performance analysis is an examination of the technical performance of a technology in regard to the criteria of reproducibility, safety, and reliability, which are expressed in terms of sensitivity and specificity. From this analysis, a receiver-operator curve can be generated that graphically displays the sensitivity of a technology as it is applied to a specific diagnostic task.

A *case series* is a collection of studies that describes the use of a particular technology for a specific patient condition, longitudinally added over time that includes all eligible patients regardless of outcome. A series may project forward or backward in time. However, a prospective study, especially if a control group (even if subjects are not randomly assigned) is included, is considered to be more reliable.

Case studies are comprehensive reviews of the medical applications of a particular technology. They include economic, legal, and ethical implications as well as clinical indications. Case studies are often presented as "state-of-the-art" documents that reflect both a synthesis of the literature as well as the expert, clinical experience of the authors.

Meta-analysis is increasingly being used as a means to combine studies of similar construction to answer questions inadequately or equivocally addressed by a single study. This technique depends on the comparability of studies and requires careful attention to the issue of selection bias due to inadequate sampling and due to the fact that studies with negative results are often not published.

Consensus development is a process whereby a panel of experts arrives at a collective opinion by using group interaction, mailings, or both. In the Delphi technique, opinions regarding a particular technology are collected, and a summary is produced after each round of opinion until a consensus report can be written. A methodology referred to as the "forum" method (short for the technology assessment and practice guidelines forum) was recently developed in response to some of the shortcomings of the National Institutes of Health consensus process. It includes some features of the Delphi technique and group process. RAND has pioneered a modified Delphi process to rate appropriateness of a large number of indications for the use of health care procedures. This process involves individual initial ratings of appropriateness, a discussion among panelists, and a revision of ratings with the goal of reaching agreement, when possible, without forced consensus.

An *opinion survey* is a technique in which participants do not interact with each other and a report is generated that reflects the collective judgment of those experts involved. There is no revision of initial opinion.

Many of these formal methodologic processes have been developed and promoted by Eddy,[36] Sackett and associates,[37] and Brook.[38] Eddy's processes involve use of explicit methods of appraising supporting data and summary reports found in literature to create "practice policies" including the assessment of technologies. Sackett and colleagues have developed criteria for evaluating diagnostic and therapeutic procedures. These criteria have been widely accepted and embraced as a yardstick for critical appraisal. These criteria lists were adopted by the commission that developed the Mercy recommendations.[39] A sequence for assessing quality of evidence can be found in Algorithm 1.

Application of the processes of technology assessment is appropriate for the chiropractic profession. Kaminski and colleagues[15] offered a sequence of steps of assessment based on criteria of science and evidence of safety and effectiveness. They also offered a lexicon that identifies the hierarchy of acceptance. Their algorithmic sequence emphasized aspects of doctor-centered clinical science, but did not assess patient-centered qualities or needs of the health care community. Although often cited, this algorithm did not enjoy full implementation in the chiropractic profession and has not stood the test of time. It served as a preliminary look into the contemporary issues of technology assessment in the late 1980s.

Now, with the evolving nature of health delivery, it is time to refocus the process to include those attributes important to the "customer." Deber and coworkers[40] offer a four-phase sequence that integrates the issues of technology assessment with customer and community needs (Table 3). In this matrix, each screen details the key questions as they reflect effectiveness, appropriateness, informed decision making, and insured services. Physician-centered criteria are contrasted to those that are patient-centered and of community value. The appreciation of "who is involved" is also noted.

With this new direction in mind, the authors offer a reworking of the previous algorithmic sequence of Kaminski and colleagues[15] for chiropractic procedures. Algorithm 2 includes sequences that consider the needs of customers and the community. It is offered as a "seed" algorithm for future comment and study. It can be used as a basis of discussion for assessing technologies in chiropractic in the arenas of education, administration, regulation, policy making, and research.

WHAT NOT TO DO

TA and accountability strategies are like everything else. They can be used appropriately, they are subject to holes and biases, and they can be misused or twisted out of context. These problems can occur in development, implementation, or both. Some common errors and abuses that can occur in TA efforts are identified in Table 4. Among these, a preconceived bias of outcome is perhaps the most substantive problem in TA. An intelligent person-with-a-mission can go through a number of steps and processes that look good superficially but, on closer examination, are seriously flawed. Problems may arise if only the literature and evidence that support one position or agenda are chosen, if a poor methodology is selected, if strong personalities or people with preconceived convictions are used in consensus efforts, if experts are used inappropriately, if guidelines are developed based on a specific belief system or for economic gain, or if there is a tendency only to consider those who sell or market devices. Obviously there are other issues and qualifications that need to be considered in the TA and guideline development processes.

The importance of proper processes has been stressed throughout health care literature, including popular and refereed chiropractic literature.[22,32,41–43] They suggest that responsibility for understanding TA and the associated processes and attributes resides with all stakeholders of health care, especially the practitioners or providers that use the technologies.[44] Thus, to assure that awareness of TA issues is

Table 3. The "four screen" model of TA

Screen	Criteria	Basis for choice: Who is involved?	Additional issues
Screen 1 Does it work? (Effectiveness)	Clinical Safety, effectiveness, efficacy, etc	Evidence based International researchers Professional organizations Providers/institutions	Burden of proof? Quality of evidence?
Screen 2 Is it needed? (Appropriateness)	Clinical Expected benefit, given clinical situation	Evidence based Providers/institutions Professional organizations (eg, guidelines) International researchers	Burden of proof? Extent of benefits?
Screen 3 Is it wanted? (Informed decision making)	Personal Match between expected outcomes and patient wishes	Value based Patients Providers	Informed patient?
Screen 4 Should the public pay? (Insured services)	Economic/political Most cost-effective option? Strong moral objections? Can society tolerate denial?	Value based Citizens Governments	Participation process? Available resources?

Source: Reprinted with permission from R.B. Deber et al., The Public-Private Mix in Health Care, in *Striking a Balance: Health Care Systems in Canada and Elsewhere,* Vol. 4, pp. 423–545, © 1998.

Table 4. Common misconceptions and/or faulty assumptions in TA

- **Ignore the literature.** Consideration of studies favorable to one's position only will undermine the integrity of any formal TA process.
- **Strength of personalities.** Consensus efforts can be overwhelmed by well-informed, articulate, or assertive individuals who may or may not have a good and unbiased grasp of the real issues. Balancing personalities and knowledgebases on sides is a must.
- **Preconceived conviction approach.** If you know you are right, no amount of evidence to the contrary will ever convince you otherwise. While this posture may be helpful for political ascendancy within a trade association, it is bad for the science and explicit process required in TA.
- **All evidence is created equal approach.** Studies can be of varying quality and type. The methodologic strength of any given study must be weighed appropriately. Thus a methodologically good study with dissenting results cannot be thrown out. Likewise, a weak methodologic study with good outcomes must be discarded.
- **Experts-R-Us.** Bringing individuals on board who have impressive degrees or credentials (provided they agree with you) is a strategy that can only backfire in the long term. Often, someone unfamiliar with the ins and outs of a particular field may be bamboozled into supporting something that looks good on the surface, but has no understanding of the substantive underlying weaknesses or issues. Ultimate credibility of a TA endeavor will rest on the process and content, not on who poses for a picture or writes a foreword in the proceedings.
- **Consensus of the congregation of true believers.** Perhaps the most common error among clinical disciplines is to assume that a fair result cannot be attained unless all parties are unequivocal supporters of the cause. For example, surgical guidelines for spinal fusion developed only by spinal fusion surgeons in isolation might meet with a serious credibility problem. Why should it be any different for chiropractors?
- **It is easy to be suckered in by a good salesperson.** Medical device developers, however well intentioned, must tend to the marketplace, recoup development costs, and show a profit. Often the concern with side effects, scientific investigation criteria, or patient outcomes can be secondary to the need to market a product. Consider the government regulations on new pharmaceuticals that have had to be put in place as a result of past eagerness to bring a drug to market before good independent safety and efficacy research is available.
- **Remain uninformed.** TA is not something just for pointy heads. Tables 3 and 5 present inventories of TA attributes and indicate which constituencies have roles to play. It is a mistake to let others (usually the loudest and slickest) do the thinking for you.

Table 5. Role of various groups in increasing practitioner knowledge regarding TA

Assessment/attributes of practitioner knowledge of TA	Individual providers	Health purchasers	MCOs	Device/procedure developers	Chiropractic colleges	Licensing boards	Professional associations
Education and training							
Level of training	X			X	X	X	X
Critical appraisal skills	X				X		X
Decision-making/analysis skills	X				X		X
Skills displacement	X		X	X	X		
Legal—regulatory							
FDA, NIH, OSHA, NIOSH	X		X		X	X	X
Patent law/intellectual	X			X			
Property rights	X			X			
Legal—malpractice							
Malpractice	X		X	X			X
Informed consent	X				X	X	X
Risk	X			X		X	
Strict liability	X			X			
Patient competency	X				X		X
Standard of care	X			X	X	X	X
Organizational							
MCO/facility accreditation (NCQA, Joint Commission)	X	X	X	X			X
Ethical							
Informed consent	X				X	X	X
Right to life/death	X			X			
Access to technology	X	X	X	X	X	X	X
Norms/standards of care	X			X	X	X	X
Allocation of community resources	X	X	X		X		X
Risks	X		X	X	X	X	X
Economic							
Cost benefit	X	X	X	X	X	X	X
Cost-effectiveness	X	X	X	X	X	X	X
Third-party payers		X	X	X			X
Allocation of economic resources	X	X	X		X		X
Personnel displacement	X		X		X		X
Safety							
Risks	X		X	X	X	X	X
Efficacy							
Risks	X		X	X	X	X	X
Cost benefit	X	X	X	X	X	X	X
Cost-effectiveness	X	X	X	X	X	X	X
Dissemination							
Adoption of technology	X	X	X	X	X	X	X
Use of technology	X	X	X	X	X	X	X
Distribution of technology	X	X	X	X	X		X
Educational/scientific constraints	X		X	X	X	X	X

FDA, Food and Drug Administration; NIH, National Institutes of Health; OSHA, Occupational Safety and Health Administration; NIOSH, National Institute of Occupational Safety and Health; MCO, managed care organization; IRB, Institutional Review Board; NCQA, National Commission on Quality Assurance; Joint Commission, Joint Commission on Accreditation of Healthcare Organizations.

Source: Reprinted with permission from G.R. Goodman, Increasing Physician Acceptance of Technology Assessment Through a Focused Training Program. International Journal of Technology Assessment in Health Care, Vol. 10, No. 2, pp. 312–316, © 1994, Cambridge University Press.

broadened and that reports of technology assessment exercises are disseminated and implemented, payers, MCOs, device developers, colleges, administrative boards, and trade associations must contribute to practitioner knowledge and understanding. Moreover, consistent with the trend toward continuous quality management, the affected parties must measure outcomes of TA as they regard public health, health care economics, and the inherent resources found in the chiropractic profession.

The attributes of practitioner knowledge of TA are listed in Table 5. In addition, the table presents a matrix of those stakeholder groups that should participate in enhancing the knowledge of practitioners. Health care providers have some obvious responsibility to obtain knowledge through self-learning opportunities. Likewise, professional associations, licensing boards, and chiropractic colleges need to provide focused learning opportunities that enhance learning and understanding. Furthermore, payer groups and MCOs have a strong financial interest to see that there is proper compliance with and favorable outcomes from technology assessment implementation. Thus, they, too, need to offer learning opportunities. Last, device developers have an important role to play because they can provide background information on the attributes of the assessment of their respective technology. A number of resources and organizations exist and are readily accessible to doctors, physician organizations, and other interested groups by telephone, mail, and internet (see Appendix I-A).

CONCLUSIONS

Times have changed in the delivery of health care. Health professionals and institutions are now held accountable for the quality of care provided and the appropriateness of the devices and procedures used. Furthermore, the competitive nature of the indemnification industry in the United States and the need for careful use of limited health care resources in virtually every society are creating demand for answers regarding which health services should be available in a given community. Health care system reform requires that systematic processes be applied to assure cost-effectiveness, safety, and efficiency of procedures and devices used on patients. TA affords a means to critically review available information, as well as to extrapolate from the consensus of representative experts and users. Some of the key issues identified in this article relative to proper application of TA include interpretation of evidence, consensus building, dissemination and implementation of TA results, and measurement of effect of the TA on health practice and on society as a whole. There is a risk of misapplying TA that can range from inappropriate use in policy and reimbursement settings to biased efforts employing a slick facade to disguise a marketer's special interest.

Today's health care system is moving toward a patient-centered, value-driven industry.[45] To navigate through this new paradigm, practitioners, academics, scientists, administrators, policy makers, patients, payers, and device developers will be watching the compass, knowing that the process is open, documented, dynamic, retrievable, and reproducible as new information and opinion yield modification and revision.

The "choice of the ages" for the chiropractic discipline appears to be whether to pursue status in the mainstream of health care or to stay entrenched as a segment of alternative health care. While legitimate science has been a part of the chiropractic "veneer" for the last couple of decades, there is significance to what has been found to be valid and publicly accepted. The public is beginning to appreciate that manipulation, the principal mode of treatment by chiropractors, replaces many of the caustic drugs and brutal surgeries that have long served as the mainstream medical alternative in mechanical spinal problems. Most insurance and reimbursement systems are evolving to include chiropractic services as a "carve-out," replacing what would have been allocated for drugs, surgery, or even hospitalization. In order for other chiropractic methods to gain similar acceptance, and for manipulation and adjusting to be embraced as reasonable alternatives in non-mechanical conditions, rigorous scrutiny through formalized TA process will be a prerequisite. Perhaps the greatest value of these efforts will lie in their ability to focus on meaningful clinical and social outcomes, thereby offering the chiropractic profession an important tool for clinical refinements that focus on quality patient care.

The tasks of the chiropractic profession in the assessment of technologies should be clearer. There should be a heightened realization that chiropractors are not in this situation alone and that their partners include patients, purchasers, MCOs, device developers, colleges, licensing boards, trade associations, and other community resources. The tough questions now being asked by the consuming public need to be answered. Awareness and action on public expectations, use of proper methodologies and processes to answer the tough questions, and broad efforts on focused learning opportunities on TA are all agenda items for a responsible place in health care.

REFERENCES

1. Patrick DL, Erickson P. *Health Status and Health Policy.* New York, NY: Oxford University Press; 1993.
2. Flesia J. Science and clinical competency. In: *Proceedings of 1995 Hawaii State Chiropractic Association Convention.* Colorado Springs, Colo: Renaissance International; 1995.
3. Eisenberg DM, Kessler R, Foster C, et al. Unconventional medicine in the United States: prevalence, costs and patterns for use. *N Engl J Med.* 1993;328(4):246–252.
4. Chiropractic treats 33% of back pain patients, study says. *Dynam Chiro.* 1994;12(19):1.
5. Mootz RD, Shekelle PG, Hansen DT. The politics of policy and research. *Top Clin Chiro.* 1995;2(2):56–70.
6. Coile RC. Chiropractic treatment: an "alternative medicine" becomes mainstream health care. *Health Trends.* 1995;7(9):1.
7. McGivney WT. Technology assessment and coverage decision making. *J Am Assoc Pref Provider Org.* Sept/Oct 1994: 11–17.
8. Ferrara EP, Servis KW. *State Task Force on Clinical Guidelines and Medical Technology Assessment.* Albany, NY: New York State Department of Health; 1994.
9. Bigos S, Bowyer O, Braen G, et al. *Acute Low Back Problems in Adults.* Clinical practice guideline no. 14. Washington, DC: US Department of Health and Human Services, Agency for Health Care Policy and Research; 1994.
10. Prescott PA. Cost effective primary care providers: an important component to health care reform. *Int J Tech Assessment.* 1994;10(2):249.
11. Owens EF. Line drawing analyses of static cervical X-ray used in chiropractic. *J Manipulative Physiol Ther.* 1992;15(7):442–449.
12. Taylor JAM. Full-spine radiography: a review. *J Manipulative Physiol Ther.* 1993;16(7):460–474.
13. Bartol KM. A model for categorization of chiropractic treatment procedures. *J Chiro Tech.* 1991;3(2):78–80.
14. Gatterman MI, Hansen DT. Development of chiropractic nomenclature through consensus. *J Manipulative Physiol Ther.* 1994;17(5):302–309.
15. Kaminski M, Boal R, Gillette R, et al. Model for evaluation of chiropractic methods. *J Manipulative Physiol Ther.* 1987;10(2):61–64.
16. Kaminski M. Evaluation of chiropractic methods. *J Chiro Tech.* 1990;2(3):107–113.
17. Boal R, Kaminski M, Peterson DH, Gillette RG. An algorithm for the analysis of chiropractic methods. In: Vear H, ed. *Chiropractic Standards of Practice and Quality of Care.* Gaithersburg, Md: Aspen Publishers; 1992.
18. ACA policies on public health and related matters. In: *ACA Membership Directory.* Arlington, Va: ACA; 1990.
19. Lamm LC, Wegner E. Chiropractic scope of practice: what the law allows. *Am J Chiro Med.* 1989;2:155–159.
20. Hansen DT, ed. *Chiropractic Standards of Practice and Utilization Guidelines in the Care and Treatment of Injured Workers.* Olympia, Wash: Chiropractic Advisory Committee, Washington State Department of Labor and Industries; 1989.
21. Bergmann TF. Proceedings of the first consensus conference on validation of chiropractic methods. *J Chiro Tech.* 1990;2(3).
22. Hansen DT, Adams AH, Meeker WC, Phillips RB. Proposal for establishing structure and process in the development of implicit chiropractic standards of care and practice guidelines. *J Manipulative Physiol Ther.* 1992;15(2):430–438.
23. Hansen DT. Prospects for the future of chiropractic guidelines. In: Lawrence D, ed. *Advances in Chiropractic.* Chicago, Ill: Mosby-Year Book; 1993;1.
24. Hansen DT, Triano JJ. Applications of quality assurance in chiropractic practice. In: Lawrence D, ed. *Advances in Chiropractic.* Chicago, Ill: Mosby-Year Book; 1993;2.
25. Cooperstein R, Schneider MS. Assessment of chiropractic techniques and procedures. *Top Clin Chiro.* 1996;3(1):44–52.
26. Shekelle PG, Adams AH, Chassin MR, et al. The appropriateness of spinal manipulation of low-back pain: indications and ratings by a multidisciplinary expert panel. Santa Monica, Calif: RAND Corporation; 1991. R-4025/2-CCR/FCER.
27. Coulter ID, Shekelle PG, Mootz RD, Hansen DT. The use of expert panel results: the RAND panel for appropriateness of manipulation and mobilization of the cervical spine. *Top Clin Chiro.* 1994; 2(3):54–62.
28. Shekelle PG, Hurwitz EL, Coulter ID, et al. The appropriateness of chiropractic spinal manipulation for low back pain: a pilot study. *J Manipulative Physiol Ther.* 1995;18:265–270.
29. Coulter ID, Hays RD, Danielson CD. The chiropractic satisfaction questionnaire. *Top Clin Chiro.* 1993;1(4):40–43.
30. Coulter TD, Danielson CD, Hays RD. Measuring chiropractic practitioners satisfaction. *Top Clin Chiro.* 1996;3(1):65–70.
31. Morton L. ACA position statement on release of AHCPR guideline no. 14 [press conference for Agency for Health Care Policy and Research]. Washington, DC: American Chiropractic Assoc; December 8, 1994.
32. AHCPR clinical guideline 14: an ICA analysis. In: Clum GW, ed. *Acute Low Back Problems in Adults: An Abridged Version with Analysis and Commentary.* San Lorenzo, Calif: Life Chiropractic College of Chiropractic–West; 1995.
33. National Board of Chiropractic Examiners. *Job Analysis of Chiropractic: A Project Report, Survey Analysis and Summary of the Practice of Chiropractic within the United States.* Greely, Colo: National Board of Chiropractic Examiners; 1993.
34. Bowers LJ, Mootz RD. The nature of primary care: the chiropractor's role. *Top Clin Chiro.* 1995;2(1):66–84.
35. O'Kane M. *1994 Standards for the Accreditation of Managed Care Organizations.* Washington, DC: National Commission on Quality Assurance; 1993.
36. Eddy DM. *A Manual for Assessing Health Practices and Designing Practice Policies.* Philadelphia, Pa: American College of Physicians; 1992.
37. Sacket DL, Haynes RB, Tugwell P. *Clinical Epidemiology.* Boston, Mass: Little, Brown; 1985.
38. Brook RH. Practice guidelines and practicing medicine: are they compatible? *JAMA.* 1989;262(21):3027–3030.
39. Haldeman S, Chapman-Smith D, Petersen D. *Guidelines for Chiropractic Quality Assurance and Practice Parameters.* Gaithersburg, Md: Aspen Publishers; 1992.
40. Deber R, Ross E, Catz M. *Comprehensiveness in Health Care: A Report of the HEAL Action Lobby.* Toronto, Ontario, Canada: Department of Health Administration, University of Toronto; 1994.

41. Brook RH, Chassin MR, Fink A, Solomon DH, Kosecoff J, Park RE. A method for the detailed assessment of the appropriateness of medical technologies. *Int J Technology Assessment Health Care.* 1986;2:53–63.
42. Audet AM, Greenfield S, Field M. Medical practice guidelines: current activities and future directions. *Ann Intern Med.* 1990;113:709–714.
43. Coulter ID, Adams AH. Consensus methods, clinical guidelines, and the RAND study of chiropractic. *J Chiro.* December 1992;29(12):52–61.
44. Goodman GR. Increasing physician acceptance of technology assessment through a focused training program. *Int J Tech Assessment.* 1994;10(2):312–316.
45. Elwood PM. Shattuck lecture—outcomes management: a technology of patient experience. *N Engl J Med.* 1988;318(23):153–155.

Algorithm 1

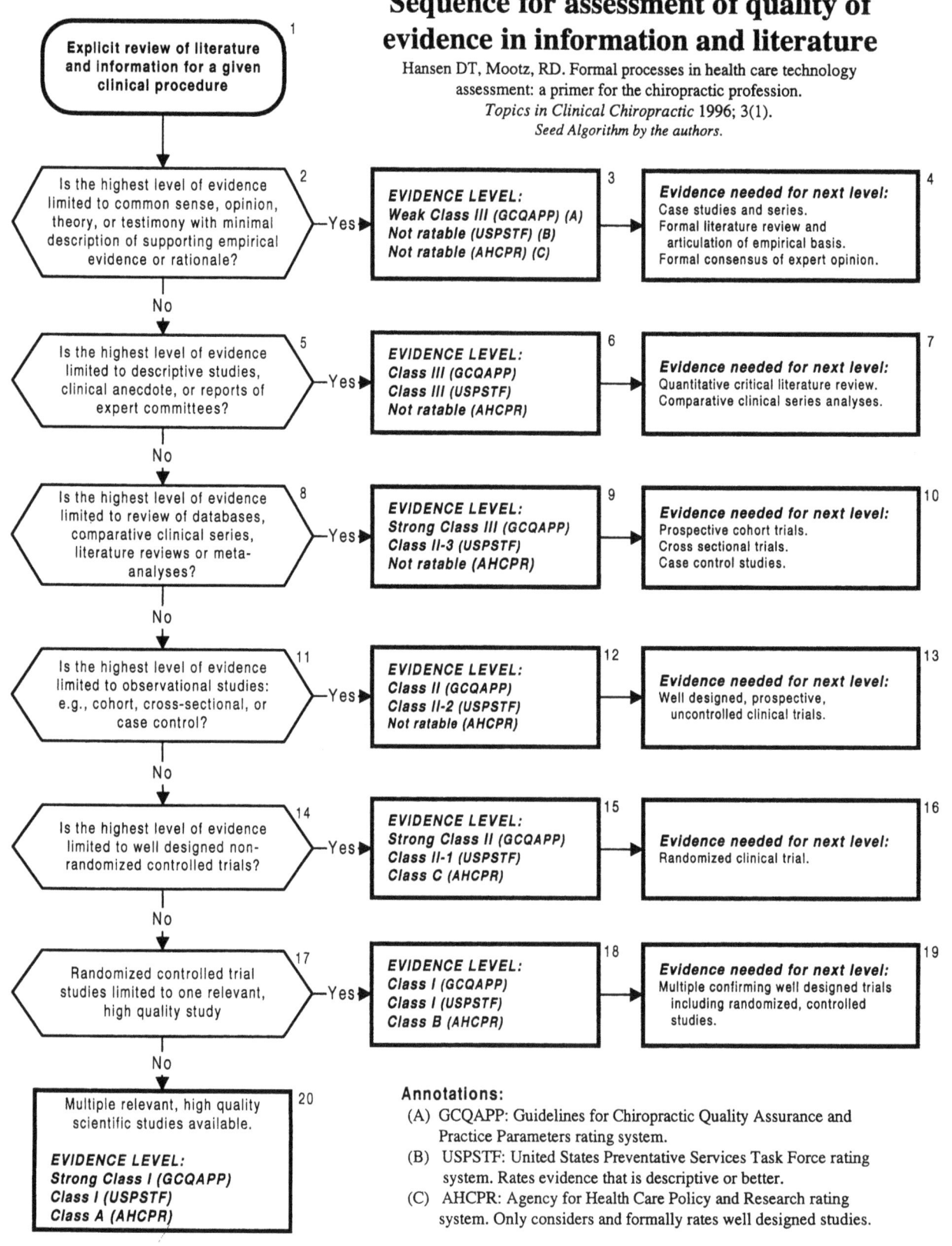

Algorithm 2

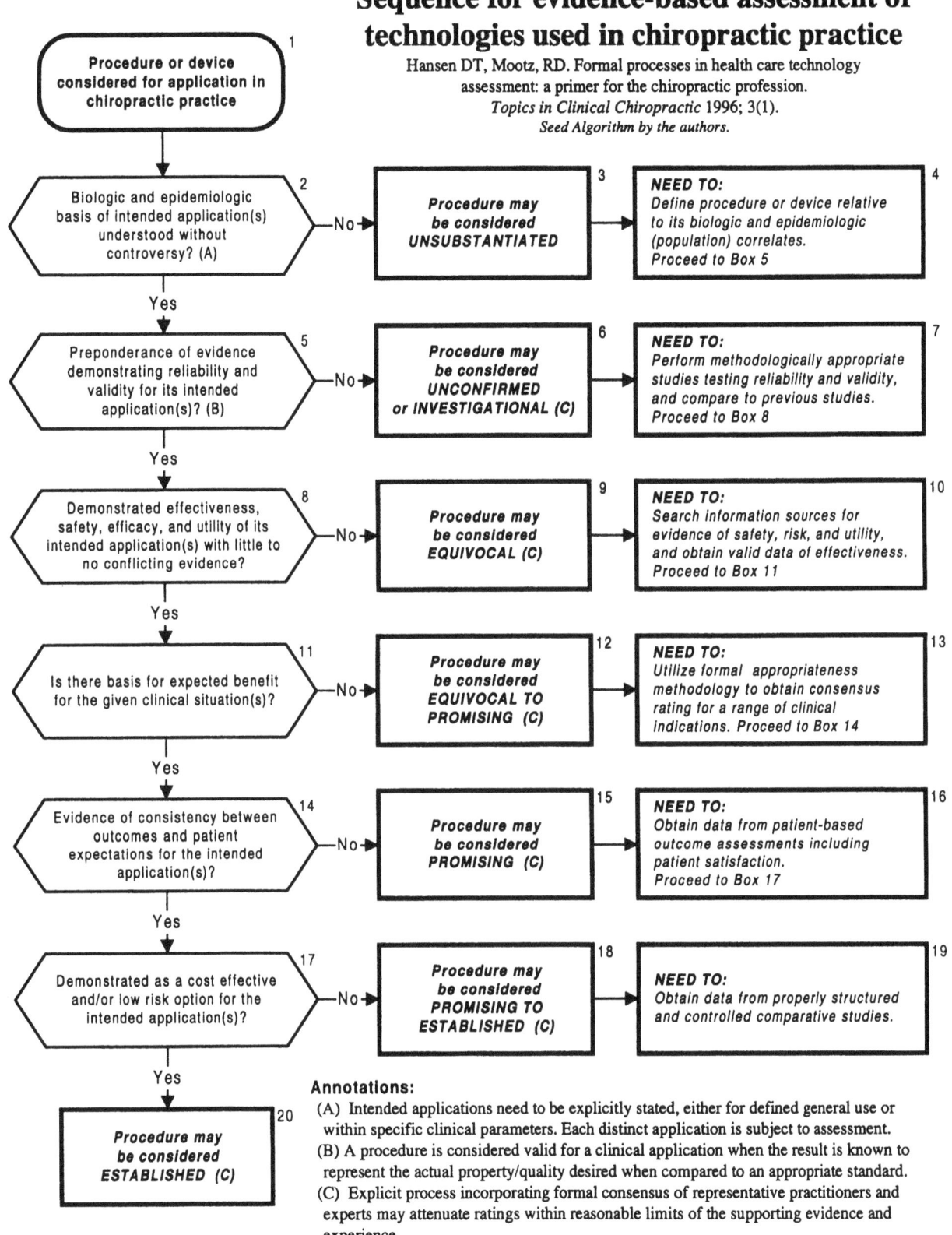

Sequence for evidence-based assessment of technologies used in chiropractic practice

Hansen DT, Mootz, RD. Formal processes in health care technology assessment: a primer for the chiropractic profession. *Topics in Clinical Chiropractic* 1996; 3(1). *Seed Algorithm by the authors.*

Annotations:

(A) Intended applications need to be explicitly stated, either for defined general use or within specific clinical parameters. Each distinct application is subject to assessment.

(B) A procedure is considered valid for a clinical application when the result is known to represent the actual property/quality desired when compared to an appropriate standard.

(C) Explicit process incorporating formal consensus of representative practitioners and experts may attenuate ratings within reasonable limits of the supporting evidence and experience.

2

Public and Occupational Health Regulations in Chiropractic Practice

David Wickes, Grant Iannelli, and John Livingston

Modern health care professionals are faced with an increasing number of state and federal regulations that influence the delivery of office-based care. In the past few years, regulations have been enacted that govern office laboratory testing, handling of biohazard materials, protection of patients and office employees from infectious and chemical agents, and mandatory reporting of sexually abused pediatric patients. Additionally, practitioners have responsibilities to the public at large regarding reporting of communicable diseases. Each of these topics is now reviewed.

OFFICE-BASED LABORATORY TESTING

Despite the widespread availability of reference laboratories, many physicians perform some type of laboratory testing in the office. Occasionally, the motivation is primarily financial, with considerable revenue generation being possible in busy offices. In other practices, the speed of obtaining results from office-based testing is the primary consideration. Regardless of the motives, all office-based laboratories were affected by the implementation of the Clinical Laboratory Improvement Act (CLIA) amendments of 1988,[1] which went into effect on February 28, 1992. CLIA is considered a procedure-specific, rather than site-specific, regulation. This means that what is regulated is the diagnostic procedure, not the location of the testing. Even the simplest of laboratory tests, such as a dipstick urinalysis, is included in CLIA, even if the physician does not charge for the procedure.

CLIA currently has four levels of complexity for laboratory tests (Table 1). The first level, referred to as waived tests, includes tests of a relatively uncomplicated nature. Waived tests are held to be unlikely to suffer from technical errors, and several are approved by the Food and Drug Administration (FDA) for home use.[2] Within this category, the dipstick urinalysis and the Wintrobe or Westergren erythrocyte sedimentation rate (ESR) are among the most often performed laboratory tests in the chiropractic office. The decision to send a urine sample to a reference laboratory for microscopic analysis or culturing is often based upon a preliminary dipstick analysis while the patient is still in the office. Because ESR studies are optimally performed on fresh specimens of whole blood, many practitioners prefer to perform these in the office rather than send them out to a reference laboratory. Pregnancy tests are sometimes done in the office before radiographs are taken on a female patient when the pregnancy status is uncertain. It should be noted that only color-comparison urine pregnancy tests are included in the waived category. Agglutination-inhibition slide and tube pregnancy tests are considered moderate complexity tests.

Practitioners wishing to perform any laboratory tests in their offices must obtain certification from the Health Care Financing Administration (HCFA). For tests in the waived category, the physician will need to apply for a certificate of waiver. This involves submitting an application listing the physician's name and tests performed plus a $100 fee. Waivers need to be renewed every 2 years. Laboratories operating with a certificate of waiver are not required to be inspected annually, but they must allow an inspection if such is desired by the regulatory agency.

The second CLIA category of tests was added to the original categories in January 1993. This category, referred to as physician-performed microscopy, allows doctors to analyze certain fresh samples immediately in their offices that would otherwise suffer from deterioration during transit and do not have controls to monitor the test process.[3] Such tests include

Adapted from *Top Clin Chiro* 1994; 1(3): 9–19
© 1994 Aspen Publishers, Inc.

Table 1. CLIA 1988 classification of laboratory tests*

Waived tests	Physician-performed microscopy	Medium complexity tests	High complexity tests
Urinalysis—dipstick or tablet 　Glucose 　Hemoglobin 　Bilirubin 　Ketones 　Nitrite 　Specific gravity 　Protein 　Leukocytes 　pH 　Urobilinogen Fecal occult blood Urine pregnancy tests (color) Blood hemoglobin (by sulfate) Blood hemoglobin (by single analyte instrument) Blood glucose† Spun microhematocrit ESR Ovulation tests (color method)	Urine sediment examination Wet mounts Pinworm examination Fern tests Potassium hydroxide preps	Urine culture Manual white blood cell count and differential‡ Rheumatoid factor (slide) Cholesterol (reagent strip) Pregnancy tests (slide) Mononucleosis screen	Pap smears Fluorescent anti-nuclear antibodies Radioimmunoassays Manual white blood cell count and differential§ Manual platelet count Manual reticulocyte count Electrophoresis procedures Sputum cytology Chromatography studies

*Lists of tests shown in medium and high complexity categories are incomplete; see references 1 and 3 for complete lists.
†On device approved by FDA for home use.
‡Without identification of atypical cells.
§With identification of atypical cells.

potassium hydroxide yeast mounts and evaluation of urine sediment. Physicians wishing to perform tests in this category must apply for a certificate, which is valid for 2 years and costs $150. Routine inspections are not required, but inspections may be held for the purpose of verifying that only registered tests are being performed. It appears that the physician must be an MD, DO, or DPM, but the regulations are somewhat vague in this regard.

The third CLIA category includes tests of moderate complexity. Such tests include microscopic studies, cultures, slide agglutination tests, blood chemistries, and blood counts. Although most chiropractic physicians do not perform microscopic studies or automated blood counts in their offices, many do perform reagent-strip cholesterol or glucose studies in the office or at health fairs, and these tests are included in this category.

The final CLIA category comprises tests of high complexity. Few chiropractic offices perform high complexity laboratory tests. Manual white blood cell differential counts with identification of atypical cells, manual reticulocyte counts, and manual platelet counts fall into this category. Any tests not specifically listed as being waived or of medium complexity become high complexity tests by default.

A fifth category has recently been proposed by the CLIA Advisory Committee and would comprise kits for which manufacturers have included all required quality control and quality assurance materials. This category has not been formally approved by the HCFA, but such is expected in the near future.

The procedure for becoming certified to perform moderate and high complexity tests is fairly complicated. For these tests, the laboratory must participate in proficiency testing three times per year for each test to be performed. Proficiency testing consists of testing unknown samples provided by an independent testing agency. The physician must have prepared written manuals covering analytic and quality control procedures. Records must be kept on test and instrument calibration, which must be performed at least semiannually. Calibration must also be done every time a reagent lot number changes. Centrifuges must be checked quarterly. Daily logs must be kept on temperature readings in refrigerators and freezers in the laboratory, and even the thermometers must be calibrated and checked periodically.[4]

Perhaps of greatest significance to the chiropractic office are the requirements regarding personnel. Laboratories providing moderate and high complexity tests must have a designated laboratory director, a technical consultant, and a clinical consultant. The director must be an MD, DO, DPM, or PhD or have a bachelor's or master's degree along with specific laboratory training. CLIA does not include the DC among those persons eligible to direct a laboratory or act as a consultant unless there has been additional training or experience in a laboratory setting. Although it might seem feasible to ask an eligible professional acquaintance to assume one of the roles in title, CLIA mandates that there be a significant degree of oversight and interaction with the laboratory. The director obviously assumes overall responsibility for compliance with the CLIA regulations. The technical consultant must also have advanced training in the specific test methodologies and must be available for consultation regarding test performance, quality assurance, and competency evaluation of test personnel. The clinical consultant must be an MD or DO and must be available for consultation regarding diagnosis, treatment, and management of patients. Neither the technical consultant nor the clinical consultant is required to be on site at all times, but both must be available on an as-needed basis. Unlike the case for waived tests, testing personnel must meet specific qualifications, consisting primarily of either an earned degree or documented training in the test procedures being performed. Registration fees for the moderate and complex categories are higher than for the simpler levels and are based on the volume and scope of testing.

With the enactment of the CLIA 1988 regulations, it has become impractical for most small chiropractic offices to perform any on-site laboratory tests other than those classified as waived. Only multidisciplinary, multispecialty offices are likely to have the required technical personnel and other resources to make performance of other laboratory tests cost efficient.

PROTECTION FROM BLOODBORNE PATHOGENS

Regulations issued by the Occupational Safety and Health Administration (OSHA) in 1992 govern the protection of health care workers from bloodborne pathogens, including the hepatitis B virus (HBV) and the human immunodeficiency virus (HIV).[5] Although most practitioners and laboratory workers long ago adopted protective measures, the OSHA regulations added further responsibilities. The major features of the regulations are outlined in Table 2.

As of May 1, 1992, every clinic where there exists the possibility of exposure of employees to blood or other potentially infectious materials was expected to have a written exposure control plan. Key elements of this plan include a copy of the OSHA standard, an explanation of the rights of employees regarding HBV vaccination and testing after accidental exposure, a description of protective physical measures in place at the worksite, procedures for dealing with accidental exposure, training opportunities, and record-

Table 2. Major components of the OSHA bloodborne pathogens standard

Written exposure control plan
HBV vaccination for employees
Protective engineering controls
Personal protective equipment
Training of employees
Exposure incident management
Written records

keeping. Sample exposure control plans, as well as copies of the standard and educational materials are available from OSHA.

The bloodborne pathogens standard applies to any employee with possible exposure to blood or other potentially infectious materials regardless of the frequency or extent of interaction. For example, even if a physician performs the venipuncture and sample collection, if an office worker is asked to centrifuge the sample or to transfer it to a laboratory pick-up bag that office worker is covered by the standard. The standard applies equally to full-time, part-time, and temporary employees.

Each employee must be offered the opportunity to be vaccinated against HBV. Employees who decide against the vaccination series must sign a formal declination statement, which must be kept on file in the office. Employees must also receive formal training, beginning within 10 days of their employment and repeated annually. Documentation of this training must also be kept on file. Employees must be provided with any necessary protective gowns and gloves. Protective devices, such as splash shields and centrifuge covers, must be utilized. Many offices have begun using self-sheathing needles to prevent accidental needlestick injuries. Separate refrigerators must be used for laboratory samples. Approved and labeled containers must be used for used needles and other sharps as well as for other blood- or fluid-contaminated waste. Regular disinfection of specimen processing work areas must be performed. Employees must be trained to clean up broken glassware and spills properly. Universal precautions, the concept of considering all laboratory samples potentially infectious, must be the standard operating procedure.

PROTECTION FROM TUBERCULOSIS

As with bloodborne pathogens safety measures, protection of health care workers from tuberculosis (TB) exposure has become increasingly regulated. In 1990, the Centers for Disease Control and Prevention (CDC) issued preliminary guidelines for prevention of transmission of TB in health care facilities.[6] A second draft was issued on October 12,

1993,[7] and a final draft is expected in 1994. Unwilling to wait for the final CDC documents, OSHA issued its own enforcement policy on October 8, 1993, which was effective immediately, and officials have been authorized to issue citations to employers for noncompliance.[8]

Five workplaces have been identified as needing TB control measures: health care settings, correctional institutions, homeless shelters, long-term care facilities for the elderly, and drug treatment centers. Health care settings include hospitals, ambulatory care facilities, and outpatient and dental clinics. Although OSHA regulations pertain solely to employers and employees, the CDC guidelines include volunteers and students. Both agencies are primarily concerned with employees who are likely to have contact with a TB patient, including first contact employees (eg, receptionists) as well as treating physicians.

The required written TB exposure control plan must address overall risk assessment at the facility, TB skin testing for employees, training of employees, a protocol for the identification of persons with active TB, and management of employees found to be infected. Although this may seem extreme for the typical chiropractic office, OSHA and the CDC do not differentiate among provider types. The CDC guidelines are applicable to all settings in which health care is provided, and OSHA is expected to adopt the final CDC guidelines when they are issued in 1994. It is likely that OSHA will initially concentrate upon those workplaces that have the greatest likelihood of TB infection, such as clinics for patients with acquired immunodeficiency syndrome (AIDS) and hospitals, but OSHA will investigate a complaint from an employee at any site.

Risk assessment includes an evaluation of the number of known TB patients seen at the clinic and any known TB skin test conversions among employees at the workplace. Sites seeing fewer than six patients per year and with no employee conversions are considered low risk. Sites with six or more TB patients per year are considered intermediate risk, and sites with evidence of employee skin test conversion or evidence of patient-to-patient transmission are considered high risk. Most chiropractic offices will probably be classified as low risk, and employees will need to have annual skin tests. Intermediate risk offices will need to provide skin testing every 6 months. It should be recognized that chiropractic physicians are being consulted by many AIDS patients for provision of alternative health care, and the incidence of TB among immunocompromised patients is rising dramatically.

An integral part of the exposure control plan is a TB educational program for workers. This training program must include information about the recognition of the signs and symptoms of TB, pathogenesis and transmission of the disease, risk reduction measures, skin testing, and responsibilities of employees. The training must be conducted for all new employees at risk and must be repeated annually for all employees at risk. Written records of these training sessions must be maintained. Regardless of whether there is an existing medical file for the employee, OSHA mandates that a separate and secure file be kept for all medical and training records pertaining to the bloodborne pathogens and tuberculosis standards.

Sample exposure control plans, compliance checklists, and educational materials for employees have not been developed by OSHA for the TB standard. At the time of this writing, besides the original OSHA memorandum, all that is available from OSHA to assist employers is a fact sheet (OSHA 93-430). It is anticipated that the other materials will be released subsequently, as was the case with the bloodborne pathogens standard.

REPORTING OF COMMUNICABLE DISEASES

All states have laws requiring the reporting of communicable disease by health care providers to local public health authorities. It is through this means that disease trends can be tracked and potentially dangerous outbreaks of infectious diseases controlled. Chiropractic physicians are required to participate in the reporting process in most states (Table 3).

Not all infectious disease must be reported, and the nature of the report varies with the specific disease. Table 4 gives a representative sample of the types of infectious diseases and conditions requiring reporting in many states. Although it is unlikely that the chiropractic physician would be the initial provider involved with many of these conditions, several reportable diseases are frequently diagnosed in the chiropractic practice, including measles, mumps, chickenpox, foodborne illnesses, streptococcal infections, and Lyme disease.

Infectious diseases posing the greatest risk of spread to the public have the most stringent reporting criteria, and often some type of confinement of the patient is required. Meningitis and foodborne illness are examples of diseases that must be reported by phone to the local health department within 24 hours. Less communicable illnesses usually have a

Table 3. Persons required to report communicable diseases to local public health authorities

Medical physicians
Osteopathic physicians
Chiropractic physicians
Podiatrists
School nurses
Dentists
Laboratory personnel
Day care personnel
Other health care practitioners

Table 4. Diseases and conditions requiring reporting in many states

AIDS/HIV infection	Intestinal worms	Rabies (human)
Amebiasis	Legionnaire's disease	Rocky mountain spotted fever
Animal bites	Leprosy	Rubella
Anthrax	Leptospirosis	Salmonellosis
Brucellosis	Lymphogranuloma	Shigellosis
Chancroid	venereum	Staphylococcal infections
Chickenpox	Lyme disease	(some)
Cholera	Malaria	Streptococcal infections
Diarrhea of the newborn	Measles	Syphilis
Diphtheria	Meningitis	Tetanus
Encephalitis	Meningococcemia	Toxic shock syndrome
Enteropathic *Escherichia coli* infection	Mumps	Trachoma
Foodborne illnesses	Ophthalmia neonatorum	Trichinosis
Giardiasis	Pertussis (whooping	Tuberculosis
Gonorrhea	cough)	Typhoid fever
Granuloma inguinale	Plague	Typhus
Hepatitis (viral)	Polio	
Histoplasmosis	Psittacosis	

reporting period of up to 1 week and can be reported by either phone or writing.

It is important for the provider to have a copy of the applicable health department regulations on the reporting of infectious diseases. Most health departments have written materials available to physicians for educational purposes as well as preprinted reporting forms. The local regulations will also state the necessary isolation requirements. In most states the licensed clinical laboratory is required to report positive test results for many infectious diseases, but this often does not eliminate the responsibility of the provider also to make notification.

MEDICAL WASTE PROCESSING

Any physician who provides in-office clinical laboratory services (including blood sample collection via venipuncture) or who generates materials contaminated with body fluids should have an answer to the question, "What do I do with medical waste (MW)?" After several New England beaches were closed during the summer of 1988 because trash washed ashore that included used needles, syringes, and blood tubes, federal legislators enacted the MW Tracking Act of 1988.[9] Although this was a 2-year pilot program involving only a limited number of states, it started the process in most other states. When the US Environmental Protection Agency formulated regulations based on the act, it shifted the majority of control for MW tracking to the individual states. At this time most states have enacted their own waste regulations. This section addresses MW issues that concern chiropractic practice and is based on existing Illinois state law. Other states' laws are similar, but readers are advised to obtain copies of the statutes specific for their state.

States define MW as they see fit and may include different waste components in the definition. Table 5 lists the components that represent MW in the state of Illinois. Additionally, states also specifically exclude certain waste from the regulations, as listed in Table 6. Among the myriad of MW regulations, the following aspects should concern chiropractic physicians: MW production, storage, transport, treatment, and disposal.

Production

Any physician who produces MW is considered an MW generator and must abide by all federal, state, and local regulations concerning the MW. In some states (eg, Illinois and Wisconsin),[10,11] small generators (producing less than 50 lb of MW per month) receive exemption from registration requirements and need no permit to operate. Other states (eg, Michigan)[12] require all generators to register and pay a fee. Also, a generator can be held responsible for its MW if an incident occurs anywhere along the MW management track,

Table 5. Types of regulated MW

Cultures
Human pathologic wastes
Human blood and blood products
Used sharps
Animal waste
Isolation waste
Unused discarded sharps

Table 6. MW excluded from regulations

Waste generated as household waste
Waste (except sharps) whose infectious potential has been eliminated by treatment
Sharps whose infectious potential has been eliminated by treatment and that have been rendered unrecognizable

from initial transport and/or treatment to the final disposal site. Generators are also required to maintain all shipping manifests indicating final disposition of the MW shipment.

Storage

Regulations prevent the storage of MW at any site other than an approved storage facility. Once enough MW has accumulated to fill a shipment container, it must be transported to a storage or treatment facility within 72 hours unless it is kept at a temperature below 45°F. In any event, MW may not be stored for more than 30 days.

Transport

MW must be transported by a state-approved MW hauler. The only exception to this requirement is when an MW generator (or its agent) transports its own MW weighing less than 50 lb between facilities or to a treatment facility. In any event, MW for transport must be placed in a container that meets the criteria listed in Table 7. Transport containers for sharps must also be puncture resistant. Packages must be labeled with the international biohazard symbol (Fig 1) and the word *biohazard* as well as with the word *sharps* if the package contains materials capable of puncturing the skin. A label must also indicate the generator's name, address, and phone number. The transporter will also label the package with its name, address, phone number, and permit number and the date on which the MW left the generator's site.

Treatment

MW treatment serves to eliminate the waste's infectious potential. It can be affected through thermal, chemical, or

Table 7. MW transport container criteria

Rigid
Leak resistant
Impervious to moisture
Strong enough to prevent tearing or bursting under normal conditions of use and handling
Sealed to prevent leakage during transport

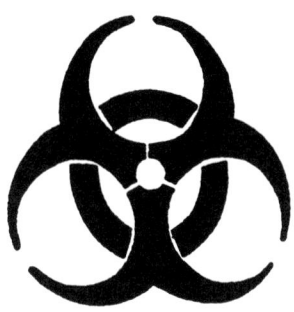

Fig 1. International biohazard symbol. It must appear on any medical waste containers.

irradiation treatment. The most common type of MW treatment is a thermal process, either incineration or autoclaving. Operators of treatment units are required to perform monthly quality control tests and to maintain records of all waste treated and its final disposition and may be required to register and obtain a permit. If less than 50 lb of MW is treated per month, no permit or registration is needed, although the other requirements must be met. Once MW has been treated, with the exception of sharps, it can be disposed of as unregulated trash. Sharps are still regulated as MW unless they are also rendered unrecognizable. This is carried out by incineration, grinding, or embedding in plastic.

Disposal

Untreated MW or recognizable sharps must be disposed of in state-approved disposal facilities. These facilities must meet stringent requirements that ensure that no leakage to the surrounding environment will occur.

Office guidelines

At the time of generation, sharps must be segregated from other waste. This is easily accomplished by using red and/or labeled polybags for nonsharp MW and rigid containers for sharps. Clinicians must remember to locate sharps containers out of the reach of children. One convenient method for treatment and disposal of MW is through the local hospital. Hospitals typically operate an MW treatment unit on site (autoclave, incinerator, etc) and are allowed to treat the MW generated by their physicians in their offices. This would be an important benefit to gaining hospital privileges. Larger reference laboratories may also be able to assist the practitioner.

Although there are a host of requirements that dictate how MW must be handled in private practitioners' offices, most physicians qualify as small generators and are exempt from the majority of regulations. By having an MW policy in place that outlines the basic procedures and identifies transport and treatment/disposal contractors/agents and then following that policy, chiropractic physicians will fulfill their MW management responsibilities.

OFFICE INFECTION CONTROL PROCEDURES

Health care practitioners must be cognizant of and practice procedures to minimize the spread of communicable disease. Most of these procedures are based on common sense, but many are required by state and local health codes.

The most basic infection control procedure is handwashing. Hands should be washed before and after every patient contact as well as at other times, as listed in Table 8. Table 9 outlines a recommended handwashing technique. At times, the lack of available plumbing, such as at a health fair or athletic event, precludes soap and water handwashing. In these instances the use of an antimicrobial foam or rinse is acceptable.

Infection control also applies to the reception area. Patients with highly communicable but not serious illnesses (eg, chickenpox or measles) should be advised not to come to the clinic while infectious unless absolutely necessary. Any patient with a suspected or known communicable disease should be taken to an examination/treatment room immediately rather than left to wait in the reception area. Tissues should be available for coughing or sneezing patients.

Patient care and diagnostic equipment must be disinfected if reused. Otoscope specula should be wiped with alcohol between patients. Diagnostic scopes and stethoscope diaphragms should be wiped with alcohol as needed. If glass thermometers are used, a disposable sheath should cover the thermometer during its use. The thermometer should be wiped with alcohol after each use. Examination and treatment tables and rehabilitation equipment that contact patients' skin should be wiped with a disposable disinfectant cloth or sprayed with a germicidal agent and wiped with disposable towels. Radiograph tables should be disinfected after use, or disposable table paper can be used (this does not interfere with the quality of the exposure). Table 10 lists several sources of infection control supplies.

A policy should exist covering the wearing of gloves. Disposable latex or vinyl gloves should be worn any time contact with body fluids is anticipated. Practitioners must decide whether gloves are to be worn during venipuncture, acupuncture needle insertion/removal, or other activities. If a glove rips during a procedure, it should be removed as soon as practical, the hands washed, and a new glove put on. Among emergency supplies should be a one-way pocket mask for artificial resuscitation, which allows for mouth-to-mask instead of mouth-to-mouth contact. Soiled gowns and towels should be kept in a covered container or bag away from the clean linens.

Consideration should be given to physiotherapy equipment and application methods. Either disposable adhesive electrode pads should be used (these may be kept in a sealed bag in the patient's file if reusable) or a disposable moist pad should be placed between the electrode and the patient's skin. Ultrasound heads should be sprayed with a disinfectant or wiped with alcohol after each use. Many local public health codes specify that lotions and gels must be kept in wide-mouthed containers to allow for periodic cleaning of the containers.

Table 8. Handwashing guidelines

Before and after patient contact
After glove removal
After using the restroom
After coughing/sneezing into the hands
After handling soiled linen

Table 9. Handwashing procedure

1. If rings cannot be removed, special attention should be paid to cleansing and drying the skin under the ring as well as the ring itself.
2. Wet hands and then apply soap. Use friction and rub all surfaces of hands and fingers.
3. Pay special attention to the thumbs and fingertips.
4. Hands should be rinsed with fingers down so that water and residue are carried away.
5. Water should be left running until hands have been dried with a paper towel so that the used towel can be used to turn the faucet off. Patting to dry rather than rubbing will lessen chapping.

Table 10. Infection control supplies

Product	Distributor	Type of product
Cal Stat®	Calgon Corp	Waterless liquid antiseptic hand cleanser
Purell®	GoJo Co	Waterless liquid antiseptic hand cleanser
Vionex®	Viro Research	Antimicrobial soap and skin wipes
Sani-Dex™	PDI	Antiseptic hand wipes
Sani-Cloth®	PDI	Disposable germicidal cloth
CPR Microshield™	MDI	Disposable cardiopulmonary resuscitation (CPR) shield
Pocket-Mask™	Laerdal Medical	Disposable CPR mask

From basic handwashing to equipment disinfection, infection control procedures are a vital component of professional health care practice. Public expectations have become great in this area, and many offices opt to perform the sanitation procedures in front of the patient to provide an additional sense of security. A disgruntled patient may prompt a surprise inspection from public health officials or a surprise lawsuit because of alleged infection. If there is any question about the applicability of these procedures to a specific situation, one should consult the city or county health department for advice.

PROTECTION FROM CHEMICAL HAZARDS

OSHA has also implemented regulations governing the management of hazardous chemicals in the workplace. Employers must have a formal hazard communication program that incorporates training of employees, labeling of hazardous chemicals, and posting of informational sheets.[13] Initially, the employer needs to make a complete survey of chemicals utilized in the office and to determine which are potentially hazardous. In general, any chemical product supplied by the manufacturer with a hazard warning label (eg, "flammable" or "causes substantial eye injury") is included in the standard. Table 11 lists some common types of office chemicals that are considered hazardous. A list of included chemicals must be kept on file and updated periodically. Chemicals intended for personal use (ie, not used in the line of duty) by the employee (eg, alcohol in the office first aid kit) are excluded from the standard.

For each hazardous chemical in the office, there must be a corresponding material safety data sheet (MSDS) available for review by employees. An MSDS provides information pertaining to the chemical and its common name, the known health hazard, precautions, emergency procedures, and measures to minimize risk. MSDSs are typically obtained from the supplier of the product. If the supplier does not provide an MSDS on the first shipment, the physician or office manager should insist that such be provided immediately. It should be noted, however, that OSHA places the responsibility for providing MSDSs on the employer, and therefore a supplier's lack of compliance in providing the necessary MSDSs should not deter the employer from obtaining the information directly from the manufacturer. For items that have been purchased in ordinary retail stores (eg, janitorial supplies), the employer will have to obtain an MSDS from the manufacturer or other source of information (MSDS information will soon become available on compact discs in reference libraries). The MSDSs must be easily accessible by the employees; most employers place them in a binder kept with other OSHA-required posters and materials.

Labeling of all hazardous chemicals is required by the standard. Labels minimally must list the chemical or the common name of the chemical agent, hazard warnings, and the manufacturer's name and address. If chemicals are transferred from an original container into secondary containers, these also must be labeled.

Employees must receive formal training about the office's hazardous chemicals, and this training must be documented. The training program should include information about the OSHA standard, the office's hazard control plan, the types of hazards present, signs and symptoms of exposure, protective measures, and the availability and use of the MSDSs. Periodic retraining is expected, and additional training is necessary whenever a new hazard is introduced.

REPORTING OF CHILD ABUSE

For centuries, general practice and child abuse have existed alongside each other as virtually distinct entities whose paths seldom knowingly crossed. As such, the medical profession has historically been in the dark concerning this delicate and sordid topic, resulting in an unnecessary blanket of ignorance among most health care practitioners. This notion changed in 1962, when Kempe and associates[14] published an article on the battered child syndrome, shedding some much-needed light on the topic of child abuse and bringing this delicate concern into the arena of health care. Today, the awareness of child abuse continues to grow, and the facts are appalling. Each year in the United States, at least 4,000 children die from physical abuse, and 10% of children younger than age 5 who are seen in emergency departments are the victims of inflicted injuries. In all, at least 1% of all children are suspected of being the victims of various forms of abuse and neglect.[15]

The role of the physician in reporting child abuse, maltreatment, and neglect must be examined on several fronts. With each instance of abuse, both the nature of the abuse and the facts surrounding it vary, such that the practitioner is often in an awkward situation of having to decipher fact from fiction. The perpetrator may be a total stranger, an acquain-

Table 11. Common office hazardous chemicals

Rubbing alcohol
Radiograph processing solutions
Iontophoresis solutions
Cleaning solutions and disinfectants
Ammonia
Laboratory reagents
Drain cleaners
Emergency oxygen
Photocopier toner
Athletic tape remover
Fluoromethane spray

tance, or, as is most often the case, a parent or legal guardian, but the physician must handle each incident with the best interests of the child in mind. A doctor who cares for a child who is severely bruised and marred from repeated falls down the stairs may be committing a major injustice because the cause of the injury may have been abusive in nature rather than accidental. That child might then face similar, repeated attacks in the future, all with deleterious effects on the child's physical and emotional well-being. It is vital for the attending physician to remain unbiased while carefully sifting through the initial evidence that has been presented and then to perform a thorough history and physical examination to determine whether the physical findings do indeed support the alleged story behind the injury.

One of the first things to keep in mind is that child abuse exists in a wide variety of forms. According to Fontana,[16] abuse may be physical, emotional, verbal, or sexual; or it may be described in terms of neglect (eg, emotional neglect or maternal deprivation), physical neglect, malnutrition, inappropriate clothing, lack of supervision, medical neglect, educational neglect, and abandonment. Each case is serious and warrants stringent consideration by any practitioner who detects such occurrences in daily contacts with patients and their children.

If, after questioning the child and performing the physical examination, the physician believes that abuse has transpired, the incident must be reported. Not only is it necessary that the case be reported to the proper authorities so that future abuses to the child are avoided, but also it is important to realize that such reporting is mandatory as required by law. Such is the case in all the 50 states as well as Canada, and professionals from many fields are involved[15] (Table 12).

If incidents are not reported, strict penalties may be warranted, such as fines and/or suspension of license. The procedure one must follow has been described by Blumberg et al[17] and consists of four general steps:

1. If the practitioner has admitting privileges, any child younger than 18 years who has allegedly been physically or sexually abused or severely neglected should be admitted to an inpatient pediatric or adolescent unit without delay.
2. The incident should be reported to the state child protective services agency (the name will vary among the different states) by a call placed to a 24-hour commission. If the practitioner has no admitting privileges, then the agency and local police will coordinate placing the child in protective custody.
3. A hospital pediatric social worker will be assigned to the child.
4. The admitting physician thoroughly examines the child for traumatic lesions and photographs any evidence of abuse for documentation.

It is vital to recognize that time is of the essence in all cases of suspected child abuse to ensure that the child receives the most prompt and proper care available, both medically and legally. What may appear to be merely a bruise on the surface may actually be a complex fracture or more severe internal injury underneath. Delayed reporting by the physician might jeopardize the child's health on a temporary, or even permanent, basis. In addition, if immediate action is not taken, documentable lesions may have a chance to heal with time, thereby eliminating the proof that the child was ever abused and diminishing the chance for legal intervention and protection for the child.

Incidents of child abuse should not be allowed to slip through the cracks and go unreported because these may scar the child physically and psychologically for life. The fact remains, however, that physicians often hesitate to report cases of abuse to the proper authorities for fear of a lack of immunity in court if the incident proves to be false and legal action is taken by the parent. Such a belief is unfounded because laws passed several years ago by all the states make reporting of abuse a mandatory obligation. Today, all reporters of suspected child abuse are granted immunity from criminal and civil liability for reports made in good faith.[15] With this in mind, the only concern practitioners should have with regard to legal prosecution lies in an act of omission (ie, failing to recognize and report incidents of child abuse).

Chiropractic physicians have become increasingly utilized sources of health care for pediatric patients. With that comes the responsibility of protecting these patients from mental and physical injuries resulting from child abuse. It is essential that the possibility of abuse be kept in mind when one is dealing with young patients with repeated or unusual types of injuries.

CONCLUSION

It is obvious that a chiropractic physician has professional responsibilities above and beyond those imposed by practice guidelines and standards of care. Local, state, and federal

Table 12. Health care professionals required to report child abuse

Medical physicians	Resident physicians	Hospital personnel
Medical examiners	Osteopathic physicians	Chiropractic physicians
Registered nurses	Podiatrists	Optometrists
	Interns	Mental health professionals

regulations have established requirements for the protection of office employees, patients, and the public. All chiropractic offices, from solo practitioners to multiphysician, multidisciplinary practices, must take the necessary steps to ensure that they are in compliance with all applicable public health, abuse reporting, OSHA, and other federal regulations and statutes.

Further information can be obtained by writing to OSHA, Room N3647 (Room N3101 for publications), 200 Constitution Avenue NW, Washington, DC 20210. The HCFA can be contacted for information about CLIA at Room 132, East High Rise Building, 6325 Security Boulevard, Baltimore, MD 21207. Appendix I–B includes a directory of state and national public health offices.

REFERENCES

1. US Department of Health and Human Services, Health Care Financing Administration. Clinical Laboratory Improvement amendments of 1988 (42 CFR Part 405 et al). *Federal Register.* February 28, 1992;57(40):7,002–7,288.
2. US Department of Health and Human Services, Centers for Disease Control. Regulations for implementing Clinical Laboratory Improvement amendments of 1988: a summary. *JAMA.* 1992;267:1,725–1,734.
3. US Department of Health and Human Services, Health Care Financing Administration. Medicare, Medicaid and CLIA programs; CLIA fee collection; correction and final rule (42 CFR Part 493) *Federal Register.* January 19, 1993;58(11):5,212–5,237.
4. Lee R. Physician office laboratory regulation: proven strategies to meet the demands of the CLIA. *Med Staff Couns.* 1993;7(3):11–26.
5. US Department of Labor, Occupational Safety and Health Administration. Occupational exposure to bloodborne pathogens; final rule (29 CFR Part 1910.1030). *Federal Register.* December 6, 1991;56(235):64,175–64,182.
6. US Department of Health and Human Services, Centers for Disease Control. Guidelines for preventing the transmission of tuberculosis in health-care settings, with special focus on HIV-related issues. *Morb Mortal Wkly Rep.* 1990;39(RR-17):1–29.
7. US Department of Health and Human Services, Centers for Disease Control and Prevention. Draft guidelines for preventing the transmission of tuberculosis in health-care facilities, 2nd edition; notice of comment period. *Federal Register.* October 12, 1993;58(195):52,810–52,854.
8. US Department of Labor, Occupational Safety and Health Administration (OSHA). *Enforcement Policy and Procedures for Occupational Exposure to Tuberculosis.* (internal memorandum). Washington, DC: OSHA; October 8, 1993.
9. Nakamura RT, Church TW, Cooper PJ. A blip on the radar screen: formulation and implementation of the Medical Waste Tracking Act. *J Health Polit Policy Law.* 1992;17(2):299–328.
10. Illinois Pollution Control Board. *Potentially Infectious Medical Waste (PIMW): Treatment, Storage, and Transfer Facilities and Transportation, Packaging and Labeling* (35 Ill Adm Code 1420, 1421, and 1422). Springfield, Ill: Illinois Pollution Control Board; 1993.
11. Wisconsin's infectious waste regulations. *Wis Med J.* 1990;6:275–278.
12. Chadzynki LS. Medical Waste Act requires physician compliance. *Mich Med.* 1991;7:41–47.
13. US Department of Labor, Occupational Safety and Health Administration. Hazard communication (29 CFR Parts 1910, 1915, 1917, 1918, 1926, and 1928). *Federal Register.* February 9, 1984;59:6,126–6,184.
14. Kempe CH, Silverman FN, Steele BF, et al. Battered-child syndrome. *JAMA.* 1962;181:17–24.
15. Gordon M, Palusci V. Physician training in the recognition and reporting of child abuse, maltreatment and neglect. *NY State J Med.* 1991;91(1):1–2.
16. Fontana V. Child abuse: the physician's responsibility. *NY State J Med.* 1989;89(3):152–155.
17. Blumberg M, Lynn D, Caldwell E, DiMaio D, Fontana V, Gold J. The physician's management of child maltreatment. *NY State J Med.* 1989;89(3):168.

3

Decision Analysis: Are Calculations and Clinicians Really on a Collision Course?

Gary D. Schultz

The drive for accountable health care practitioners has created sweeping changes in the business of providing chiropractic services including a number of reimbursement review and cost containment strategies. Practitioners may often feel like pinballs in a busy arcade as they maneuver through the prerequisites to reimbursement. While these maneuvers go by a number of names, they all emanate from the boiling cauldron of clinical decision making (and demonstration of the same).

In a perfect world, infinitely wise practitioners make clinical decisions based on perfect evidence, and these decisions are made in sufficient quantity to define optimally and treat the patient's problem. The problem with this "reference standard practitioner" is that he or she does not exist, nor does the perfect information, nor the perfect and uniform patient, nor the perfectly definable patient disorder. Alas, the practitioner is confronted with uncertainty.

The mere exclamation "It works! It really, really works!" no longer serves as adequate documentation of the effectiveness of chiropractic diagnosis and treatment. Unfortunately, the chiropractic adjustment sometimes works less effectively than other therapies, and sometimes it does not work at all. In an era where maximization of benefit per dollar expended has become a national imperative, someone is going to have to wield the "big stick" and decide what is and is not worth the expense or risk.

Enter technology assessment—the process of objectively, fairly, and thoroughly evaluating the capability of a device, procedure, or idea to identify or alleviate patient problems. Technology assessment is but a piece of the decision analysis pie. *Decision analysis* is the process of explicitly (using data rather than intuition) determining what is wrong with the patient and which of the available means to treat and predict the expected course of disorders is most appropriate. Because it is explicit, decision analysis uses quantified (numeric) information and a systematic process to provide certainty rather than intuition or person-centered experience (anecdote).

For better or for worse, doctors are not numbers, and most are not very comfortable with using them to the exclusion of intuitive judgment.[1] The idea of using mathematical models to determine what is next clinically is inherently unpopular in the "trenches," and it is probably untenable as the sole basis for decision making in the clinical arena (ie, replacing intuitive decision making). Along the way, decision analysis as an adjunct for deciding the next move has acquired a bad reputation. This prejudice is probably based on ignorance of the intent of decision analysis and periodic experiences of an inappropriate application of decision analysis concepts as cost-saving strategies within certain managed care organizations. Ever-dwindling physician autonomy becomes a point of rabid contention as doctors take issue with "formulary" or "cookbook" health care.

The doctor-patient interaction is complex. At one end of the spectrum of interactions are purely physician-centered decisions and actions; at the other end are purely patient-mediated decisions. Complex combinations of the two exist between, coupled with beliefs, experiences, and biases from both spectrum extremes. These interactions are important when dissecting the doctor-patient interaction.

Conceptually, clinical decisions must consider the doctor, the patient, the disorder (the reason the doctor and the patient meet in the first place), and the tools that will be employed to define and treat the problem. In addition, no discussion of the clinical decision-making process can responsibly ignore money, because the desire to keep it and the desire to get it can become central in the decision path. This chapter describes some of the rudiments of each of the above from a decision analysis perspective in order that the precepts of decision analysis will become better understood and more often applied.

Ethically, the fundamental goal of formal decision analysis principles is to assist the doctor in making the best decisions.[2] The best decisions afford the most benefit to the patient (and hence society), the least harm, are just, and they demure to the informed autonomy of the patient, wherever possible. Ethical decision analysis recognizes the duty of the professional to meet or exceed the reasonable expectations of the patient and society.

Decisions are expected to be paternalistic in some instances (doctor as the patient's agent, because the patient is incapable of responsibly making the decision) and informed in all others.[3] In short, appropriately performed decision analysis is the embodiment of ethical behavior—to not use decision analysis of some type is *unethical*. The ethical practitioner attempts to use all information available to him or her in order to provide health care as efficiently and effectively as possible.

If using decision analysis is an ethical imperative, then why are formalized approaches so unpopular? The answer may be the lack of familiarity of understanding of the process of decision analysis. Understanding the variables is one way to reduce some of the mysticism that often accompanies complex formulas and a dialect of the English language known as statistics (as cryptic as a foreign language to many clinicians). Often, a lack of understanding or interest in mathematics creates a barrier to acknowledging the abundant common ground that lies within familiar, comfortable decision processes and the less familiar, quantitative approaches to the same situation.[2] Often, intuitive conclusions are no different than the formal, quantitative conclusions to a clinical problem. In short, the purpose of formal decision making is to support and assist the clinician when he or she is uncertain, not to dictate procedure or process despite the certainty the clinician might have.

DECISION MAKING: THE GROUNDWORK

Physician behaviors

Application of decision-making principles requires some knowledge of how clinicians know and learn in the clinical setting. There are three methods commonly employed by clinicians when establishing a diagnosis: (1) pattern recognition, (2) expert algorithms, and (3) the hypothetico-deductive method.[5]

Pattern recognition

Pattern recognition might also be termed the "Aunt Minnie approach." Just as we know Aunt Minnie when we see her because she is Aunt Minnie, has always been Aunt Minnie, and to call her anything else would be absurd, pattern recognition relies on instantaneous identification of the problem. Usually this ability is the result of mentors pointing to a distinctive presentation, identifying that process with a name, and reinforcing that knowledge with facts and other data that support the conclusion.[4]

Bolstered with experience, this method of decision processing becomes quick and impressive, frequently resulting in the exact diagnosis in short order. It is not flawless, however. Not every patient with swollen ankles has congestive heart failure, and failure to consider deep vein thrombosis could prove a deadly oversight. Moreover, pattern recognition becomes problematic when one encounters the atypical example of a disease, or is faced with a stage in the natural history of the condition not previously witnessed. If a physician has been trained to call neck pain with radiation into the shoulder a disc protrusion, he or she might fail to associate the trigger point deep in the trapezius muscle as a potential cause of the very same presentation and subsequently incur great expense and inconvenience to the patient chasing the nonexistent disc lesion in the neck.

Expert algorithms

Algorithms are classically flow diagrams that guide the clinician through a series of steps designed to lead to the appropriate clinical conclusion. They typically use the best available evidence coupled with the opinions of experts in the area of the clinical problem. They are most effective when applied to a condition infrequently seen in practice, or when the clinician is inexperienced. They serve as a generic "expert at your fingertips."

While quite effective in improving accuracy of diagnosis,[5] care must be exercised in the application of expert algorithms. Simplicity of the algorithm[6] and failure to include atypical or subtle signs of disease can hamper the utility of the algorithm as a replacement for additional consultation. Also, there is the potential problem of the expert's bias in evaluating the condition. Who is to say that the expert is perfectly efficient and correct?[7]

Another problem with algorithmic evaluation of a condition is the potential to force a clinician through an unnecessary series of steps, which reduces efficiency and potentially increases cost and risk to the patient.[8] In short, algorithms, regardless of precision and efficiency, are no replacement for intimate contextual knowledge of the whole clinical circumstance. Optimally, the algorithm is constructed in a way that allows the clinician to bypass patently unnecessary steps and serves as a resource (rather than replacement) for clinical decision making.

Hypothetico-deductive decision making

The hypothetico-deductive method strikes a balance between the Aunt Minnie approach and the rigid application of an expert algorithm. This method of investigation allows the physician to establish a list of likely contenders (hopefully less than six) for the diagnosis and to choose selectively the best studies or maneuvers to attain the correct diagnosis. This method is commonly employed when the diagnosis is not immediately recognized, or when an algorithm (cognitive or flow diagram) is not available to apply to the condition. It is in these circumstances of uncertainty that decision analysis is of greatest assistance to the clinician.

Decision analysis might involve simply attaining demographic and epidemiologic data about the differential list of diagnostic possibilities. For example, if a clinician is faced with a patient who has inflammatory arthritis of the sacroiliac joints, he or she might entertain a differential diagnosis of ankylosing spondylitis, psoriatic arthritis, or infection. Clinically, this patient is a young male and his sacroiliitis is bilateral and relatively symmetric, and there are no other sites of involvement. Understanding that the therapy and prognosis for each differential possibility are significantly different, the practitioner is compelled to attain more certainty about which is the correct diagnosis.

Epidemiologic data reveal that infection of the sacroiliac joints is nearly always unilateral and is seen predominantly in immunosuppressed populations (eg, patients with the acquired immunodeficiency syndrome or long-term intravenous drug abusers). Based on this knowledge, the clinician can confidently rule out infection. By learning that psoriatic arthritis typically occurs in middle-aged individuals, is unusual in the spine without hand disease, is very unusual in the absence of skin lesions and pitting of the fingernails, and, when it occurs in the sacroiliac joints, is usually bilateral but visibly asymmetric, the probability of psoriatic arthritis becomes quite low. The more confident clinician now learns that ankylosing spondylitis is most frequently encountered in young males and is bilateral and symmetric in the sacroiliac joints. Hence, the diagnosis is established. As demonstrated, epidemiologic data used in diagnostic decision making to reduce uncertainty avoid expense and time and allow the more important issue (of how best to assist the patient) to ensue.

Integration of approaches

Experienced clinicians often employ parts of all three types of evaluation when proceeding with the investigation of a clinical problem. The combination of intuitive and quantitative information is often used by highly skilled and experienced clinicians. Interestingly, expert clinicians frequently need less data to establish a correct diagnosis than nonexperts.[9] It is highly likely that this superior performance is the result of smooth integration of existing knowledge to establish more quickly what data are needed to reduce uncertainty and greater ability to discriminate and eliminate superfluous information that may lengthen the investigation or mislead the doctor. In short, experienced clinicians are more efficient in a clinical sense and are more able to focus on the important facets of investigation.

Mental processing errors

> Always go to other people's funerals, otherwise they won't come to yours.
> —Yogi Berra[10(p17)]

Mistakes occur, and they are not rare. Under the best of circumstances, errors occur and are unimportant for therapy and thus go unnoticed. Under the worst scenario, the patient suffers or even dies as a result of the error. For this reason, it is important to acknowledge that errors occur, understand how they occur, and, most important, implement strategies designed to minimize their impact. Errors of judgment or thinking are frequently the result of oversimplification.[11] Other general cognitive mistakes result from assuming a static problem when it is dynamic, viewing only part of the patient's problem (ie, ignoring the psychosocial aspects of a chronic condition), and assuming that the perceived problem is not a part of a multifactorial or multilevel clinical dilemma.[12,13]

Specifically, errors of clinical cognition fall into three categories: (1) disease misclassification, (2) information gathering errors, and (3) errors of information integration. Errors of disease classification involve thinking of one disease to the exclusion of the correct diagnosis. This error could be the result of bias arising out of pattern recognition or misinterpreting the probability of a disease. Overestimating the prevalence of a disease is one such possibility. The probability of Cushing's syndrome in a patient with truncal obesity and hypertension is quite low, despite the fact that these signs are classic of the disease. The reason that Cushing's syndrome is unlikely is simply that it is a rare disease, and these signs are not exclusive to Cushing's syndrome. Last, errors of classification can result from attaching significance to a finding when, in fact, it is simply a variation of the spectrum of normal.

Errors in information gathering involve obtaining too much, too little, or simply obtaining the wrong information. "Defensive medicine" (covering one's derriere) is a prime example of obtaining too much clinical data. It is interesting to note that tendencies toward excessive test acquisition in practice parallel attitudes toward clinical uncertainty and tolerance for ambiguity.[14–16]

Not obtaining enough information is often related to pattern recognition and overconfidence in one's conclusions. Failure to seek reference material to ensure consideration of all the reasonable possibilities is a part of this error chain. Clinicians are most likely to seek information from readily available sources such as colleagues, easily accessed experts, and general texts. "Hold the X-rays closer to the phone, Doc, I can't quite see them from here" is a glib reminder of the radiologist's dilemma in confirming or denying the clinician's concerns about a radiograph over the telephone. Clinicians are less willing (or unable) to consult subspecialty texts, databases, and journal articles, presumably because of the effort necessary to obtain them quickly in the clinical setting.[17]

Another shortcoming in the clinical setting relates to failure to integrate all data into a cogent continuum. Principle in this error is failure to revise the likelihood of the differential diagnostic possibilities as new data are acquired. This error assumes that the most likely culprit for the patient's problem will remain the most likely item in the differential until it is convincingly ruled out. This stance all but ignores the changing probabilities of the other items in the differential diagnosis as the investigation progresses.

Reducing errors in practice

> I was under medication when I made the decision not to burn the tapes.
> —Richard Nixon[10(p72)]

Despite all the possible ways to err, clinical thinking is overall quite sound. Errors are abundant, but usually they are small and innocuous.[13] Improvements in clinical accuracy and efficiency can be made by first acknowledging the presence of errors. Having established a culture for improvement, clinicians need to improve the frequency and intensity of available evidence used to assist, modulate, and guide the real-time decision process.

In addition, mere practice needs to be replaced with practice with meaningful reflection. Practice with meaningful reflection is termed *praxis*. The absence of praxis in clinical practice, particularly early on, all but guarantees perpetuation of errors and reaction to error, rather than prevention. Introspection and retrospection are important components of refining skills such as spinal adjusting. These processes should thus be employed to improve the quality and efficiency of a diagnostic approach. Last, examining the culture in which health care is delivered must be evaluated. The current "more is better" philosophy of risk management and financially motivated practitioners in health services delivery need reconciliation with case managers' perspectives on cost containment, appropriateness, and common sense.

The diagnostic test

> Free cholesterol testing will be offered at 10 this morning. The cost is $6.
> —Notice in the Hammond, Indiana, *Times*[10(p280)]

Clinicians use history, examination, and diagnostic testing to reduce clinical uncertainty and establish an understanding of the disease process. These procedures serve their purpose, but they do so imperfectly. Just as a clinician is capable of error, so too is the diagnostic test. In establishing greater precision through decision analysis, it is important to establish how imperfect a test is. Precisely how much can clinicians depend on the results obtained from the test (ie, knowing the probability that the patient actually has the disease that the test indicated was present)? What is the likelihood that the test was wrong (ie, falsely proclaiming disease when none was present, or falsely proclaiming normality when the patient was, in fact, diseased)?

A number of tests are available for nearly any clinical problem. To wit, myelography, discography, computed tomography (CT), magnetic resonance imaging (MRI), and CT myelography are all available to evaluate the low back of an individual suspected of having a clinically significant disc protrusion. Which test should be used? Which test is the best? The perfect diagnostic test is able to distinguish nondiseased from diseased populations 100% of the time, and to distinguish normal from diseased populations 100% of the time. Table 1 lists the performance characteristics commonly used to characterize the ability of a test to help in a clinical situation.

A word about test characteristics; they are often better in print than they are in practice. This discrepancy is due to careful selection of the diseased (they are selected because they are moderately to severely affected, leaving no question about the fact that they are diseased) and normal populations (they are selected because they are really normal, with no questionable characteristics) to be tested. In addition, the best test interpreters available are usually employed to interpret the test results, and frequently their performance is far superior to that which could be expected outside the laboratory. In short, what is published in the critically reviewed literature is the best possible expectation, or optimistic assessment, of the abilities of the test.

It is valuable to know how well a test detects disease and differentiates normal from abnormal. These qualities help in selecting a test; however, the real clinical value of a test is not exclusively in its performance characteristics. To the clinician, tests are only useful if they provide some assurance that if the test is positive the patient has the disease and, conversely, if the test is negative that the patient does not have the disease. This characteristic is *predictive value*. Predictive value, which is mathematically described in Table 2, uses the test performance characteristics in addition to prevalence of disease.

Positive predictive value is the percentage of positive test results that will actually turn out to be diseased patients. Negative predictive value is the percentage of patients with a negative test who are actually nondiseased. Of interest is the dependence of predictive value on prevalence of disease (the rate of disease in the population tested). If the prevalence of disease is only 1%, then no matter how good the test is (short of perfection) there will be a low predictive value. In other words, the test is most useful when the tested population is screened to increase the number of diseased people in the population. If radiography is used to screen for fracture in the cervical spine of the general population, less than 1% will have a fracture. For every false positive (thinking there was a fracture when none existed) there is a reduction in the ability to rely on the true-positive assessments. However, if the same test is applied to a population of individuals sustaining neck injuries in high-speed automobile accidents, then the prevalence of fractures might increase to 25%. Intuitively one can see the increase in the ability to rely on the result.

Choosing a test should be the result of obtaining an answer to the question "Is the test any good at finding the kind of problem I suspect?" This question begs answers to the parameters listed in Table 1. The second question, which relates to the parameters listed in Table 2, asks, "How much can I rely on the answers I get from the test?" Often, obtaining evidence to answer these two questions will give a sense as to whether a test is not only useful for a specific problem, but also helpful in giving a sense of how credible the data regarding the overall applicability of the modality in practice are. This simple "separating the wheat from the chaff" process is critical for the cost-conscious practitioner who needs certainty, not higher costs and more questions.

The disease

> I wouldn't say Joe has a sore arm, per se, but his arm is kind of sore.
> —Weeb Ewbank, New York Jets Coach on Joe Namath's absence from practice[10(p356)]

Disease follows a course in time. At the beginning, most conditions are subclinical. Certainly the subclinical component of a fracture is quite brief; for all intent and purposes, it is nonexistent. However, the common cold has a subclinical origin, which gradually gives way to a typical prodrome that then manifests as the viral illness we all know and disdain. Some diseases are self-limiting and resolve spontaneously, while others are cyclic. Still others are progressive and lead to death. Fig 1 diagrammatically illustrates the natural histories of different conditions. Of interest is the fact that a practitioner might encounter any of the conditions at any point in time.

If each disease has a natural history, then it stands to reason that at some point the organism suffering from the disorder will begin to diverge from normal. It is also reasonable to assume

Table 1. Choosing a test: Characteristics to look for

Test characteristic	Definition	Example
Reliability	Ability to get the same result at multiple measures	Two radiologists arrive at the same diagnosis from films
Validity	Ability to be correct as compared to "gold standard"	The radiologists' answer matches the pathology report
Sensitivity	Number of times a test is positive in a population with confirmed disease	90 out of 100 ankylosing spondylitis patients have a positive HLA-B27 test
Specificity	Number of times a test is negative in a population of confirmed normals	75 out of 100 normal patients have a negative HLA-B27 test

Table 2. Interpreting a test: Characteristics to look for

Test characteristic	Definition	Impact
Positive predictive value [(+)PV]	$\dfrac{\text{prevalence} \times \text{sensitivities}}{(\text{prevalence} \times \text{sensitivity}) + [1 - \text{specificity}) \times (1 - \text{prevalence})]}$	Percent of people with a positive test that will actually have the disease (true positives)
Negative predictive value [(−)PV]	$\dfrac{(1 - \text{prevalence}) \times \text{specificity}}{[(1 - \text{prevalence}) \times \text{specificity}] + [\text{prevalence} \times (1 - \text{sensitivity})]}$	Percent of negative tests that will be normal (true negatives)
Receiver-operator characteristic curve	Curve obtained by plotting false positive rate (1 − specificity) vs true positive rate (sensitivity) on a graph	Allows check of where test optimizes sensitivity and where specificity is optimized based on different cut-off values for abnormal test result

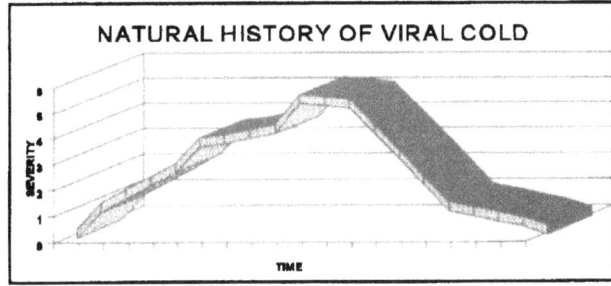

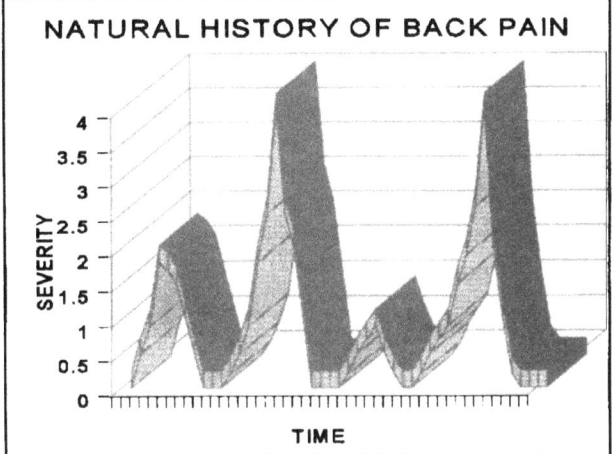

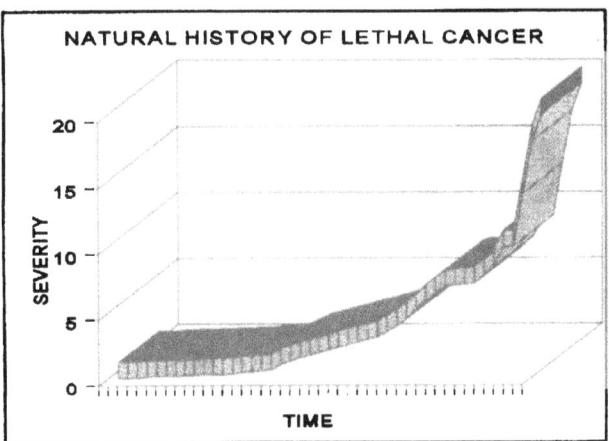

Fig 1. Natural history of diseases.

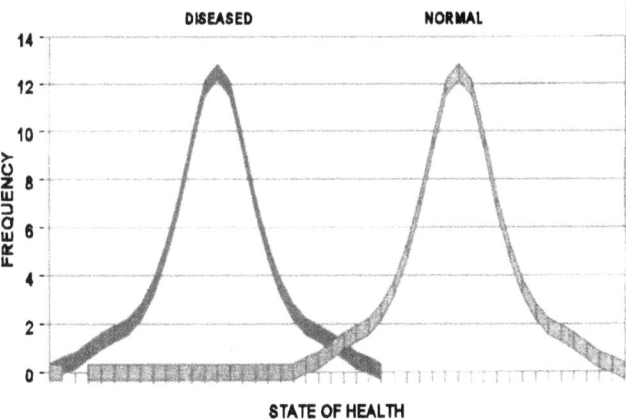

Fig 2. Overlapping populations.

that the spectrum of normal demonstrates some overlap with the spectrum of disease. Fig 2 demonstrates the potential overlap of normal populations with the spectrum of diseased individuals for a condition. Where on the spectrum the disease is encountered will usually determine how easy it is to detect and isolate it as the cause of the patient's problem. Some conditions demonstrate a considerable amount of similarity to normal, and others diverge from normal early in their course. The key to diagnosis is to choose tests that are good at distinguishing the normal from the abnormal and to encounter the problem at a stage where differentiation is possible.

BAYESIAN ANALYSIS

Bayesian analysis is a method of decision making that establishes a probability for each condition that could exist in a clinical situation on a spectrum from no probability (0% probability) to certain probability (100% probable). The probability of each differential diagnostic item is adjusted following input of new data.[18] Chang has conceptualized this model by creating a probability spectrum for each condition in the differential diagnosis, allowing for modification of the probability of disease for each new step in the work-up.[19]

Understanding that total certainty (achieving 0% or 100% probability of a diagnosis) is not reasonably possible in prospective settings, the clinician is left to "manage uncertainty" and its risks. For this reason, points are established on the spectrum of probability that reflect a clinician's willingness to "go with" or "exclude" a diagnosis.

Exclusion threshold (ET) is the point at which the probability of the disease is so low that it is no longer considered as part of the differential diagnosis. In other words, we no longer test the patient for the possibility of that condition. Action threshold (AT) is the point at which there is enough certainty about the condition's presence that we decide to treat on the premise of its presence. Once the AT has been achieved for a condition, we should begin treatment for that condition, unless there is a compelling differential diagnosis that has not been driven to the ET. ATs and ETs apply only to a condition that might warrant therapy. In other words, time and resources are not spent on a condition that will require no therapy.

Prior probability (PP) is the critical link in using Bayesian analysis. PP is the point on the probability scale that describes the clinician's estimate of how likely the disease is.

This scale is constantly changing as the clinical evaluation progresses. Revision of the PP is essential to reach therapeutic or exclusion thresholds in Bayesian analysis (Fig 3).

As one completes the chief complaint and present illness of a new patient in the hypothetico-deductive model of cognition, a few thoughts for diagnosis enter the clinician's mind. The examination will likely be tailored to confirm or eliminate these possibilities. At this point, a PP of each differential diagnostic possibility exists, and it will change as a result of the clinical examination and orthopaedic/neurologic/chiropractic examinations. Examination procedures should be performed that have the greatest potential to change all of the prior probabilities the most.

A hypothetical application without numeric application will assist in demonstrating the power and utility of Bayesian analysis in practice. The hypothetical patient is a 30-year-old male with low back pain of 6 months' duration. The chosen differential diagnostic possibilities in this case are: degenerative joint disease (DJD)/mechanical back pain, herniated nucleus pulposus, and ankylosing spondylitis (AS). These differential diagnostic possibilities are sufficiently diverse that their therapies are different and their prognoses are unique.

The history is focused on delineating the epidemiologic and clinical factors that would point toward one of the possibilities, and hopefully, away from the others. The posthistory prior probability (hypothetically) for each of these conditions is provided in Fig 4. Note that the probability of AS is low, but that the ET and therapeutic threshold are closer to 0% and 100%, respectively. These probabilities reflect the fact that AS would be rare compared to the other diagnostic hypotheses (lower prevalence)[20] but its presence might render chiropractic adjustments contraindicated (highly clinically significant). Therefore greater certainty is needed about whether it is (or is not) present before proceeding from the diagnostic phase of the case.

The clinical/orthopaedic/neurologic/chiropractic assessments would further delineate and distinguish if the characteristics associated with each of the conditions are present. In this situation, negative findings are just as important as positive findings. If the orthopaedic/neurologic evaluation found no root signs or intrathecal pressure signs, no radiation of pain, no neurologic deficits or alterations, and normal reflexes, the probability of a disc protrusion would drop dramatically. Conversely, these negative findings might also help to improve the probability of degenerative disease/mechanical dysfunction. These findings would have little impact on the prior probability of AS.

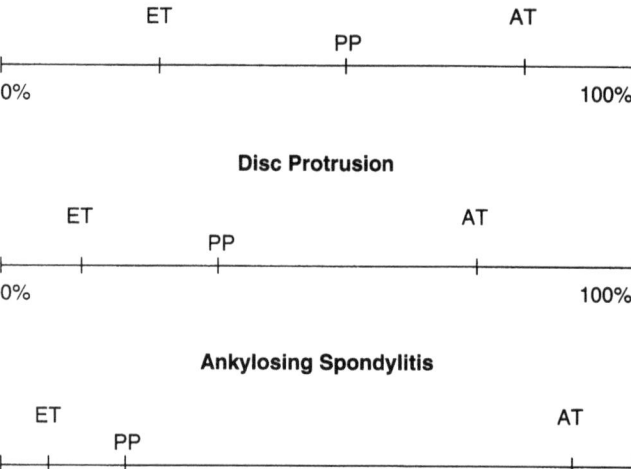

Fig 4. Posthistory Bayesian probability scales. ET = exclusion threshold; AT = action threshold; PP = prior probability.

If the chiropractic examination revealed reduced, but not absent, ranges of motion and muscle tenderness with articular stiffness and tenderness of the sacroiliac joints and lower lumbar facet articulations, greater evidence would be garnered for the articular dysfunction hypothesis without dramatically altering the protrusion hypothesis. It would also slightly lower the prior probability of the AS hypothesis due to the mild nature of the findings.

Fig 5 illustrates how the revised probabilities for the hypotheses might look following the examination procedures. Note that the probability of a disc protrusion has dropped below the exclusion threshold—it is no longer a part of the differential diagnosis.

The differential diagnosis still contains two important conditions, one (DJD/mechanical dysfunction) is supported with nearly enough certainty to begin therapy. However, while there is growing certainty that it is not AS, this diagnosis is still possible primarily because of the duration of symptoms and the presence of some stiffness in the examination. (Recall it is possible that AS is presenting at an early stage, when it bears resemblance to normal individuals, yet is still abnormal.) A test is needed that will provide certainty (high positive and negative predictive values) about the presence of AS. Two diagnostic procedures might be helpful: laboratory analysis to include erythrocyte sedimentation rate (ESR) with or without HLA-B27 and plain film radiography of the low back or sacroiliac joints or both. In reality, there are many more diagnostic procedures possible but, for the sake of brevity, only these are discussed.

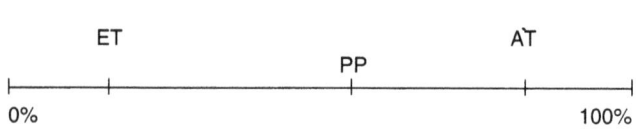

Fig 3. Bayesian probability scale for any disease. ET = exclusion threshold; AT = action threshold; PP = prior probability.

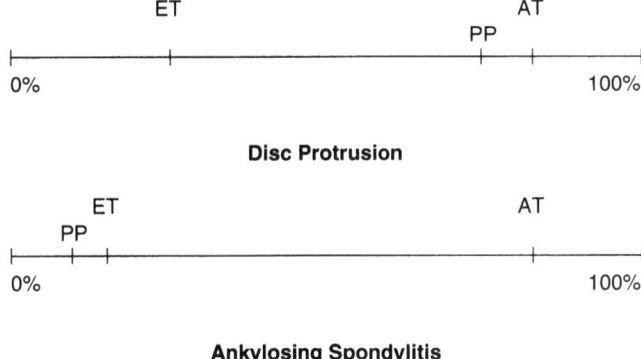

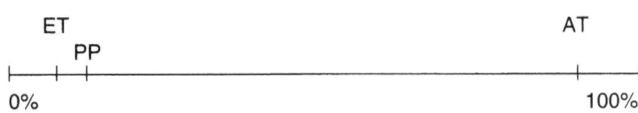

Fig 5. Postexamination Bayesian probability scales. ET = exclusion threshold; AT = action threshold; PP = prior probability.

Decision analysis principles will be needed to assist in determining which of the tests is more appropriate since a high degree of certainty is required and one condition is not encountered often. Explicitly evaluating the best next step (with the actual predictive values, sensitivities and specificities, and so forth) is well advised when the clinician is inexperienced.

In keeping with the non-numeric promise of this case, the assessment is conceptualized as follows. The ESR is very sensitive for AS, but very poorly specific; its predictive value is low when not correlated with other tests.[21,22] HLA-B27 is highly sensitive, but moderately specific.[23,24] Plain film radiography is moderately sensitive and highly specific.[25–28] The performance characteristics might point to the need for the HLA-B27 or radiographs in this instance; however, they define only one part of the clinician's decision to use the test.

It is important that consideration of the safety and cost of the test be evaluated in the decision process. ESR is the least expensive and has almost no risk (venipuncture is safe). Radiography (posteroanterior and lateral views) has intermediate cost, but a small amount of risk. HLA-B27 has low risk, but a high cost.

What comes next? Reams of analysis have been summarized, and still there is no decision. Given the low probability of AS at this point, one should proceed with as inexpensive and low risk an evaluation as possible to rule out AS. The cheapest option is ESR only, ruling in mechanical dysfunction by default. The most certainty would be obtained from radiography, because it would not only provide certainty about the absence of AS, but also provide information about degenerative disease and intersegmental relationships.

HLA-B27 would be helpful, especially in conjunction with ESR because it combines sensitivity and specificity and keeps risk extremely low, but incurs additional cost; DJD/mechanical dysfunction could be established by default. Combining radiography and ESR adds a small risk and more cost (slightly less than ESR with HLA-B27), but the combination yields very high sensitivity and high specificity.

Which selection is right? More important, which is wrong? The answer is that no option is wrong, and all are imperfect. The appropriate choice depends on the physician's characteristics. An extremely risk-averse clinician (low comfort with uncertainty) would not feel guilty about exposing the patient to the risk and cost of all the tests before proceeding with a management plan. An extremely risk-tolerant (high degree of comfort with clinical uncertainty) clinician would be satisfied with the cheapest, safest, appropriate test (ESR only). Most clinicians would probably opt for radiography and the ESR.

CAVEATS FOR DECISION ANALYSIS CONVERTS

> Caution: Cape does not enable user to fly.
> —Instructions on a Batman costume[10(p301)]

It is important to note that in using a Bayesian model, the particular idiosyncracies of the physician, the patient, and the context of the case must be considered. If the example above is complicated by a litigious patient or severe financial hardship, or worst, both, even the most certain of physician personalities would be compelled to alter his or her clinical choices. This fact is both the bane and boon of the Bayesian model.

Using this type of model in a hypothetico-deductive cognitive approach, the clinician is called on to inspect all decisions and perceptions and to weigh the significance of each and every finding. Frequent alteration of the prior probability will occur if Bayesian analysis is properly applied. Furthermore, the clinician is obligated to acknowledge his or her uncertainty honestly and forthrightly. False bravado (I'm lost, but I'm going to speed-up) and clinical paranoia (I'm going to consult the road map to get to the same store I've been going to for years) are the most pernicious ways to circumvent the value of Bayesian analysis.

So, Bayesian analysis can be very heavy and cumbersome in the clinical setting. It requires the clinician to have a thorough grasp of information-seeking methods and a willingness to take the time to use them. It also requires that biases such as financial gain or habit be purged from the clinical regimen. Sometimes these old habits are deeply engrained and die hard. Practice and praxis are necessary to overcome these "clinical demons."

In practice, bits and pieces of Bayesian ideology are often applied intuitively. A practitioner who consults the literature regarding the utility of a diagnostic test before proceeding with the application of a recommended test in an algorithm, or a clinician who asks "Could there be something I'm missing here?" after making a pattern diagnosis are demonstrating the use of the questions mandated in Bayesian analysis.

CONCLUSIONS

Uncertainty is everywhere, and decision analysis exists to assist the clinician in reducing this uncertainty for the benefit of his or her patients in a repeatable, defensible manner. Good decision making is a combination of knowledge, intuition, error detection, communication, and common sense. Unskilled physicians will (and rightly so) rely on more knowledge and critical appraisal than intuition and common sense compared to experienced clinicians. In essence, unskilled physicians will need more data to attain the same levels of certainty in the clinical arena. Experience is a great teacher, but a merciless taskmaster.

The utility of explicit methods lies not in dictation of what is appropriate or inappropriate, but rather in quantifying the benefits and shortcomings of decision options. Applying decision analysis does not guarantee precision, but failure to use decision analysis of some type does raise the likelihood of mistakes substantially.

REFERENCES

1. Schmidt H, Norman G, Boshuizen H. A cognitive perspective on medical expertise: theory and implications. *Acad Med.* 1990;65:611–621.
2. Bergus G, Hamm R. Clinical practice: how physicians make medical decisions and why medical decision making can help. *Med Decis Making.* 1995;22(2):167–180.
3. Obergfell AM. Ethics in imaging and therapy. In: Obergfell AM, ed. *Law and Ethics in Diagnostic Imaging and Therapeutic Radiology.* Philadelphia, Pa: W.B. Saunders; 1995.
4. Sackett D, Haynes R, Tugwell R. *Clinical Epidemiology: A Basic Science for Clinical Medicine.* Boston, Mass: Little, Brown; 1985.
5. McNutt R, Selker H. How did the acute ischemic heart disease predictive instrument reduce unnecessary coronary care unit admissions? *Med Decis Making.* 1988;8:90–94.
6. Abernathy C, Hamm R. *Surgical Scripts.* Philadelphia, Pa: Hanley and Belfus; 1994.
7. Heckerling P, Conant R, Tape T, et al. Clinical prediction rule for pulmonary infiltrates. *Ann Intern Med.* 1990; 113:664–670.
8. Abernathy C, Hamm R. *Surgical Intuition.* Philadelphia, Pa: Hanley and Belfus; 1994.
9. Shanteau J. How much information does an expert use? Is it relevant? *Acta Psychol.* 1992;81:75–86.
10. Petras R, Petras K. *The 365 Stupidest Things Ever Said: The 1996 Calendar.* New York, NY: Workman Publishers; 1995.
11. Cook R, Woods D. Operating at the sharp end: the complexity of human error. In: Bogner S, ed. *Human Error in Medicine.* Hillsdale, NJ: Erlbaum; 1994.
12. Feltovich P, Spiro R, Coulson R. Learning, teaching and testing for complex conceptual understanding. In: Fredericksen N, Mislevy R, Bejar I, eds. *Test Theory for a New Generation of Tests.* Hillsdale, NJ: Erlbaum; 1993.
13. Hamm R, Zubialde J. Physicians' expert cognition and the problem of cognitive biases. *Med Decis Making.* 1995;22(2):181–212.
14. Nightingale S. Risk preference and laboratory use. *Med Decis Making.* 1987;7:168–172.
15. Ornstein S, Johnson A, Markert G, et al. Association between family medicine residents' personality and laboratory test ordering for hypertensive patients. *J Med Educ.* 1987; 62:603–605.
16. Yarnold P, Nightingale S, Curry R, et al. Psychological androgyny and preference in loss-framed gambles of medical students: possible implications for resource utilization. *Med Decis Making.* 1991;11:176–179.
17. Curley S, Connely D, Rick E. Physicians' use of medical knowledge resources: preliminary theoretical framework and findings. *Med Decis Making.* 1990;10:231–241.
18. Glasziou P. Probability revision. *Med Decis Making.* 1995;22(2):235–246.
19. Chang R. Bayesian analysis: a radiologist's survival guide. *Am J Roentgenology.* 1989;152:721–727.
20. Lawrence J. The prevalence of arthritis. *Br J Clin Pract.* 1963; 17:699–705.
21. Resnick D, Niwayama G. Ankylosing spondylitis. In: Resnick D, Niwayama G, eds. *Diagnosis of Bone and Joint Disorders.* 2nd ed. Philadelphia, Pa: W.B. Saunders; 1988.
22. Tilkian S, Conover M, Tilkian A. *Clinical Implications of Laboratory Tests.* 3rd ed. St Louis, Mo: Mosby; 1983.
23. Calin A. Spondyloarthropathy in caucasians and non-caucasians. *J Rheumatol.* 1983;10:16–19.
24. Armstrong R, Panayi G, Welsh K. Histocompatibility antigens in psoriasis, psoriatic arthropathy and ankylosing spondylitis. *Ann Rheum Dis.* 1983;42:142–146.
25. Hollingsworth P, Cheah P, Dawkins R, et al. Observer variation in grading sacroiliac radiographs in HLA-B27 positive individuals. *J Rheumatol.* 1983;10:247–254.
26. Wilkinson M, Bywaters E. Clinical features and course of ankylosing spondylitis as seen in a follow up of 222 hospital referred cases. *Ann Rheum Dis.* 1958;17:209–228.
27. Polly H, Slocumb C. Rheumatoid spondylitis. A study of 1035 cases. *Ann Intern Med.* 1947;26:240–256.
28. Rosen P, Graham D. Ankylosing (Strumpell-Marie) spondylitis: a clinical review of 128 cases. *Am J Roentgenology.* 1962;5:158–211.

4

Technology Assessment of the Chiropractic Subluxation

Paul J. Osterbauer

The concept of vertebral subluxation has been deified and demonized from within and without the chiropractic profession.[1] This debate in part stems from the difficulty the profession has in realistically characterizing the disorder that it professes to correct. A variety of measures has been undertaken in an effort to describe the vertebral subluxation and the effects it might have on human biology. This effort has been increasingly manifest through the use of modern technology, in attempts to assess and objectify functional and physiologic effects of subluxation. However, unsubstantiated use of technology risks professional credibility in an age of increasing provider accountability. Assessment of technologies that might be used to assess subluxation, as well as its relationship to health, is at least as important as the effort to define it operationally. It is only through credible evidence and process that a reasonable picture of this clinical entity will emerge.

VERTEBRAL SUBLUXATION UNDEFINED

At the turn of the century, the healing arts were being transformed by the application of scientific principles based on observation. Significant advances were made in many disciplines, especially surgery because gross pathology was easily identified and treated.[2] For example, in the case of low back pain, Mixter and Barr[3] implicated disc herniation as the major cause of lower back and sciatic pain. This theory took hold in such a way as to dominate the concept of back pain for nearly 60 years. Competing theories of back pain (including referred pain syndromes) were not taken seriously by the majority of US medical practitioners.

This diagnostic tunnel vision was perhaps due in part to the training and background of the practitioner making the diagnosis.[4] As a matter of survival, the emerging chiropractic profession stressed its uniqueness, identifying a disease entity to "hang its hat on."[5] Allopaths have been frustrated by patients with subclinical conditions such as simple mechanical low back pain, the cause of which is not detectable by any "objective" diagnostic test.[6] Chiropractors often have conveyed a great deal of confidence in that regard.[6] The concept of vertebral subluxation has provided the chiropractor and the patient with an entity that can be identified and "corrected." Earlier in the profession's history such an explanation for ill health lent itself to deductive reasoning, which did not require direct experimentation, and measurements were limited by lack of technology.[7]

The appeal of new technology pervades western health care. It is viewed as an important tool to approach diagnosis and treatment more objectively, educate patients on the ongoing need for care, and support claims made to third-party payers. Furthermore, contemporary patients may tend to equate high technology with better quality of care.

It is ironic that advances in technology have resulted in the ability to detect physiologic variants to such a degree as to suffer from false positive findings.[8] For example, Boden and associates[9] reported that 10% to 30% of healthy asymptomatic people exhibit disc herniation on magnetic resonance imaging (MRI) scans. The critical question is: When is a disc bulge significant enough to warrant some type of intervention?

Some consider the subluxation an anachronism.[10] While it may serve as a model for dysfunction, the term itself can be problematic because it means different things to different people. When communicating with other disciplines, unclear terminology leads to misunderstandings (eg, subluxation in the medical profession means a partial dislocation).[11] Some define it as a physiologic entity while others assign it metaphysical attributes that cannot be tested.[7] The resulting confusion over terminology has inhibited acceptance by policy makers who control access to large blocks of potential patients who could benefit from chiropractic care.[12]

SUBLUXATION DEFINED: CRISIS IN MEASUREMENT

Since the beginnings of the chiropractic profession, technologic innovations have been applied to identify and characterize subluxation. For example, chiropractors were among the first health care providers to attempt to use radiographic examinations on their patients.[13] Elaborate methods of analysis were developed including ways to position patients to minimize errors. Postural patterns and malpositions of vertebra were sought as indicators of subluxation, and they are used to this day as a diagnosis prerequisite for Medicare reimbursement.[14] These efforts stand as a historically significant contribution to health care. Another example of a technologic innovation was the neurocalometer (a thermocouple device) that measured the paraspinal temperature gradient. However, in recent times both these methods have been overshadowed by more dynamic concepts of dysfunction.[15]

A more practical approach is to think of the vertebral subluxation in terms of observable components (testable pieces; Table 1).[16] The various components included here for the purpose of discussion include functional ones such as limited gross range of motion (ROM)/intersegmental ROM, pain (global) or palpatory tenderness, tissue compliance, postural/static malpositions, physical performance, and so forth. Physiologic disturbances have also been explored such as blood pressure, pupil size, white blood cell respiratory burst, blood flow, red reaction of the skin, visual field disturbance, force expiratory volume, leg length inequality, isolation testing (tonic neck reflexes), and manual muscle testing.[1] In recent times, a spectrum of assessment methods has been available including motion palpation, leg length assessment, and radiographic marking systems, not to mention a variety of expensive diagnostic equipment such as electromyography (EMG), electrogoniometry, videofluoroscopy, and high-tech functional capacity evaluation devices. More emphasis is frequently placed on the mechanics of how to use these devices to objectify the need for ongoing care than on understanding the clinical usefulness or necessity of the devices.

A CONTEMPORARY CHIROPRACTIC MANAGEMENT SCENARIO

The following scenario illustrates potential difficulties that may arise when faced with indiscriminate use of common assessments in the current marketplace.

A chiropractor practicing in a rural mining community mostly treated patients with chronic low back pain. She graduated from chiropractic school in the mid-1970s and, at that time, the main emphasis on documenting ongoing care was to use the static radiographic listings she learned in chiropractic college. At that time it was professed that a joint malposition indicated that a subluxation was present and that the only way to restore the patient's health was to adjust the listing. A patient was managed on the basis of noting changes in listings.

For as long as she could remember this practitioner was taught that in order to be successful, patients must be taught that "pain is the last to show and the first to go." Therefore, her patients were educated that when their pain subsided they should continue care until the listings were deemed normal. Furthermore, she explained to patients that periodic examinations would be useful in preventing further episodes of low back pain and degenerative changes.

Recently, though, her claims were met with resistance when she submitted a report to justify care on a recent case of low back pain. The state workers' compensation board had denied a full year of care amounting to nearly $5,000. In order to defend her patient's case, she summarized her findings, which consisted of an initial examination and one at every 12 visits including pre-post radiograph sets, which by this time included several sets of radiographs.

When preparing for the hearing she was frustrated to discover the evidence supporting the validity of the radiographic analysis to substantiate the need for care was lacking. Reliability data suggested only low to moderate agreement, and no credible evidence was available linking positive findings on radiograph with poor health and low back symptoms. The arbitrator ruled against her and, as a result, she was reimbursed at the greatly reduced rate of $950.

With this case still fresh in her mind, she became interested in outcome measures such as the visual analog scale (VAS) and Oswestry index, and she began tracking patients in preparation for educating them as well as their insurance companies. By integrating the outcome forms with her clinical findings and objectively noting continued perceived improvement by the patients, she noticed reduced hassle when settling future cases.

This scenario might be modified to illustrate any of 20 common chiropractic methods for detecting subluxations.

Table 1. Quantifying outcomes measurement for articular dysfunction

a. Self-report instruments (eg, pain questionnaires, function questionnaires)
b. Physiological measurement (eg, range of motion, provocative testing)
c. Physical capacity assessment (eg, observe and document ability, task duration, functional capacity testing)

AN INTEGRATED MODEL: A SYSTEMATIC APPROACH

Recently work has been done to characterize component pathologic parts of the chiropractic lesion into histopathology, myopathology, and kinesiopathology.[17] Yet, very few parts have been effectively associated with clinically meaningful terms.

Pain

Pragmatically, the reason patients choose to see a doctor is to control pain and disability, not to reduce a subtle mechanical dysfunction or misalignment. As a result, assessing a patient's pain status, and how the patient responds to intervention, can be a meaningful clinical attribute for both the patient and the health services purchaser.

One of the simplest and most common ways of assessing perceived pain intensity is the VAS.[18] It may be useful to have patients rate their pain intensity three times per assessment: when it is at its worst, at its best, and at the time of assessment. Even though self-reported pain levels have been criticized for potential influence by psychosocial factors, studies have shown that individual ratings are internally consistent.[19,20]

In people with chronic neck pain, the VAS has been shown to be quite stable on repeated testing over a 10-week period.[19] Furthermore, it has been shown to be responsive to various treatment interventions for low back pain and other conditions.[20] Its usefulness in practice should be considered in the context of all the information available to the clinician. If values are not consistent with history and examination findings, the scores should be considered suspect and noted accordingly in the file.

Palpatory tenderness

Palpatory tenderness is one of the oldest assessments for locating segmental abnormality. Often, a distinction is made between pain over bony prominences such as the spinous processes of vertebra and tenderness in muscles. Examiners have been reported to locate lumbar tenderness on groups of patients and controls reliably.[21,22] However, other evidence has suggested slight to poor reliability in the cervical spine.[23]

Pressure pain threshold has also been assessed using an algometer. Sensitivity of algometry to identify people with neck symptoms has been investigated by Levoska and coworkers[23] and found to be poor, while responsiveness of algometry has been reported to be good for some patients with neck pain and headaches.[24] Difficulties in achieving consistent objectivity for this subjective examination procedure continue.

Pain provocation tests

Many standard clinical assessment strategies incorporate orthopaedic tests such as lumbar flexion and sacroiliac tests to identify and monitor certain aspects of subluxation pain syndromes.[25] However, a battery of provocation tests, over and above routine examination procedures, was unable to distinguish patients with lower back complaints from asymptomatic subjects.[26] The usefulness of these tests awaits further study using more rigorous designs such as blinding and randomization. Prospective experimental methods involving controls such as double-blinded selective nerve blocks might help elucidate the real value of these kinds of assessment methods.

Physical function

Perceived level of function has been measured using a variety of questionnaires such as the Roland-Morris[27] and Oswestry[28] low back pain questionnaires. These assessments have yielded consistent results with a variety of patients. The neck disability index,[29] which is patterned after the Oswestry, also showed stability over a 10-week period in subjects with chronic neck pain.[19] The ability of these procedures to detect meaningful changes has also been useful to track the effects of treatment.[20,29]

Gross ROM

Active ROM has been used to assess patients with lumbar and cervical spine disorders. Some evidence[30] suggests that flexion is the biggest predictor of recovery for low back pain, following spinal manipulation. More work is necessary to standardize the way lumbar ROM is measured.

In the cervical spine, reliability of ROM has been suggested by Dvorak[31] and Youdas[32] and their associates. The authors also attempted to catalog normative data that assess the stability of cervical ROM in patients seeking care. Cassidy and colleagues[33] reported on the responsiveness of this measure to manipulation. While they did not find the cervical spine to be more mobile after manipulation, a trend was reported toward an increase in ROM. The sensitivity and specificity of ROM to distinguish between injured versus noninjured patients have been reported by Osterbauer and coworkers[34] to be 76% and 84%, respectively, when using an abnormality cutoff of greater than one standard deviation below the mean.

Dvorak and associates[31] and Nansel and Szlazak[35] looked at passive ROM suggesting that it provides more information about the status of muscle tone. Nansel and Szlazak identified lateral flexion asymmetries in asymptomatic subjects. They arbitrarily chose a threshold of greater than 15° as abnormal. In this "abnormal" sample it was demonstrated that after-manipulation increases in ROM were side specific and that there was a refractory period in patients with chronic neck pain. While this model is an interesting one with which to compare interventions and determine soft tissue behavior, it has yet to be applied to symptomatic patients and tied to additional outcomes.

One of the limitations of active and passive ROM is that these measures do not describe the quality and character of the movements. The quality of movement depends on the coordination of various muscles under voluntary and involuntary control to perform a given task. For example, a patient with a mild acute whiplash injury may be able to look down without significant limitation, yet the region where the motion occurs may be located high in the spine, or low in the spine, and it is next to impossible to record such a difference without the aid of sophisticated technology. Methods have been devised to monitor the motions in all planes while performing various ROM tasks. However, few studies are available on the usefulness of these data in solving clinical problems.

A more precise method of assessing three-dimensional movements of the neck is by calculating the three-dimensional helical axis of the head during different tasks using motion analysis equipment. These data may offer an improvement over planar head movement; because they indicate where rotation would be occurring as if about and along a fixed axis.[36] Preliminary data suggest that sensitivity of the instantaneous helical axis (IHA) is 77% and specificity is 82% for a composite of different parameters.[34] Generalizability has also been shown over a period of 10 weeks in patients with mild chronic neck pain suggesting its usefulness as an outcome measure.[19] Work is ongoing to determine its ability to identify patients with a variety of neck complaints.[37]

Intersegmental ROM

Segmental end ROM can be estimated using the instantaneous center of rotation (ICR). This procedure, however, is prone to error as noted by Woltring and associates.[36]

The clinical utility of calculating the ICR has been investigated to determine its ability to identify hypermobile segments. Amevo and colleagues[38] found they could discriminate between symptomatic and asymptomatic subjects based on ICR data. However, an overlay procedure providing similar information was found to be inadequate in identifying segmental hypermobility, especially in cases where motions were small.[39]

Another approach to intersegmental ROM is motion palpation (ie, passively palpating the patient's joints and stressing them at their end range to note the presence or absence of joint play and/or to assess the character of "end feel"). Reviewing the studies of these procedures turns up modest reliability at best.[21,22] Notably, no studies have been performed associating changes in patient outcome over time with this method.

Static postural assessment/misalignments

Posture can be assessed by using a plumb line and noting deviation from an "ideal" position. Forward head posture, for example, has been related to pain syndromes such as temporal mandibular joint (TMJ) syndrome.[40] Work is needed to determine whether it is worthwhile to screen and correct postural variants. Similarly, vertebral misalignments have been implicated in subluxation, causing some to focus their care on muscles thought to be responsible to effect a change in the malposition. Left unhindered it is theorized that these lesions lead to early degenerative changes or chronic subluxation. This notion remains unsubstantiated clinically.

Dynamic spinal loading

Current technology is being borrowed from the field of structural testing and applied to the spine. For example, the mechanical integrity of a bridge can be tested by applying sudden loads (impulsive loads) and measuring vibrational response. In the same way, the concept of impulsive loads is being applied to the spine.[41]

As stiffness increases, the frequency of the output increases. As such, this analysis may provide a way to assess muscle spasm indirectly where a high frequency response is expected to sudden loading in much the same way as a guitar string's pitch (frequency) increases as it is tightened. In recent work, a significant difference was noted between vibrational response of patients with degenerative spondylolisthesis and healthy subjects.[41] Further work is necessary to determine the usefulness of this method to assess clinically the mechanical properties of the spine in patients.

Tissue compliance

Tissue compliance, used to assess a combination of muscle and soft tissue stiffness, has been measured by noting the displacement per unit of force applied to a probe. While some have found this technique to provide reliable information,[42] others have found the intra- and interexaminer reliability to be poor.[43]

Electromyography (EMG)

Muscle tone has also been assessed using EMG, which is complicated due to the limitations inherent in obtaining accurate measurements. It is not possible to assess a single muscle without using needle probes. The reliability of scanning (surface) EMG as a diagnostic test of intersegmental muscle spasm secondary to vertebral subluxation is not well supported.[44] EMG has been used to determine the degree of neuromuscular coordination and remains a tool mainly for research purposes due to its complexity.[44]

Reactive leg length discrepancy

Prone leg alignment analysis has been used by many as an indicator of paraspinal muscle imbalance and/or pelvic torsion. Changes observed in leg alignment (reactivity) following various stimuli (isolation or pressure tests) have been reported; they are thought to be related to tonic neck reflexes.[45]

Although these procedures are widely used, little is known about the normative behavior of this phenomenon, let alone its true clinical utility. Reliability studies indicate poor to moderate agreement and have suffered from a variety of design flaws in terms of subject spectrum, blinding, randomization, and analysis. As with most assessments, these procedures await further investigation.

Examples of spectrum bias are found in studies of this phenomenon. Youngquist and colleagues[46] assessed the ability of two observers to obtain the same findings of C-1 subluxation. They included an equal number of patients who had a history of C-1 abnormality based on the prone leg check along with those who consistently had C-1 problems. Moderate reliability was reported. A criticism was raised because the doctor was told ahead of time which leg was the short leg.

Haas and associates[47] included mostly asymptomatic students in their trial of the prone leg check and isolation tests. They concluded that the prone leg check was essentially useless, noting that perhaps the phenomenon of reactivity they were after was undetectable. Further studies using an appropriate spectrum of subjects are necessary to understand this technique fully.[47]

Table 2. Reliability of various subluxation assessment methods

Method	Reliability	Rating
Chiropractic method*		
Osseous pain	0.55–0.90	Fair to excellent
Soft tissue pain	0.40–0.78	Fair to good
Prone leg check	0.28–0.55	Poor to moderate
Thermal devices	0–0.5	Poor to moderate
Active motion palpation	0–0.47	Poor to moderate
Misalignment palpation	0–0.28	Poor
Radiographic analysis†		
Scoliosis	0.33–0.43	Fair to moderate
Spondylolysis	0.17–0.63	Poor to good
Osteophytes	0.58–0.64	Moderate to good

Adapted with permission from *Osterbauer PJ, Fuhr AW, Keller TS. Description and analysis of Activator methods chiropractic technique. In: Lawrence DJ, Cassidy JD, McGregor M, et al, eds. *Advances in Chiropractic*. St Louis, MO: Mosby-Year Book; 1995;2. Copyright © 1995 W.B. Saunders Co. †Designing studies of diagnostic tests for low back pain or radiculopathy. *Spine*. 1994;19(18S):2057S–2073S. Copyright © 1994 Lippincott Williams & Wilkins.

Physical performance measures

Many types of physical performance measures are available to assess patients including isometric, isokinetic, and isoinertial strength testing.[16] These procedures require strict adherence to testing protocols to ensure reliable results. Normative databases to identify abnormalities are still in developmental stages, limiting their usefulness at the present time.

Physiologic measures: Windows to autonomic function

There are many physiologic methods available that may have the potential to assess autonomic function. Some have suggested pupil diameter[48] and field of view[49] as indicators of dysfunction. Analysis of the vascular bed includes thermography, blood pressure, skin red reaction following palpation, and Doppler ultrasound. Spirometry can also be used to observe the respiratory system, and galvanic skin response can be used to assess sweat gland activity.

One of the most intriguing and carefully studied indicators of autonomic function is white blood cell metabolic activity.[50] It has been studied using chemoluminescence to monitor respiratory burst activity. Threshold effects of applied loads to the spine have been attempted and demonstrated in preliminary studies.[48]

WHAT DOES IT ALL MEAN?

In the past decade, a flurry of research activity has attempted to determine the reliability of various methods of chiropractic analysis with mixed results. Table 2 summarizes some of these results. Investigations to evaluate this large array of strategies to objectify clinically attributes of vertebral subluxation have yielded some pilot information indicating potential clinical usefulness. However, this information remains quite limited; many require more rigorous study to determine the precise extent of clinical utility. It must also be highlighted that studies to evaluate the reproducibility of measurements of perceived attributes of vertebral subluxation do not address the construct validity of subluxation models themselves.

These results need to be interpreted carefully with regard to the designs in each case. To put the reliability of chiropractic procedures in perspective, Table 2 also compares chiropractic procedures with the reliability of identifying common radiographic findings. Future work is needed to improve the research design and analysis methodology based on the previous work. In order to provide recommendations to improve practice, it is essential that investigators understand the intricacies of not only the diagnostic procedures themselves, but also the appropriateness and limitations of experimental methodologies to evaluate them.

In the absence of adequate information, practitioners are urged to be bold in patient care, yet cautious in making claims for a given procedure, depending on the available evidence. This balance is best accomplished by weighing the evidence using one's best clinical judgment and engaging the patient in the decision-making process. In this way, the art of chiropractic is practiced; patients receive the best care based on evidence; and, when evidence is not available, the best choices are presented to the patient based on the insights of practitioners.

TECHNOLOGY ASSESSMENT ISSUES FOR CHIROPRACTIC'S FUTURE

Recent attention to lowering health care costs has resulted in keen interest in the topic of technology assessment.[8,51,52] Identification of "gold standards" to locate lesions such as subluxation is a pressing issue in chiropractic education and in the marketplace. Widespread acceptance and access of patients to chiropractic care hinge on credibility. In order to conduct an assessment properly several issues must be considered.[8] These considerations are summarized in Table 3.

Specificity and sensitivity

How well is the procedure able to identify correctly the target lesion? This issue may be thought of as the gold standard in terms of the sensitivity (PiD or positive in disease) and specificity (NiH or negative in health).[51] In most cases it is impossible to be 100% accurate even under the best of circumstances. If a gold standard is not available, then a bronze standard will have to do, especially in the early stages of a disease process.[8]

Table 3. Design considerations for studying a diagnostic test

Test comparisons
1. Was the test independently compared with an appropriate "gold standard" for the diagnosis?
2. Was the test assessed blindly relative to the gold standard or competing tests?
3. Was the "final diagnosis" established without the results of the test being evaluated?
4. Was the reproducibility of the test determined (intra- and interobserver variability)?
5. Was the test described in a reproducible manner?
6. Were sensitivity and specificity calculated for comparing the test with the final gold standard diagnosis?

Study population
1. Did the patient sample include an appropriate spectrum of mild and severe, treated and untreated disease, as well as patients with different, but easily confused, conditions?
2. Were the study setting and referral pattern for study subjects described?

Strategies for use
1. If the test is part of a group or sequence of tests, was its contribution to the overall validity of the sequence determined?
2. Was the utility of the test determined, in terms of actual effects on patient care or outcomes?

Reprinted with permission from Designing studies of diagnostic tests for low back pain or radiculopathy. *Spine.* 1994;19(18S):2057S–2063S. Copyright © 1994, Lippincott Williams & Wilkins.

Blinding

Blinded interpretation of tests is important in order to minimize observer bias. Without blinding the clinician may favor one test over another and his or her decision-making process cannot be understood. Would the same result be obtained without all the additional information? For example, how well could a team of clinicians (blinded to diagnostic tests such as computed tomography and MRI) identify patients with stenosis compared to a team that was not?

Reproducibility

Reproducibility of test interpretation deals with how well two or more practitioners agree on the same test for the same patient. The preferred statistics for assessing concordance are the Kappa statistic or interclass correlation coefficients. Goals should be made to identify reasons for poor concordance in order to see if it is possible to improve the findings. For elusive subclinical disturbances such as subluxation in the patient on maintenance, it may be difficult to distinguish the patient who could benefit from care (true positives) from those who would not (false positives).

Sample selection

A major issue to consider when designing and interpreting reliability and validity studies is the size and composition of the sample. In order to determine the appropriate sample size, a good sense of the normal variability in the target group is necessary. Also, the group should contain an appropriate spectrum of subjects, possibly extending all the way from not affected to mildly affected to severely affected. The sample should also be described carefully so that readers have a clear understanding of the subjects involved and can replicate the study.

Consistency of application

Implementation of diagnostic tests or sequencing of tests refers to the effects the order of testing plays in the decision-making process. A doctor who palpates a patient first and then looks at the radiographs may arrive at a different impression than one who performs this analysis in reverse.

CONCLUSIONS

Interest in criteria for assessing clinical methods is accelerating. Scientific strategies have been developed in other disciplines, and only recently applied in a meaningful manner to clinical medicine. Awareness of these procedures should result in an expanded application to chiropractic questions. Such studies help provide a means to gauge

Table 4. Usefulness of selected subluxation assessment procedures

Measure	Severity	Prognosis	Responsiveness	Reliability
VAS	+	+	+	+
NDI	+	+	+	+
Roland-Morris	+	+	+	+
EMG	?	?	?	?
LL reactivity	?	?	?	?
Motion palpation	?	?	?	?
Misalignments				

VAS = visual analog scale; NDI = neck disability index; EMG = electromyography; LL = leg length
+ = Solid studies support recommendation.
? = Research of equal quality exists with opposing conclusions or there is no solid research.

---

present knowledge of clinical utility and guide clinical decision making. Table 4 contrasts various clinical measures and how they apply to practice based on the literature.

Difficulties in reaching consensus on the definition of the chiropractic lesion have been fueled by several factors. Within the profession some may feel that the term is outdated while others may assert that subluxation is the Holy Grail of health and disease. Since the term was first applied to chiropractic by D.D. Palmer, a significant amount of new information has become available regarding the assessment of subluxation and its relationship to health and disease. More has to be done to characterize the properties of the lesion and its relative importance clinically. Today, multiple models more consistent with contemporary understandings of spinal biomechanics and neurophysiology have been proposed, including integrated models that consider the lesion as a problem of movement (opposed to a "malposition"). Whatever models and definitions continue to evolve, it seems the only way to determine the existence of such a pathophysiologic entity is to measure the physiologic components determined to be abnormal.

The extent to which abnormalities can be defined will depend on proper design and analysis, as outlined in this article. In the interim, reliable, valid methods are available to clinicians to address the complaints of patients and help guide care. Regardless, most of chiropractic's rich heritage of approaches to patient care, like most of medical care, remains in the realm of art.

REFERENCES

1. Gatterman MI. *Foundations of Chiropractic: Subluxation.* St Louis, Mo: Mosby; 1995.
2. Anderson R. Diagnosis and treatment of low back pain since 1850. In: White AH, Anderson R, eds. *Conservative Care of Low Back Pain.* Baltimore, Md: Williams & Wilkins; 1990.
3. Mixter WJ, Barr JS. Rupture of the intervertebral disc with involvement of the spinal canal. *N Engl J Med.* 1934; 211:210–215.
4. Bergmann TF. Chiropractic technique: an overview. In: Lawrence DJ, ed. *Advances in Chiropractic.* St Louis, Mo: Mosby-Year Book; 1995;2.
5. Keating JC. Science and politics and the subluxation. *Am J Chiro Med.* 1988;1:107–110.
6. Cherkin DC, MacCormack FA, Berg AO. The management of low back pain—a comparison of the beliefs and behaviors of family physicians and chiropractors. *West J Med.* 1988;149:475.
7. Keating JC. *Toward a Philosophy of the Science of Chiropractic.* Stockton, Calif: Stockton Foundation for Chiropractic Research; 1993.
8. Deyo RA, Haselkorn J, Hoffman R, Kent DL. Designing studies of diagnostic tests for low back pain or radiculopathy. *Spine.* 1994;19(18S):2057S–2065S.
9. Boden SD, Davis DO, Dina TS, et al. Abnormal magnetic resonance scans of the lumbar spine in asymptomatic subjects: a prospective investigation. *J Bone Joint Surg (Am).* 1990;15:571–576.
10. Bryner P. Isn't it time to abandon anachronistic terminology? *J Aust Chiro Assoc.* 1987;17:53–58.
11. Gatterman MI. Advances in subluxation terminology use. In: Lawrence DJ, ed. *Advances in Chiropractic.* St Louis, Mo: Mosby-Year Book; 1995;2.
12. Mootz R, Shekelle P, Hansen D. The politics of policy and research. *Top Clin Chiro.* 1995;2:56–70.
13. Canterbury R, Krakos G. Thirteen years after roentgen: the origins of chiropractic radiology. *Chiro History.* 1986;6:25–29.
14. Peterson DH, Bergmann TF. Joint assessment principles and procedures. In: Bergmann TF, Peterson DH, Lawrence DJ, eds. *Chiropractic Technique.* New York, NY: Churchill-Livingstone; 1993.
15. Lantz CA. A review of the evolution of chiropractic concepts of subluxation. *Top Clin Chiro.* 1995;2:1–10.
16. Triano JJ. The subluxation complex outcome measures of chiropractic diagnosis and treatment. *J Chiro Tech.* 1990;2:114.
17. Lantz CA. The vertebral subluxation complex: 2. The neuropathological and myopathological components. *Chiro Res J.* 1990;1:19–37.
18. Huskisson EC. Measurement of pain. *Lancet.* 1974;2:1127–1131.
19. Osterbauer PJ, Patterson LJ, Petermann EA, et al. Generalizability of selected patient outcome measures in volunteers with chronic neck

pain. In: *The Proceedings of the Chiropractic Centennial Foundation.* Davenport, IA: CCF; 1995.

20. Triano JJ, McGregor M, Hondras M, et al. Manipulation therapy vs education programs in chronic low back pain. *Spine.* 1995;20:948–955.

21. Keating JC, Bergmann TF, Jacobs GE, et al. Interexaminer reliability of eight evaluative dimensions of lumbar segmental abnormality. *J Manipulative Physiol Ther.* 1990;13:463–470.

22. Boline PD, Haas M, Meyer JJ, et al. Interexaminer reliability of eight evaluative dimensions of lumbar segmental abnormality: II. *J Manipulative Physiol Ther.* 1993;16:363–374.

23. Levoska S, Kiukaanniemi-Kienänen S, Bloigu R. Repeatability of measurement tenderness on the neck and shoulder region by a dolorimeter and manual palpation. *Clin J Pain.* 1993;9:229–235.

24. Vernon HT, Aker P, Burns S, et al. Pressure pain threshold evaluation on the effect of spinal manipulation on the treatment of chronic neck pain. *J Manipulative Physiol Ther.* 1990;14:404–415.

25. Osterbauer PJ, DeBoer KF, Widmaier R, Petermann EA, Fuhr AW. Treatment and biomechanical assessment of patients with chronic sacroiliac syndrome. *J Manipulative Physiol Ther.* 1993;15:82–90.

26. Triano JJ, McGregor MM, Doyne M, et al. Criterion-oriented validity of manual diagnostic maneuvers. In: *The Proceedings of the Chiropractic Centennial Foundation.* Davenport, IA: CCF; 1995.

27. Roland M, Morris R. A study of the natural history of back pain: development of a reliable and sensitive measure in low back pain. *Spine.* 1983;8:141–144.

28. Fairbank JCT, Couper J, Davies JB, et al. The Oswestry low back pain disability questionnaire. *Physiotherapy.* 1980;66:271–273.

29. Vernon HT, Mior S. The neck disability index: a study of reliability and validity. *J Manipulative Physiol Ther.* 1991;14:409–415.

30. Cassidy JD, Balageorge D, Kim P, et al. A longitudinal study of impairment and disability in low back pain patients. In: *The Proceedings of the International Society for the Study of the Lumbar Spine.* Chicago, IL: ISSLS; 1994.

31. Dvorak J, Antinnes JA, Panjabi M, et al. Age and gender related normal motion of the cervical spine. *Spine.* 1992;17(10S):S393–S398.

32. Youdas JW, Garret TR, Suman VJ, et al. Normal range of motion of the cervical spine: an initial goniometric study. *Phys Ther.* 1992;72:770–780.

33. Cassidy JD, Quon JA, LaFrance LJ, et al. The effect of manipulation on pain and range of motion in the cervical spine. *J Manipulative Physiol Ther.* 1992;15:495–500.

34. Osterbauer PJ, Koepsell T, Ribaudo TA, et al. Validity estimation of three dimensional head kinematics and cervical range of motion in the diagnosis of patients with acute neck injuries. In: *The Proceedings of the International Conference on Spinal Manipulation.* Sunnyvale, Calif: Consortium for Chiropractic Research; 1994.

35. Nansel DD, Szlzak M. Findings on the relationship between spinal manipulation and cervical passive end-range capability. In: Lawrence DJ, eds. *Advances in Chiropractic.* St Louis, Mo: Mosby-Year Book; 1994;1.

36. Woltring HJ, Long K, Osterbauer PJ, Fuhr AW. Instantaneous helical axis estimation from 3D video data in neck kinematics for whiplash diagnostics. *J Biomech.* 1994;27:1415–1432.

37. Osterbauer PJ, Patterson LJ, Petermann EA, et al. Generalizability of selected 3D helical axis parameters of the head in volunteers with chronic neck pain. In: *The Proceedings of the Chiropractic Centennial Foundation.* Davenport, IA: CCF; 1995.

38. Amevo B, Worth D, Bogduk N. Instantaneous axes of rotation of the typical cervical motion segments: a study in normal volunteers. *Clin Biomech.* 1991;6:111–117.

39. McGregor M, Mior S, Shannon H, et al. The clinical usefulness of flexion-extension radiographs in the cervical spine. *Top Clin Chiro.* 1995;2:19–28.

40. Curl DD. The temporomandibular joint. In: Lawrence DJ, ed. *Advances in Chiropractic.* St Louis, Mo: Mosby-Year Book; 1995;1.

41. Nathan M, Keller TS. Measurement and analysis of the in vivo posteroanterior impulse response of the human thoraco-lumbar spine. A feasibility study. *J Manipulative Physiol Ther.* 1994;17:431–441.

42. Nansel DD, Waldorf T, Cooperstein R. Effect of cervical spine adjustments on lumbar spine muscle tone: evidence for facilitation of intersegmental tonic neck reflexes. *J Manipulative Physiol Ther.* 1993;16:91–95.

43. Kawchuk G, Herzog W. The reliability and accuracy of a standard method of tissue compliance assessment. *J Manipulative Physiol Ther.* 1995;18:298–301.

44. Meyer JJ. Clinical electromyographic and related neurophysiologic responses. In: Lawrence DJ, ed. *Advances in Chiropractic.* St Louis, Mo: Mosby-Year Book; 1994;1.

45. Osterbauer PJ, Fuhr AW, Keller TS. Description and analysis of activator methods chiropractic technique. In: Lawrence DJ, ed. *Advances in Chiropractic.* St Louis, Mo: Mosby-Year Book; 1995;2.

46. Youngquist MW, Fuhr AW, Osterbauer PJ. Interexaminer reliability of an upper cervical isolation test. *J Manipulative Physiol Ther.* 1989;12:93–97.

47. Haas M, Peterson D, Panzer D, et al. Reactivity of leg alignment to articular pressure testing: evaluation of a diagnostic test using a randomized crossover trial clinical trial approach. *J Manipulative Physiol Ther.* 1993;16:220–227.

48. Briggs L, Boone WR. Effects of chiropractic adjustment on changes in pupillary diameter: a model for evaluating somato-visceral response. *J Manipulative Physiol Ther.* 1988;11:181–189.

49. Gorman RF. Monocular visual loss after closed head trauma: immediate resolution associated with spinal manipulation. *J Manipulative Physiol Ther.* 1995;18:308–314.

50. Brennan PC, Kokjohn K, Kaltinger CJ, et al. Enhanced phagocytic cell respiratory burst induced by spinal manipulation: potential role of substance P. *J Manipulative Physiol Ther.* 1991;14:399–408.

51. Sackett DL, Haynes RB, Guyatt GH, Tugwell P. *Clinical Epidemiology: A Basic Science for Clinical Medicine.* 2nd ed. Boston, Mass: Little, Brown; 1991.

52. Haldeman S, Chapman-Smith D, Petersen D. *Guidelines for Chiropractic Quality Assurance and Practice Parameters.* Gaithersburg, Md: Aspen Publishers; 1993.

Appendix I-A

Resource List for Technology Assessment in Health Care

Hansen DT, Mootz, RD. Technology assessment in health care: A primer for the chiropractic profession.
Topics in Clinical Chiropractic 1996; 3(1).

FEDERAL GOVERNMENT SOURCES

National Information Center on Health Services Research and Health Care Technology (NICHSR)
This is the federal government's central source for publicly funded scientific and technical information, including databases, internet Grateful Med, publications; outreach and training; and research and development programs.

National Information Center on Health Services Research
and Health Care Technology (NICHSR)
National Library of Medicine
8600 Rockville Pike
Building 38A, Mail Stop 20
Bethesda, MD 20894
(301) 496-0176
FAX: (301) 402-3193
E-mail: nichsr@nlm.nih.gov
Web: www.nlm.nih.gov/nichsr/

Agency for Health Care Policy & Research (AHCPR)
AHCPR supports and conducts research on health services, clinical practice guideline development, and technology assessment. The agency disseminates its information to practitioners, policymakers, researchers and consumers.

Department of Health & Human Services
Agency for Health Care Policy & Research
2101 E Jefferson St.
Rockville, MD 20852
(301) 594-1364
Web: www.ahcpr.gov

To order publications:
AHCPR Publications Clearinghouse
PO Box 8547
Silver Spring, MD 20907
(800) 358-9295

Health Care Financing Administration (HCFA)
HCFA is responsible for the Medicare program, federal participation in the Medicaid program, and other health care quality-assurance programs. It has a number of individual agencies and bureaus to obtain information.

Office of Research and Demonstrations (ORD) - HCFA
Oak Meadows Building, Room 2230
6325 Security Blvd.
Baltimore, MD 21207
(410) 966-6584
Fax: (410) 966-6511

Office of Statistics and Data Management (OSDM) - HCFA
Security Office Park Building, Room 3B-8
6325 Security Blvd.
Baltimore, MD 21207
(410) 597-3933
Fax: (410) 597-3675 or (410) 597-2128

Health Resources and Services Administration (HRSA)

Bureau of Health Professions (HRSA)
This bureau's mandate is to produce reports and publications on issues, developments, trends, and projections concerning health care personnel in the U.S.

Office of Health Professions Analysis and Research
Bureau of Health Professions (HRSA)
Parklawn Building, Room 8-47
5600 Fishers Lane
Rockville, MD 20857
(301) 443-6936
Fax: (301) 444-8003

National Center for Health Statistics (NCHS)

This agency collects, analyzes, and disseminates health statistics on vital events and health activities. The agency prints an annual compilation of U.S. health trends, titled *Health United States*, a must for every researcher.

Scientific and Technical Information Branch
Division of Data Services
National Center for Health Statistics
6525 Belcrest Rd., Room 1064
Hyattsville, MD 20782
(301) 436-8500

ASSOCIATIONS, INSTITUTES, FOUNDATIONS

American Managed Care and Review Association (AMCRA)

This association represents the full spectrum of managed care programs including HMOs, IPAs, PPOs, etc. and conducts research projects ranging from cost studies to CEO surveys.

American Managed Care and Review Association
1200 19th St. NW, Suite 200
Washington, DC 20036-2437
(202) 728-0506
Fax: (202) 728-0609

Consortial Center for Chiropractic Research (CCCR)

The CCCR is a Research Center for the National Center for Complementary & Alternative Medicine (NCCAM) and a part of the National Institutes of Health (NIH). It consists of faculty and administrators from five chiropractic institutions, the University of Iowa, and Kansas State University. This organization provides an infrastructure to examine the potential effectiveness and validity of chiropractic health care and to provide the appropriate clinical, scientific, and technical assistance to chiropractic researchers in developing high quality research projects.

Consortial Center for Chiropractic Research
Palmer Center for Chiropractic Research
741 Brady Street
Davenport, IA 52803
(319) 884-5162
Fax: (319) 884-5227
E-mail: info@c3r.org
Web: www.palmer.edu

Institute of Medicine (IOM), National Academy of Sciences

The IOM is an invitation-only membership organization chartered by the National Academy of Sciences (NAS) to enlist distinguished health professionals to examine policy matters pertaining to public health. Its reports are published by the National Research Council.

Reports and Information Office
Institute of Medicine
National Research Council
National Academy of Sciences
2101 Constitution Ave., NW
Washington, DC 20418
(202) 334-2352
Fax: (202) 334-1412
Publication information:
National Academy Press
2101 Constitution Ave., NW
PO Box 285
Washington, DC 20055
(202) 334-3313
(800) 624-6242

International Society of Technology Assessment in Health Care (ISTAHC)

The Society is primarily concerned with emerging medical technologies as they are developed, produced, disseminated, applied and costed. Major issues of concern include: safety and efficacy; cost and cost-effectiveness; ethics; quality of care; access to health care; appropriateness of application; legal and regulatory considerations; and competing technologies.

ISTAHC Membership Office
Cambridge University Press
40 West 20th Street
New York, NY 10011-4211

National Health Policy Forum

This forum is a nonpartisan, educational program serving congressional, White House, and executive agency specialists in health affairs with the objective of improving the process of federal health policy decision-making.

National Health Policy Forum
2021 K St., NW, Suite 800
Washington, DC 20006
(202) 872-1390
Fax: (202) 785-0114

RAND Corporation
This private research institute's focus is on health care financing and quality of care.

The Health Sciences Program
RAND Corporation
PO Box 2138
1700 Main St
Santa Monica, CA 90407-2138
(310) 451-7002
Fax: 451-6915
E-mail: info@rand.org
Web: www.rand.org

Robert Wood Johnson Foundation
This research foundation has a mission to improve health and health care to all Americans by assuring access to basic health care, improving the way health services are organized and delivered to those with chronic conditions, and addressing the problem of escalating health care costs.

Robert Wood Johnson Foundation
Route 1 and College Road East
PO Box 2316
Princeton, NJ 08543-2316
(609) 452-8701
E-mail: mail@rwjf.org

Workers Compensation Research Institute
This organization reports on significant ideas, issues, research studies, and data of interest to those involved in workers' compensation.

Workers' Compensation Research Institute
101 Main St.
Cambridge, MA 02142
(617) 494-1240
Fax: (617) 494-5240

PERIODICALS

American Journal of Public Health
APHA Publication Sales
1015 15th St., NW, Suite 300
Department 5037
Washington, DC 20061-5037
(202) 789-5600
Fax: (202) 789-5661

Health Affairs
Project Hope
7500 Old Georgetown Rd., Suite 600
Bethesda, MD 20814-6133
(800) 825-0061
(301) 656-7401
Fax: (301) 654-2845

Health Care Financing Review
Office of Research & Demonstrations
Health Care Financing Administration
Oak Meadows Building, Room 1-A-9
6325 Security Blvd.
Baltimore, MD 21207
(410) 966-6572
Fax: (410) 966-6511
Subscriptions:
Government Printing Office
(202) 512-1800

Healthcare Trends Report
Health Trends
4405 East-West Highway, Suite 406
Bethesda, MD 20814
(800) 945-8816
Fax: (301) 907-6790

Health Services Research Journal
Health Services Research Foundation of the American
    College of Health Care Executives
1951 Cornell Ave.
Melrose Park, IL 60160
(708) 450-9952
Fax: (708) 450-1618

International Journal of Technology Assessment in Health Care
Cambridge University Press
110 Midland Ave.
Port Chester, NY 10573

Journal of Health Politics, Policy and Law
Journals Department
Duke University Press
PO Box 90660 College Station
Durham, NC 27708-0660
(919) 687-3600

Quality Management in Health Care
QMHC
Aspen Publishers, Inc.
7201 McKinney Circle
Frederick, MD 21701
(800) 234-1660

Report on Medical Guidelines and Outcomes Research
Capitol Publications
PO Box 453

1101 King St., Suite 444
Alexandria, VA 22314
(800) 655-5597
Fax: (703) 739-6517

Statistical Bulletin
Metropolitan Life Insurance Co.
1 Madison Ave.
New York, NY 10016
(212) 578-5014
Fax: (212) 213-0577

Topics in Clinical Chiropractic
(TICC)
Aspen Publishers, Inc.
7201 McKinney Circle
Fredrick, MD 21701
(800) 234-1660

ONLINE HEALTH DATABASES

Federal Online Databases

National Library of Medicine (NLM)
MEDLARS is the computerized system of databases and databanks offered by the National Library of Medicine.

For information on accessing NLM's online databases and or obtaining a NLM use code, contact:

MEDLARS Management Section
National Library of Medicine
8600 Rockville Pike
Bethesda, MD 20894
(800) 638-8480
Fax: (301) 496-0822
E-mail: mms@nlm.nih.gov

For information on the content of NLM databases contact:

National Information Center for Health Services Research
   and Health Care Technology (NICHSR)
National Library of Medicine
8600 Rockville Pike
Bethesda, MD 20894
(800) 272-4787
Fax: (301) 402-3193
E-mail: nichsr@nlm.nih.gov

User Interfaces for NLM Databases:

Grateful Med
National Technical Information Service
US Department of Commerce
5285 Port Royal Road
Springfield, VA 22162
(800) 423-9255
E-mail: gmhelp

Internet Access
NLM provides many services using the capabilities of the Internet. These can be accessed using such tools as Gopher Servers or Mosaic for World Wide Web servers. Connection can be accomplished through direct network connections or through dial-up Internet services such as PRODIGY, CompuServe, or America Online.

World Wide Web:
   NLM's Home Page: http://www.nlm.nih.gov

Gopher Servers:
   From gopher server to NLM's gopher.nlm.nig.gov

List of NLM Online Databases and Databanks:
   BIOETHICSLINE (Bioethics on Line)
   DIRLINE (Directory of Information Resources onLine)
   HEALTH (Health Planning and Administration)
   HSRPROJ (Health Services Research Projects in
      Progress)
   HSTAR (Health Services/Technology Assessment
      Research)
   HSTAT (Health Services/Technology Assessment Text)
   MEDLINE (MEDlars onLine)
   POPLINE (Population information online)

Other Federal Online Databases
   Thomas World Wide Web Server
      http://thomas.loc.gov
   White House World Wide Web Server
      http://www.whitehouse.gov
   National Technical Information Services (NTIS)
      http://www.fedworld.gov/

ONLINE INFORMATION SOURCES

Discussion and Information Listservers

Office of Technology Assessment (OTA)
This Congressional office maintains a free electronic mailing list known as OTANEWs, which allows anyone with access to e-mail on the Internet to receive notices of OTA reports. To subscribe, address an e-mail message to listserver@ota.gov, leaving the subject line blank. Questions can be posted by e-mail at postmaster@ota.gov.

QP-HEALTH E-mail Discussion List
A list for discussion of Quality-related Issues for Professionals in Health care. Discussions revolve around topics such as

the dimensions of quality as defined by the Joint Commission for Accreditation of Healthcare Organizations, medical ethics, competency, internal and external customer satisfaction, multidisciplinary and cross-functional approaches to process assessment and improvement, utilization of statistical process control and quality tools, integration of Deming's 14 points into healthcare organization culture, and achieving and measuring continuous quality improvement. To subscribe, address an e-mail message to majordomo@quality.org, leaving the subject line blank with only the following in the body of your message: *subscribe qp-health*.

World Wide Web Sites (WWW)
RAND Corporation
  http://www.rand.org
National Commission on Quality Assurance (NCQA)
  http://www.ncqa.org
Health Care Financing Administration (HCFA)
  http://hcfa.gov
National Library of Medicine
  http://www.nlm.nih.gov
Center for Evidence-Based Medicine
  http://cebm.jr2.ox.ac.uk
Centers for Disease Control and Prevention
  http://www.cdc.gov/epo/mmwr/mmwr.html
Cochrane Collaboration
  http://hiru.mcmaster.ca/cochrane/default.htm
Council of State Governments
  http://www.csg.org
Robert Wood Johnson Foundation for State Health Policy
  http://www2.umdnj.edu/shpp/homepage.html
Health Services Research Journal
  http://www.xnet.com/~hret/hsr.htm
United Kingdom National Health Service Health Technology Assessment Programme
  http://www.soton.ac.uk/~hta/index.htm
Netting the Evidence (Introduction to Evidence Based Practice on the Internet)
  http://www.shef.ac.uk/~scharr/ir/netting.html

Adapted with permission from *Healthcare Trends Report 1995 Sourcebook*, Health Trends, Bethesda, MD, (800) 945-8816.

Appendix I–B

Directory of State and National Public Health Offices

ALABAMA
Department of Public Health
434 Monroe Street
Montgomery, AL 36130
(205) 242-5052

ALASKA
Division of Public Health
Department of Health and Social
 Services
PO Box H
Juneau, AK 99811
(907) 465-3090

ARIZONA
Department of Health Services
1740 W Adams Street
Phoenix, AZ 85007
(602) 542-1024

ARKANSAS
Arkansas Department of Health
4815 W Markham Street
Little Rock, AR 72205
(501) 661-2111

CALIFORNIA
Department of Health Services
714 P Street
Sacramento, CA 95814
(916) 657-1425

COLORADO
Department of Health
4210 E 11th Avenue
Denver, CO 80220
(303) 331-4600

CONNECTICUT
Department of Health Services
150 Washington Street
Hartford, CT 06106
(203) 566-2038

DELAWARE
Division of Public Health
Department of Health and Social
 Services
PO Box 637
Dover, DE 19903
(302) 739-4701

FLORIDA
Health Office
Department of Health and
 Rehabilitative Services
1323 Winewood Boulevard,
 Building 1
Tallahassee, FL 32301
(904) 487-2705

GEORGIA
Division of Public Health
Department of Human Resources
878 Peachtree Street
Atlanta, GA 30309
(404) 894-7505

HAWAII
Department of Health
1250 Punchbowl Street
PO Box 3378
Honolulu, HI 96801
(808) 586-4410

IDAHO
Division of Health
Department of Health and Welfare
450 West State Street
Boise, ID 83720
(208) 334-5945

ILLINOIS
Department of Public Health
535 W Jefferson Street
Springfield, IL 62761
(217) 782-4977

INDIANA
Board of Health
1330 W Michigan Street
PO Box 1964
Indianapolis, IN 46206
(317) 633-8400

IOWA
Department of Public Health
Robert Lucas State Office Building
East 12th and Walnut Streets
Des Moines, IA 50319
(515) 281-5605

KANSAS
Department of Health and
 Environment
900 SW Jackson
Topeka, KS 66612
(913) 296-1522

KENTUCKY
Department for Health Services
Cabinet for Human Resources
275 E Main Street
Frankfort, KY 40621
(502) 564-3970

LOUISIANA
Department of Health and Hospitals
PO Box 629
Baton Rouge, LA 70821
(504) 342-9500

MAINE
Bureau of Health
Department of Human Services
State House Station 11
Augusta, ME 04333
(207) 289-2736

MARYLAND
Department of Health and Mental
  Hygiene
201 W Preston Street
Baltimore, MD 21201
(410) 225-6500

MASSACHUSETTS
Department of Public Health
150 Tremont Street
Boston, MA 02111
(617) 727-2700

MICHIGAN
Department of Public Health
3423 North Logan Street
Lansing, MI 48909
(517) 335-8024

MINNESOTA
Department of Health
717 Delaware Street, SE
PO Box 9441
Minneapolis, MN 55440
(612) 623-5460

MISSISSIPPI
Department of Health
2423 North State Street
PO Box 1700
Jackson, MS 39215
(601) 960-7634

MISSOURI
Department of Health
PO Box 570
Jefferson City, MO 65102
(314) 751-6001

MONTANA
Department of Health and
  Environmental Sciences
Cogswell Building
Helena, MT 59620
(406) 444-2544

NEBRASKA
Department of Health
301 Centennial Mall South
PO Box 95007
Lincoln, NE 68509
(402) 471-2133

NEVADA
Health Division
505 E King Street
Carson City, NV 89701
(702) 687-4740

NEW HAMPSHIRE
Division of Public Health Services
Health and Welfare Building
Hazen Drive
Concord, NH 03301
(603) 271-4500

NEW JERSEY
Department of Health
CN 360
Trenton, NJ 08625
(609) 292-7837

NEW MEXICO
Department of Health
1190 St. Francis Drive
Santa Fe, NM 87503
(505) 827-2613

NEW YORK
Department of Health
Tower Building
Empire State Plaza
Albany, NY 12237
(518) 474-2011

NORTH CAROLINA
Division of Health Services
Department of Environment, Health
  and Natural Resources
PO Box 27687
Raleigh, NC 27611
(919) 733-4984

NORTH DAKOTA
Department of Health and
  Consolidated Laboratories
State Capitol, Judicial Wing
600 East Boulevard
Bismarck, ND 58505
(701) 224-2372

OHIO
Department of Health
246 North High Street
Columbus, OH 43266
(614) 466-2253

OKLAHOMA
Department of Health
1000 NE 10th Street
PO Box 53551
Oklahoma City, OK 73152
(405) 271-4200

OREGON
Health Division
Department of Human Resources
1400 SW 5th Avenue
Portland, OR 97201
(503) 229-5032

PENNSYLVANIA
Department of Health
PO Box 90
Harrisburg, PA 17108
(717) 787-6436

RHODE ISLAND
Department of Health
Cannon Health Building
3 Capitol Hill
Providence, RI 02908
(401) 277-2231

SOUTH CAROLINA
Department of Health and
  Environmental Control
2600 Bull Street
Columbia, SC 29201
(803) 734-4880

SOUTH DAKOTA
Department of Health
445 E Capitol
Pierre, SD 57501
(605) 773-3361

TENNESSEE
Department of Health
344 Cordell Hull Building
Nashville, TN 37247
(615) 741-3111

TEXAS
Department of Health
1100 W 49th Street
Austin, TX 78756
(512) 458-7111

UTAH
Department of Health
288 N 1460 W
PO Box 16700
Salt Lake City, UT 84116
(801) 538-6111

VERMONT
Department of Health
60 Main Street
PO Box 70
Burlington, VT 05402
(802) 863-7280

VIRGINIA
Department of Health
PO Box 2448
Richmond, VA 23218
(804) 786-3561

WASHINGTON
Department of Health
112 SE Quince Street
Olympia, WA 98504
(206) 753-5871

WEST VIRGINIA
Bureau of Public Health
Building 3, Capitol Complex
Charleston, WV 25305
(304) 348-2971

WISCONSIN
Division of Health
Department of Health and Social
  Services
PO Box 309
Madison, WI 53707
(608) 266-1511

WYOMING
Department of Health
Hathaway Building
Cheyenne, WY 82002
(307) 777-7656

AMERICAN PUBLIC HEALTH ASSOCIATION
1015 15th Street NW
Washington, DC 20005
(202) 789-5600

OCCUPATIONAL SAFETY AND HEALTH ADMINISTRATION
200 Constitution Avenue, NW
Room N3647
Washington, DC 20210
(202) 219-7075

Appendix I–C

Public Health Resources on the Internet

Centers for Disease Control and Prevention

Agency for Toxic Substances and Disease Registry
atsdr1.atsdr.cdc.gov:8080/

Centers for Disease Control and Prevention
www.cdc.gov

Epidemiology Program Office
www.cdc.gov/epo

Morbidity and Mortality Weekly Report
www.cdc.gov/epo/mmwr/mmrw.html

National Center for Chronic Disease Prevention and Health Promotion
www.cdc.gov/nccdphp/nccdhome.htm

National Center for Environmental Health
ww.cdc.gov/nceh/ncehhome.htm

National Center for Health Statistics
www.cdc.gov/nchswww/nchshome.htm

National Center for HIV, Sexually Transmitted Diseases, and Tuberculosis
www.cdc.gov/nchstp/od/nchstp.html

National Center for Infectious Diseases
www.cdc.gov./ncidod/ncid.htm

National Institute for Occupational Safety and Health
www.cdc.gov/niosh/homepage.html

Department of Agriculture

Animal & Plant Health Inspection Service
www.aphis.usda.gov

Department of Agriculture
www.usda.gov

Food and Consumer Service
www.usda.gov/fcs/fcs.htm

Grain Inspection Packers & Stockyards Administration
www.usda.gov/gipsa

National Agricultural Library
www.nalusda.gov

Department of Health & Human Services
www.os.dhhs.gov/

Administration for Children and Families (ACF)
www.acf.dhhs.gov

Administration on Aging (AoA)
http://www.aoa.dhhs.gov

Agency for Health Care Policy and Research (AHCPR)
www.ahcpr.gov/

Agency for Toxic Substances and Disease Registry (ATSDR)
atsdr1.atsdr.cdc.gov:8080/

Centers for Disease Control and Prevention (CDC)
www.cdc.gov

Food and Drug Administration (FDA)
www.fda.gov

Health Care Financing Adminstration (HCFA)
www.hcfa.gov

Health Resources and Services Administration (HRSA)
www.os.dhhs.gov/hrsa

Indian Health Service (IHS)
www.tucson.ihs.gov

National Institute of Health (NIH)
www.nih.gov/

Program Support Center (PSC)
www.psc.gov/

Substance Abuse and Mental Health Services Administration (SAMHSA)
www.samhsa.gov/

National Clearinghouse for Alcohol and Drug Information (Prevention Online)
www.health.org

National Health Information Center
nhic-nt.health.org

Office of Disease Prevention and Health Promotion
odphp.oash.dhhs.gov/

Office of Minority Health
http://www.os.dhhs.gov/progorg/ophs/omh

Office of Public Health and Science
www.osophs.dhhs.gov/ophs/

Public Health Service
phs.os.dhhs.gov/phs/phs.html

Secretary of Health and Human Services
phs.os.dhhs.gov/progorg/ospage.html

Food and Drug Administration

Center for Devices and Radiological Health
www.fda.gov/cdrh/index.html

Center for Drug Evaluation and Research
www.fda.gov.cder

Center for Food Safety and Applied Nutrition
vm.cfsan.fda.gov/list.html

FDA *Consumer*
www.fda.gov/fdac

Food & Drug Administration
www.fda.gov

MEDWATCH
www.fda.gov.medwatch/

National Institutes of Health
www.nih.gov/

Magnuson, Warren Grant Clinical Center
www.cc.nih.gov

National Cancer Institute
nci.nih.gov

National Center for Complementary and Alternative Medicine
altmed.od.nih.gov/nccam/

National Center for Human Genome Research
www.nchgr.nih.gov

National Center for Research Resources
www.ncrr.nih.gov

National Eye Institute
www.nei.nih.gov

National Heart, Lung, and Blood Institute
www.nhlbi.nih.gov

National Institute of Allergy and Infectious Diseases
www.niaid.nih.gov

National Institute of Arthritis and Musculoskeletal and Skin Diseases
http://www.nih.gov/niams

National Institute of Child Health and Human Development
http://www.nih.gov/nichd

National Institute of Diabetes and Digestive and Kidney Diseases
www.niddk.nih.gov

National Institute of Dental Research
www.nidr.nih.gov

National Institute of Environmental Health Sciences
www.niehs.nih.gov

National Institute of General Medical Sciences
www.nih.gov/nigms

National Institute of Mental Health
www.nimh.nih.gov/home.htm

National Institute of Neurological Disorders and Stroke
www.nih.gov/ninds

National Institute of Nursing Research
www.nih.gov/ninr

National Institute on Alcohol Abuse and Alcoholism
niaaa.nia.gov

National Institute on Drug Abuse
www.nida.nih.gov

National Institutes of Health
www.nih.gov

National Institutes of Health Research Grants Division
www.drg.nih.gov

National Library of Medicine
www.nlm.nih.gov

Other Selected Government Agencies and Independent Agencies

American Cancer Society
www.cancer.org/bottom.html

American Diabetes Association
www.ada.org/

American Heart Association
www.amhrt.org/

American Lung Association
www.lungusa.org/

American Public Health Association
www.apha.org/

American Red Cross
crossnet.org/

Arthritis Foundation
www.arthritis.org

Asthma and Allergy Foundation of American
www.aafa.org

Consumer Information Center
www.pueblo.gsa.gov

Consumer Product Safety Commission
ww.cpsc.gov

Department of Veterans Affairs
www.va.gov

Environmental Protection Agency
www.epa.gov

Federal Emergency Management Agency
www.fema.gov

Federal Trade Commission
www.ftc.gov

General Accounting Office
www.gao.gov

General Services Administration
www.gsa.gov

Government Printing Office
www.access.gpo.gov

Health People 2010
web.health.gov/healthypeople/

Library of Congress: Links to State and Local Government Web Sites
lcweb.loc.gov/global/state/stategov.html

National Kidney Foundation
kidney.org/

Occupational Safety and Health Administration
www.osha.gov

Pan American Health Organization
www.paho.org/

Persian Gulf Veterans' Illness
www.va.gov/health/environ/persgulf.htm

Social Security Administration
www.ssa.gov

Veterans Affairs Medical Center
pet.med.va.gov:8080

World Health Organization
www.who.int

Part II

Diagnostic Technologies

5

Improving the Clinician's Use of Orthopedic Testing: An Application to Low Back Pain

Kevin A. McCarthy

Throughout much of its history, the practice of chiropractic has focused primarily on the use of radiographs, instrumentation, and various forms of palpation to determine the presence of spinal subluxation. The clinician's skill was measured largely on his or her ability to find and reduce the spinal subluxation and to produce a satisfactory patient outcome. Diagnostic skills were mostly used for ruling out patients with certain pathologies. Although often in the minority, some clinicians attempted to identify the relationship between the subluxation and known pathology. These pathologies, for the most part musculoskeletal, were identified by the clinician applying various orthopedic testing procedures to diagnose the condition. Students of chiropractic were trained to memorize a multitude of orthopedic maneuvers in the hope of learning how to diagnose various conditions.

As understanding of musculoskeletal pain syndromes has increased, and as the development of other diagnostic procedures has flourished (such as magnetic resonance imaging [MRI]), the use and reliance upon many of these procedures to reach diagnostic conclusions have been questioned. What useful information can we gain in the performance of these procedures? How many tests are worth performing, and what types of conclusions should the clinician draw from their outcomes? This chapter addresses the use (and misuse) of orthopedic testing procedures in chiropractic practice. Key concepts in the evaluation of patients with low back pain are applied; algorithms to outline an approach for clinical decision making can be found in Algorithms 1 and 2.

THE CHANGING FACE OF CLINICAL PRACTICE

Several developments over the last few decades have had a dramatic effect on the landscape of chiropractic practice. The elements making up the foundation for change are many, but perhaps none is more significant than the recent appreciation of research and critical appraisal of the clinical literature to chiropractic practice. This change may be viewed in context with the overall developments in health care research. Randomized clinical trials, rare in health care in the early 1960s, are now a cornerstone for providing evidence of efficacy of care. Metaanalysis is gaining in acceptance as another method of analyzing data from randomized trials and will provide valuable input into the development of treatment protocols. The use of expert panels to review procedures and to establish a baseline for clinical consensus has also gained in acceptance, as seen by the recent Rand studies.[1,2] The use of a consensus conference to establish guidelines for practice (eg, the Mercy Document[3]) has stimulated significant and productive dialogue in the area of practice parameters. Over the past 10 years a steady increase in the development of tools to measure functional outcomes of patients (the Roland Morris, Oswestry, and Rand SF 36) has provided practitioners with reliable methods to measure the effectiveness of various forms of care.[4] All these processes are based on the need to objectively assess which procedures are good for patients.

Changes in chiropractic education can also be seen over the past 20 years. There is an increased understanding and appreciation of the type of knowledge required to guide clinical practice in the future. Previously, emphasis was placed on generating an understanding of basic mechanisms of disease and pathology, passing on the unsystematic observations of experienced clinicians, and developing an appreciation of the art and philosophy of chiropractic. With these

Adapted from *Top Clin Chiro* 1994; 1(1): 42–50
© 1994 Aspen Publishers, Inc.

skills, the clinician was thought to have sufficient ability to evaluate new tests and treatments and to generate adequate guidelines for clinical practice. Emphasis was placed on the handing down of experiences and the relaying of values regarding testing and treatment procedures. Today, with large amounts of clinical information more readily available, new skills are required. Clinical judgment can no longer be generated from single events. Documenting, measuring, and systematically observing clinical events are now crucial abilities of the competent clinician. The ability to read the relevant literature and to understand basic rules of interpretation is also important if one is to make clinical decisions regarding the utility of testing procedures and the efficacy of treatment protocols. Clinicians today must put far less value on authority and far greater value on developing the skills needed to make reasoned assessments of clinical evidence.

AN APPROACH TO DATA COLLECTION AND INTERPRETATION

The use of diagnostic terminology to describe the origin of low back pain may help the clinician improve treatment protocols and better predict prognosis, but it may have little or no relationship to any actual pathology.[5] The clinician is often compelled to place all patients into a classification pattern of syndromes, yet this can be dangerous. Although some patients present with similar signs and symptoms and appear to be easily diagnosed, experience allows the clinician to recognize subtle differences in pattern. Diagnosis and classification should be approached with caution. Rather than expanding knowledge and modifying protocols, the clinician may find himself or herself using a few favorite historic questions and examination procedures that are unreliable. This may bias clinical judgment and limit clinical effectiveness.

All clinicians need to be efficient, seeking to gain the maximum amount of reliable information in an appropriate period of time. The reliability of a given diagnostic test needs to be known for the physician to apply it in a meaningful fashion. Without acceptable reliability, a test may give illusory information and compound confusion. Although reliability measurements provide the clinician with an indication of a test's reproducibility, measures of validity can help determine whether the test or procedure is actually measuring what it is proported to measure. Many common procedures in both medical and chiropractic practice remain untested in terms of their validity and reliability. An understanding of any procedure's limitations will assist the clinician in the interpretation of its results.

The clinician should standardize and organize his or her thought process. In this way clinical patterns are more readily identified, and efficiency is increased. Clinical algorithms can help organize and direct clinical problem solving. Webster's defines an algorithm as a set of rules for solving a particular problem within a finite number of steps. Algorithms can be used to help develop a systematic approach to patients presenting with various types of complaints. Algorithms 1 and 2 present assessment of low back pain patients. The reader is encouraged to modify, update, and develop other clinical algorithms to assist in evaluating other specific conditions.

DETERMINING THE SOURCES OF LOW BACK PAIN

Low back pain is the most common complaint presenting to the doctor of chiropractic. It is estimated that 70% of all adults will be affected by low back pain during some part of their lives but that only 14% will have episodes that last more than 2 weeks. About 1.5% have episodes where sciatica is a major component of the complaint.[5,6] The proportion of low back pain attributable specifically to prolapsed lumbar intervertebral discs is unknown. Various data do suggest a large burden to society from lumbar disc prolapse, particularly in people with back pain of long duration. Based on studies, it is estimated that between 1 and 5 persons per 1,000 population per year in the age range of 20 to 64 years develop new lumbar disc prolapse,[7] yet the proportion of all persons with low back pain who undergo surgery for disc lesion is about 2%.[5] In primary care, about 4% of patients who report with back pain will have compression fractures, 3% will have spondylolisthesis, and 0.3% will have ankylosing spondylitis (AS). Spinal stenosis has only been recognized as a unique clinical entity over the past 15 years. It is most common in adults, but its prevalence is unknown.[8]

Several texts dedicated to orthopedic testing procedures and methods of examination exist. Although these present an array of testing procedures, little information is provided about the reliability or validity of the procedures. In his text on orthopedic testing, Cipriano[9] recommends an approach to the orthopedic evaluation of low back pain. Beginning with range of motion and spinal percussion, the system outlines procedures to identify the presence of a radicular component. Twenty named orthopedic testing procedures are presented for the low back, the majority of which are provocative for sciatic nerve involvement or a space-occupying lesion. In their new text on orthopedic testing, Gerard and Kleinfield[10] present 52 named orthopedic testing procedures for the lumbar spine with an additional 15 for the sacroiliac joint. Algorithms are presented for patients presenting with lumbar spine and sacroiliac pain (assuming that historic information would allow one to differentiate between these conditions) without any reference to the relative reliability of the procedures. For example, the jar drop test is considered pivotal in leading to the discovery of visceral conditions referring pain to the low back. The foundation and relative reliability of the examination is not given, and the clinician may overinterpret the relative significance of a positive or negative finding. Although these approaches represent an important effort to organize clinical reasoning, they also point out the potential for overreliance upon procedures that may be limited in their reproducibility (reliability).

RULING OUT TUMORS, INFECTIONS, AND VISCERAL REFERRAL IN PATIENTS WITH LOW BACK PAIN

The clinician must rule out the potential of malignant, infectious, and visceral diseases before proceeding to search out possible origins of muscular, ligamentous, or mechanical pain. Algorithm 1 summarizes an approach to ruling out these sources of low back pain.

Cauda equina is a rare condition that represents the only surgical emergency of the low back.[11] Pressure on the caudal sac may cause bilateral sciatica, saddle anesthesia, and bladder and bowel incontinence in addition to low back pain. Deyo et al[8] report that the most consistent finding is urinary retention with a sensitivity of 0.90. Assuming a specificity of about 95%, the predictive value of a negative test (no urinary retention) would be almost 0.99. Therefore, a patient without urinary retention, or incontinence, is unlikely to have this condition. Deyo et al[8] also report a relatively high sensitivity for sciatic leg pain, a positive straight-leg raise (SLR) test, sensory and motor deficits, and saddle anesthesia in patients with cauda equina. Although immediate surgical decompression is recommended to stop progression of neurologic symptoms, the potential for reversal of neurologic loss is slight.

Less than 1% of all low back pain is caused by cancer. Primary neoplasms (such as multiple myeloma) of the spine are rare and account for less than 10% of all bone tumors. Metastatic lesions make up the majority of the tumors, especially in the older population. Approximately 80% of patients with metastatic lesions are over the age of 50. In addition to characteristic low back pain, Weinstein and McLain[12] found a relatively high incidence of neurologic abnormalities. They recommended that any patient with a neurologic deficit and back pain receive a careful radiographic evaluation before the diagnosis of herniated nucleus pulposus is established. In their series, 99% of all tumors could be identified on the initial radiographs obtained. Deyo et al[8] report that a previous history of cancer has such high specificity (0.98) that patients with a positive history should be considered to have cancer until proven otherwise. Other common symptoms include unexplained weight loss, pain duration of greater than 1 month, and failure to improve with conservative care. All are moderately specific. Most patients report pain that does not improve with bed rest. This finding is highly sensitive; a negative response most probably rules out the condition's existence, but it also can be found in many other conditions and is therefore not specific.[13] The physical examination is less useful in the early detection of systemic causes of low back pain. In a study of 2,000 walk-in clinic patients, Deyo[14] found that every patient with cancer had at least one of the following four clinical findings: age greater than 50, history of cancer, unexplained weight loss, and failure to improve with conservative therapy. No physical examination findings were significantly more common among patients with an underlying malignancy than those without.

Infections of the lumbar spine are an uncommon source of low back pain. The primary signs and symptoms vary and depend on the causative organism. Bacterial infections are more aggressive and can cause acute toxic symptoms; fungal and tuberculous infections are often silent and slowly progressive. Approximately 40% of patients with vertebral osteomyelitis have an unequivocal extraspinal source of infection. The usual locations are the genitourinary tract, skin, and respiratory tract.[15] Intravenous drug abusers, elderly patients, and patients with compromised immune systems are at risk. Patients will have low back pain that may be intermittent or constant, may be present at rest, and may radiate into the hip and cause a decreased range of motion. Laboratory findings may include elevated erythrocyte sedimentation rate (ESR), positive blood cultures, or a positive tuberculin test. Radiographic findings often lag behind clinical symptoms, sometimes by as much as 2 months. Bone scans will demonstrate abnormalities much earlier, and MRI has greater sensitivity than either plain films or computed tomography.[16] Spine tenderness to percussion has a sensitivity of 0.86 for bacterial infection, but specificity is poor (again, it is found in many conditions).[8]

It is beyond the scope of this article to attempt an extensive review of the causes of low back pain referred from visceral pathology. Disorders of the vascular, genitourinary, and gastrointestinal systems can cause stimulation of sensory nerves with resultant perception of pain by the patient in both the primary area and the corresponding spinal levels of the low back. Such referred pain is often sharp and well localized and may be associated with reflex muscle contraction and hyperalgesia.[16]

EVALUATION OF MECHANICAL BACK PAIN

The algorithm provided in Algorithm 2 reviews the musculoskeletal, ligamentous, and nonorganic sources of low back pain. This algorithm illustrates a method for a systematic evaluation of patients with low back pain that has already been determined to have a mechanical origin. This approach seeks to identify patterns of signs and symptoms and examinations that may help the clinician in developing a consistent approach to reaching a diagnostic conclusion. The validity of this seed algorithm remains to be tested, but the importance in having a systematic, consistent approach cannot be overstated.

SCIATIC LEG PAIN

The clinical finding of sciatica is highly sensitive in screening for patients with lumbar disc herniation. Therefore, the likelihood of a clinically significant disc lesion being found in a patient without sciatica is remote (1 in 1,000).[8] Most patients with disc lesions have a history of chronic intermittent back pain. There are usually several previous attacks of back pain without leg pain, but no common characteristics in these episodes of back pain have been found.[17] The pain is often characterized as a sharp, burning pain that overshadows the patient's back pain. It traverses the posterior or lateral leg and is often accompanied by paresthesia or numbness of the distal aspect of the L-5 or S-1 nerve root. The patient's pain is often aggravated by coughing, sneezing, or straining at stool (Dejerine's triad).

Examination of patients with sciatic neuropathy relies mostly upon the findings of the SLR and crossed straight-leg raise, often called the well-leg raise (WLR). The angle of the hip at the time of pain reproduction is important. A finding between 15° and 30° is considered reliable for the presence of disc herniation. A finding after 60° is thought to be clinically insignificant. Kosteljanetz and colleagues[18] found that, although there was variation, the variations were usually less than 10°. The WLR test is less sensitive than the SLR, but it is highly specific.[8] One can therefore assume that a patient with a positive WLR has a disc lesion. In the important study by McCombe et al,[19] which evaluated the reliability of various testing procedures, the WLR and SLR tests were found to be potentially reliable for reproducing patient symptoms. The SLR reproducing back and leg pain was found to be reliable. If the foot is dorsiflexed during the SLR, true sciatic pain will radiate below the knee at a lesser angle. The bowstring test or sign is potentially reliable for reproduction of leg pain.

In that 98% of all disc lesions occur at the L4-5 or L5-S1 disc spaces,[7] neurologic impairments are most likely to affect the L-5 or S-1 nerve roots. The most common neurologic deficits elicited are from the Achilles reflex. Motor examination should include ankle dorsiflexion, great toe extension, and plantar flexion of the foot. Hamstring or hip extension strength also may be checked. A loss of pain sensation is most commonly found at the distal portion of the nerve roots, the dorsum, and the lateral portion of the foot. McCombe et al[19] found that buttock wasting, toe standing, and heel standing were unreliable signs. They also found poor agreement for patellar reflexes, but the Achilles reflex was potentially reliable. All tests for muscle wasting and weakness were also found to be potentially reliable. Examination for sensory deficit is reliable.[19] Weakness in ankle dorsiflexion rarely occurs alone and is commonly found with weakness in great toe extension or sensory deficits.[20]

Two percent of lumbar disc lesions arise from higher lumbar nerve roots. This should be suspected in any patient with back pain and anterior hip or thigh numbness that is more prominent than calf symptoms. Testing includes the femoral nerve stretch (found to be potentially reliable[19]) with patellar reflexes and motor testing of the quadriceps and psoas muscles. Sensory examination includes the anterior and lateral upper leg and medial foot. The overall accuracy of neurologic findings for the diagnosis of disc lesion is moderate. Considering combinations, a finding of decreased ankle reflexes with weak foot dorsiflexion would have a sensitivity of almost 90% for patients with surgically proven disc herniations.[8]

Combinations of a positive SLR with neurologic findings will increase the probability that a disc lesion will be found at surgery.[21] In a recent study by Bush et al,[22] 86% of patients with clinical sciatica and radiologic evidence of nerve root entrapment were treated successfully by aggressive conservative management (including epidural injections). This corresponds to the reported finding of Weber[23] and Saal et al.[24] Bush et al[22] also noted a strong correlation between the clinical findings and the radiologic evidence of nerve root compression. A striking clinical feature of this study was the high percentage of disc lesions that showed partial or complete resolution within 1 year. The investigators note that this would seem to support the suggestion made by Cyriax[25] and suspicion by others that herniated nuclear material is subjected to gradual enzymatic degradation and shrivels up over time.

Piriformis syndrome is thought to cause sciatic neuritis secondary to entrapment and irritation as the nerve traverses under the muscle. Symptoms are usually characterized by minimal back pain (if any) and significant pain in the gluteal region. The patient's sciatic neuropathy can usually be reproduced by the SLR. Internal rotation of the leg during the SLR is thought to bowstring the muscle over the nerve and to cause a reproduction of leg pain at a lower angle. Resisted hip external rotation is thought to compress the muscle over the nerve. McCombe et al[19] found this procedure to be potentially reliable. No neurologic deficits are usually found with this condition. Diagnosis is often accomplished by palpation of myofascial trigger points over the muscle, but one must always be aware that lumbar disc lesions and piriformis syndrome are frequently concurrent disorders.[26]

Spinal stenosis has only been recognized as a significant clinical entity for the last 15 years. It often causes unilateral or bilateral pain that does not follow a specific dermatome pattern. It is classically found in patients over the age of 55 with a chronic history of low back pain. Patients also may exhibit symptoms of claudication. Neurogenic claudication is characterized by symptoms of increasing leg pain upon standing in one spot or ambulating that is relieved within 15 to 20 minutes of rest. The rapid relief of symptoms with rest and the palpation of abnormal arterial pulses found in vascular claudication help differentiate it from neurogenic claudication. The cycling and walking tests are often cited as methods to differentiate between neurogenic and vascular claudication. By using forward flexion to increase space in the intervertebral foramen and canal, the patient should be able to walk and cycle farther if he or she has neurogenic claudication. A small study by Dong and Porter[27] of 19 patients with neurogenic claudication and 11 with intermittent claudication found cycling and walking to be insensitive tests to distinguish between neurogenic and intermittent claudication. Neurogenic claudication is a mildly common symptom of canal stenosis (sensitivity of 0.60),[28] but when found it is probably strongly specific for the presence of stenosis.

DIAGNOSING LOW BACK PAIN WITH REFERRED LEG PAIN

Facet syndrome is often referred to as a distinct clinical entity, but studies of direct injections into this joint under fluoroscopy have yielded mixed results. Mooney[29] reports injecting saline solution into the facet joints of individuals. The onset of pain was usually within seconds and was relieved immediately by injection of local anesthetic. Clinically, Mooney found pain reproduced in the back, buttock, and leg. He also found that the facet joint could be the source of pain in a wide array of clinical settings, even causing calf pain and diminished reflexes in a few individuals. McCombe et al[19] found that the often referred to extension catch showed doubtful reproducibility. Mooney[29] in part concludes that in individuals with back and leg pain without radiculopathy one is justified in making the potential diagnosis of facet syndrome.

With the mixed clinical results found in the application of facet injections, a few investigators have tried to create more selective criteria the better to identify patients with purely facet-initiated pain. Lippitt[30] proposed a clinical syndrome that, based primarily on intuitive concepts, suggests facet syndrome. The criteria included symptoms of low back pain, hip and buttock pain, cramping leg pain above the knee, low back stiffness especially in the morning, and absence of dysesthesia in the limbs. Using these criteria, 66% of patients responded at all to injection. Helbig and Casey,[31] in a further attempt to formulate criteria for accurate diagnosis of facet syndrome in the lumbar spine, developed the following scoring system: back pain associated with groin or thigh pain, 30 points; well-localized paraspinal tenderness, 20 points; reproduction of pain with extension-rotation (Kemp's), 30 points; corresponding radiographic changes, 20 points; and pain below the knee, –10 points. Of the 22 patients examined, all with a score of 60 points or more had a prolonged positive response to facet joint injection. Seven of 9 patients with scores of 40 points or more had a prolonged response, but 4 patients with scores below 40 points also had a prolonged response.

These studies suggest that facet syndrome does not cause a pain pattern that is discernible enough to be of any diagnostic value. A major problem in identifying the potential benefits of any form of treatment for facet syndrome is the lack of methods to establish a definitive diagnosis. None of the studies reviewed identified one clinical finding that alone was discriminative for the diagnosis. It appears that the clinician must develop a clinical approach to facet syndrome that looks for a combination of clinical findings suggesting the diagnosis. In this way, therapeutic trials will be more likely to provide the clinician with valuable predictive and prognostic views of the patient's clinical picture.

Sacroiliac syndrome is a commonly referred to clinical entity with a poorly defined set of clinical findings. As with many other causes of mechanical low back pain, the pathology of the condition is poorly understood. Although some clinicians in the medical field have denied that the joint has any role in the production of low back pain, others believe that this joint may be responsible for a large number of patients presenting with low back pain. In a retrospective study by Bernard and Kirkaldy-Willis,[32] 23% of patients presenting to their clinic over a 12-year period were given this diagnosis.

Cassidy and Mierau[33] describe the classic patient as presenting with low back pain that may or may not radiate into the leg. Pain is often localized over the posterosuperior iliac spine and buttock. It may refer into the groin and lower extremity in a nondermatome pattern. Pain on walking referring to the hip and knee may cause some diagnostic confusion, and such patients should receive appropriate examination of both areas. There is evidence that the problem is more common in women, especially during pregnancy and lactation because of hormonal influences during these periods. On examination, Cassidy and Mierau report, unilateral lumbar paraspinal muscle spasms and gluteal trigger points are often present. SLR may be reduced by associated back pain and hamstring tightness. Signs of nerve root tension and neurologic deficit do not occur. Although the patient may complain of paresthesias of the lower limb, sensory evaluation is usually normal.

A number of clinical tests are described in orthopedic texts.[9,10] Cassidy and Mierau[33] list Gaenslen's, Faber-Patrick, and the extension test as being most useful and report that two of three of these procedures are found to be positive in most cases of sacroiliac syndrome. In that these tests (along with Yeoman's test) place stress on the sacroiliac joint through leverage applied to the hip, it is important to screen the patient for possible hip joint pathology before interpreting the findings. Potter and Rothstein[34] found good to moderate intertester reliability for the sacroiliac stress test (iliac gapping) and the iliac compression test. Laslett and Williams[35] report that the pain provocation tests of distraction (sacroiliac stretch test), compression (iliac compression or pelvic rock test), and pelvic torsion (Gaenslen's) were all found to be moderately reliable or better.

The most commonly used test to check for sacroiliac joint mobility is the Gillet or step test. Herzog et al[36] found this test to be reliable and concluded that their results indicated some evidence that the procedure may help a trained chiropractor arrive at the same diagnostic conclusions for the same problem. Most procedures seeking to identify motion dysfunction in the sacroiliac joint have yet to demonstrate validity, and the clinician must be careful of overinterpretation. For decades chiropractic clinicians have applied spinal manipulative therapy to the sacroiliac joints to remove joint dysfunction. Clinical experience has usually been that patients respond favorably to this form of treatment for various types of low back pain. The chiropractic clinician should establish a protocol that includes several provocative tests to determine the possible source of low back pain. In conjunction, the clinician should use various procedures to reach a working impression regarding sacroiliac mobility, the Gillet test being the most common, to identify the appropriateness of spinal manipulative therapy.

DIAGNOSING MUSCLE PAIN

Pain originating from the musculature of the low back may account for a significant percentage of low back pain in patients. Graded as mild, moderate, or severe, these conditions are usually accompanied by a patient history indicating an overload, overwork, or overstretching of the musculature. Pain may be localized or may radiate in characteristic pain patterns, as seen in myofascial trigger points. Examination of these patients relies upon palpation in combination with active, passive, and resistive ranges of motion. The classic characteristic is pain found on active motion, relieved by passive motion, and made worse by resistive motion. McCombe et al[19] found palpation for paravertebral and buttock tenderness to be unreliable, but it was recommended that, being more specific when describing palpatory pain, it would help increase reliability.

Myofascial trigger points are reportedly found in an estimated 12% to 30% of the general population.[37] Usually a regional problem, the condition is characterized by local zones of pain in the belly of the muscle. Pain can be referred in characteristic referred patterns. Palpable pain with the characteristic jump sign and a response to physical methods such as spray and stretch are hallmarks of the examination. Localized pain, absence of fatigue, and lack of pain at the muscle-tendon junction usually help differentiate this condition from fibromyalgia.[38] As previously noted, myofascial trigger points are often found concurrently with other conditions such as disc lesions, and the clinician needs to ensure that other sources of primary pathology have been ruled out.

In 1990 the American College of Rheumatology established criteria for the classification of fibromyalgia (often termed fibrositis or myofibrositis). These include the findings of pain on both sides of the body and above and below the waist, pain in the axial spine, and pain on digital palpation in 11 of 18 prescribed tender point sites.[39] Reports on the presence of fibromyalgia in rheumatology clinics have varied from 5% to 20% and in general medical clinics from 3% to 5%.[36] This condition is characteristically chronic and should be considered in patients with diffuse areas of heightened tenderness of greater than 3 months' duration. Patients often complain of fatigue and stiffness and may have specific sleep disturbances. Research indicates that a relationship between chronic fatigue syndrome and fibromyalgia exists. In one study, 70% of patients with chronic fatigue syndrome met the criteria for fibromyalgia.[36] Although debate exists about the etiology of fibromyalgia and chronic fatigue syndrome, an increase in the number of investigations in the last 2 years continues to provide further understanding of the relationship of these conditions. The clinician needs to be aware of the current diagnostic criteria to judge best the effectiveness of therapeutic trials in clinical practice.

RULING OUT RHEUMATIC CONDITIONS

Patients with spondyloarthropathy often present with significant morning pain and stiffness. Although it is not unusual to encounter patients with this symptom, patients with inflammatory arthropathies experience a significant amount of pain or stiffness that takes a period of a few hours of activity to relieve. They also often experience night pain and some relief of stiffness with exercise. One would expect these symptoms to be relatively sensitive but nonspecific. The Schober test is commonly described as an effective method for measuring lumbar flexion. McCombe et al[19] found this procedure to be reliable, but a positive finding is nonspecific in that it is found in many low back conditions. Inflammatory arthropathies are rare, and attempts at developing screening procedures for them have yielded poor results. These conditions are most often not diagnosed at the initial patient presentation and usually are identified after a failure to respond to an initial trial of conservative therapy.

To aid in diagnosis, the clinician should look for patterns of common symptoms of these conditions. Clinical features of AS include patients with chronic low back pain that started before the age of 40, which often exacerbates and remits, and has stiffness progressing up the spine. Decreased chest expansion may be seen. Although decreased chest expansion is reported to be highly specific, it is not sensitive in early cases of AS.[39] Reiter's syndrome is found more commonly in young men and primarily affects the low back and lower extremities. The syndrome consists of symptoms of conjunctivitis, urethritis, and arthritis. The urethritis is usually a mild mucopurulent discharge with dysuria in men and asymptomatic vaginitis in women. The conjunctivitis consists of redness and crusting of the eyelids. Arthritis will usually occur 1 to 3 weeks after the initial infection and is characterized by asymmetric involvement of the knees, ankles, feet, or sacroiliac joints. Involvement of the sacroiliac joint is the most common cause of back pain.[15]

Besides physical examination, an ESR and radiographs are appropriate in the evaluation of these patients. Increased ESR is common, especially during active inflammatory phases. The HLA-B27 is not diagnostic of AS. The B27 antigen is found in a majority of white AS patients, but it can be absent in nonwhite individuals. Also, a number of HLA-positive patients will never develop AS. One must be aware that HLA-B27 is found in other inflammatory arthropathies as well. There is a striking association between HLA-B27 and Reiter's syndrome, and it is found in 80% of patients with sacroiliitis and spondylitis associated with psoriatic spondyloarthropathy. It is also found in 53% of patients with Crohn's disease-associated spondylitis.[40]

THE APPROACH TO PATIENTS WITH POSSIBLE SOMATIZATION DISORDERS

Concern must be shown by the clinician for patients with chronic pain. Patients who have faced unemployment, family issues, financial stress, and changes in social aspects of their lives may have resultant somatic amplification of their symptoms. The patient seeking financial gain in instances of litigation represents a challenge to the most skilled clinician. Waddell and associates[41] proposed 5 categories of inappropriate patient responses found during examination that may indicate nonorganic low back pain: distraction, stimulation, tenderness, regional disturbances, and overreaction. A positive finding in three or more categories is considered clinically significant and may indicate somatizing on the part of the patient. Waddell et al[41] reported high precision with these tests, but subsequent studies by McCombe[19] and Fishbain[42] and their colleagues indicate poor precision in the regional disturbance category.

Distraction may be accomplished by applying variations on ankle dorsiflexion and plantar flexion during the SLR. The same types of maneuvers also may be performed in the sitting position. The patient providing unexpected responses (flip test) would indicate a positive test in the distraction category. Simulation tests are used to give the patient the sense that a particular procedure is being carried out when in fact it is not. Axial loading, rotation, and O'Donoghue's lumbar maneuver are examples of this. These tests are positive if the patient reports low back pain on axial loading or demonstrates increased pain on passive motion. Nonorganic tenderness may be superficial, the skin being tender to a light pinch over a wide area of the lumbar spine, or nonanatomic, where deep tenderness is felt over a wide area and is not localized to one structure. Regional disturbances involve weakness or sensory disturbances that are found over a widespread region of neighboring parts, such as the leg below the knee, the entire leg, or a quarter of the body. Overreaction signs may take the form of disproportionate verbalization, facial expression, muscle tension and tremor, collapsing, or sweating. Other orthopedic tests such as Libman's and Mankof's may provide additional information in evaluation of the potential nonorganic pain patient. Before one reaches a conclusion of malingering, a complete review of records along with a complete physical examination must be undertaken. Although it may be tempting to categorize the patient as malingering (a nonpsychologic disorder), care must be taken to understand the complex picture that may exist in patients with true psychologic difficulties. A further detailed picture of the somatic patient is provided by Milus.[43]

The objective pain patient, as described by Hendler,[44] has good premorbid (prepain) adjustment, normal response to chronic pain relative to the length of time that the pain has been present, and a definable organic lesion (objective findings). In contrast, the undetermined pain patient has good premorbid adjustment, a normal response to chronic pain, and an absence of objective physical findings. This patient requires careful study by a multidisciplinary team of clinicians to reach appropriate diagnostic and case management decisions.

CONCLUSIONS

Nelson and colleagues[45] in 1979 reflected upon the difficult situation the clinician faces in the evaluation of patients with low back pain. They concluded that the examination should be limited and carefully refined to minimize the introduction of items that are in fact associated with a high observer error. The clinician can collect vast amounts of information from a large number of named orthopedic testing procedures as long as he or she is willing to appreciate that much of it will be unreliable. On the other hand, the clinician may focus attention to a limited number of questions and procedures to increase the reliability of information obtained. In this way the clinician will more likely be a self-learner, expanding and improving on his or her ability to provide quality patient care.

Although the algorithms presented attempt to be comprehensive, they may not be applicable to all possible patient situations. They represent an example of one method of clinical reasoning and organization. Clinicians need to update their practices of examination as new information becomes available, and they must be willing to modify their procedures as the patient's condition warrants. The problem-solving axiom of Cutler[46] should be kept in mind: (1) Common conditions present commonly, (2) uncommon presentations of common conditions are still more common than common presentations of uncommon conditions, and (3) no condition is rare to the person who has it.

REFERENCES

1. Shekelle PG, Adams AH, Chassin MR, et al. *The Appropriateness of Spinal Manipulation for Low-Back Pain, Indications and Ratings by a Multidisciplinary Expert Panel*. Santa Monica, CA: Rand; 1991.
2. Shekelle PG, Adams AH, Chassin MR, et al. *The Appropriateness of Spinal Manipulation for Low-Back Pain, Indications and Ratings by an All-Chiropractic Expert Panel*. Santa Monica, CA: Rand; 1992.
3. Haldeman S, Chapman-Smith D, Petersen DM. *Guidelines for Chiropractic Quality Assurance and Practice Parameters*. Gaithersburg, MD: Aspen Publishers: 1993.
4. Deyo RA. Measuring the functional status of patients with low back pain. *Arch Phys Med Rehabil*. 1988;69:1,044–1,053.
5. Deyo RA, Tsui-Wu JY. Descriptive epidemiology of low-back pain and its related medical care in the United States. *Spine*. 1987;12:264–268.
6. Deyo RA, Loeser JD, Bigos SF. Herniated lumbar intervertebral disk. *Ann Intern Med*. 1990;112:598–603.
7. Kelsey JL, Golden AL, Mundt DJ. Low back pain/prolapsed lumbar intervertebral disc. *Rheum Dis Clin North Am*. 1990;16:699–712.
8. Deyo RA, Rainville J, Daniel KL. What can the history and physical examination tell us about low back pain? *JAMA*. 1992;268:760–765.
9. Cipriano JJ. *Photographic Manual of Regional Orthopaedic and Neurological Tests*. Baltimore, MD: Williams & Wilkins; 1991.
10. Gerard JA, Kleinfield SL. *Orthopaedic Testing—A Rational Approach to Diagnosis*. New York, NY: Churchill Livingstone; 1993.
11. Floman Y, Wiesel SW, Rothman RH. Cauda equina presenting as a herniated lumbar disk. *Clin Orthop*. 1980;147:234–237.
12. Weinstein JN, McLain F. Primary tumors of the spine. *Spine*. 1987;12:843–851.
13. Deyo RA, Diehl AK. Cancer as a cause of back pain: frequency, clinical presentation, and diagnostic strategies. *J Gen Intern Med*. 1988;3:230–238.
14. Deyo RA. Early detection of cancer, infection, and inflammatory disease of the spine. *J Back Musculoskeletal Rehabil*. 1991;1:69–81.
15. Waldvogel FA, Vasey H. Osteomyelitis: the past decade. *N Engl J Med*. 1980;303:360–370.
16. McCowin PR, Borenstein D, Wiesel SW. The current approach to the medical diagnosis of low back pain. *Orthop Clin North Am*. 1991;22:315–325.
17. Weber H. Natural history of the herniated disc. In: Winstein J, Wiesel S, eds. *The Lumbar Spine*. Philadelphia, PA: Saunders; 1990.
18. Kosteljanetz M, Flemming B, Schmidt-Olsen S. The clinical significance of straight-leg raising in the diagnosis of prolapsed lumbar disc. *Spine*. 1988;13:393–395.
19. McCombe PF, Fairbank JCT, Cockersole BC, Pynsent PB. Reproducibility of physical signs in low-back pain. *Spine*. 1989;14:908–918.
20. Blower PW. Neurologic patterns in unilateral sciatica. *Spine*. 1981;6:175–179.
21. Morris EW, DiPaola M, Vallance R, Waddell G. Diagnosis and decision making in lumbar disc prolapse and nerve entrapment. *Spine*. 1986;11:436–439.
22. Bush K, Cowan N, Katz DE, Gishen P. The natural history of sciatica associated with disk pathology. *Spine*. 1992;17:1,205–1,212.
23. Weber H. Lumbar disc herniation: a controlled prospective study with ten years of observation. *Spine*. 1983;8:131–140.
24. Saal JA, Saal JS, Herzog HJ. The natural history of lumbar disc extrusions treated non-operatively. *Spine*. 1990;15:683–686.
25. Cyriax J. *Textbook of Orthopaedic Medicine*. London, England: Bailliere Tindall; 1984;1.
26. Steiner C, Staubs C, Ganon M, Buhlinger C. Piriformis syndrome: pathogenesis, diagnosis and treatment. *J Am Osteopathic Assoc*. 1987:318–323.
27. Dong GX, Porter RW. Walking and cycling tests in neurogenic and intermittent claudication. *Spine*. 1989;14:965–969.
28. Turner JA, Ersek M, Herron L, Deyo R. Surgery for lumbar spinal stenosis: attempted meta-analysis of the literature. *Spine*. 1992;17:1–8.
29. Mooney V. Facet syndrome. In: Winstein J, Wiesel S, eds. *The Lumbar Spine*. Philadelphia, PA: Saunders; 1990.
30. Lippitt AB. The facet joint and its role in spinal pain: management with facet joint injections. *Spine*. 1984;9:746–750.
31. Helbig T, Casey KL. The lumbar facet syndrome. *Spine*. 1988;13:61–64.
32. Bernard TN, Kirkaldy-Willis WH. Non-specific low back pain. *Clin Orthop*. 1987;217:266–272.
33. Cassidy JD, Mierau DR. Pathophysiology of the sacroiliac joint. In: Haldeman S, ed. *Principles and Practice of Chiropractic*. East Norwalk, CT: Appleton & Lange; 1992.
34. Potter NA, Rothstein JM. Intertester reliability for selected clinical tests of the sacroiliac joint. *Phys Ther*. 1985;65:1,671–1,675.
35. Laslett M, Williams M. The reliability of selected pain provocation tests for sacroiliac joint pathology. In: Vleeming A, Mooney V, Snijders C, Dorman T, eds. *First Interdisciplinary World Congress on Low Back Pain and Its Relationship to the Sacroiliac Joint*. San Diego, CA: Rotterdam: ECO;1992.
36. Herzog W, Read LJ, Conway JW, Shaw LD, McEwen C. Reliability of motion palpation procedures to detect sacroiliac joint fixations. *J Manip Physiol Ther*. 1989;12:86–92.
37. Goldenberg DL. Fibromyalgia, chronic fatigue syndrome, and myofascial pain syndrome. *Curr Opin Rheumatol*. 1991;3:247–258.
38. Bennet J. Beyond fibromyalgia: ideas on etiology and treatment. *J Rheumatol*. 1989;16(suppl 9):185–191.
39. Wolfe F, Smythe HA, Yunus MB, et al. The American College of Rheumatology 1990 criteria for the classification of fibromyalgia. *Arthritis Rheum*. 1990;33:160–172.
40. Benoist M, Jayson MI. Inflammatory disorders. In: Winstein J, Wiesel S, eds. *The Lumbar Spine*. Philadelphia, PA: Saunders; 1990.
41. Waddell G, McCulloch JA, Kummel E, Venner RM. Nonorganic physical signs in low back pain. *Spine*. 1980;5:117–125.
42. Fishbain DA, Goldberg M, Rosomoff RS, Rosomoff H. Chronic pain patients and the nonorganic physical sign of nondermatomal sensory abnormalities (NDSA). *Psychosomatics*. 1991;32:294–302.
43. Milus TB. Somatization: psychologic considerations in chiropractic practice. *Topics Clin Chiro*. 1994;1(1):13–25.
44. Hendler N. *Diagnosis and Nonsurgical Management of Chronic Pain*. New York, NY: Raven; 1981.
45. Nelson MA, Allen P, Clamp SE, De Dombal FT. Reliability and reproducibility of clinical findings in low back pain. *Spine*. 1979;4:97–101.
46. Cutler P. *Problem Solving in Clinical Medicine*. Baltimore, MD: Williams & Wilkins; 1985.

Algorithm 1

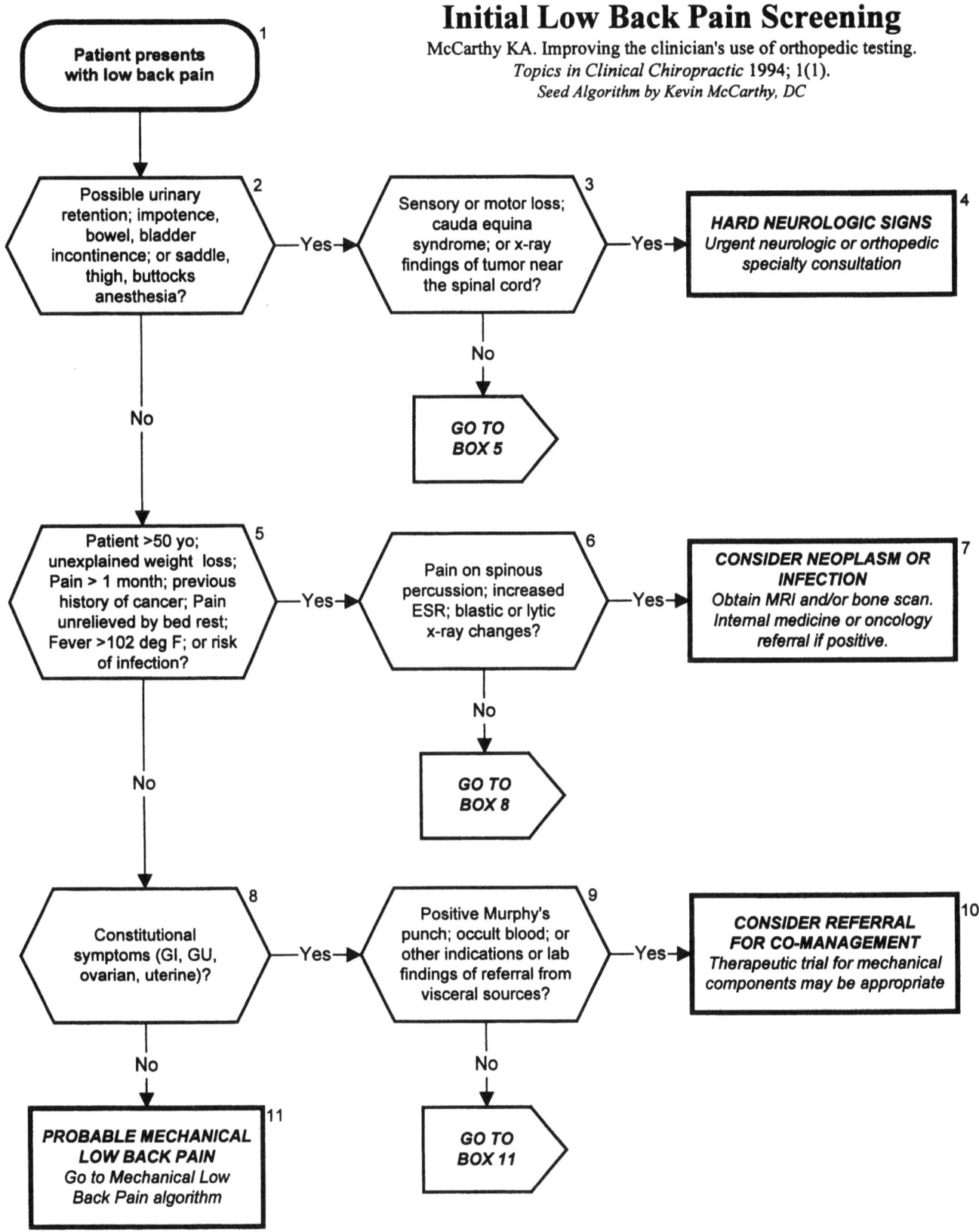

Algorithm 2

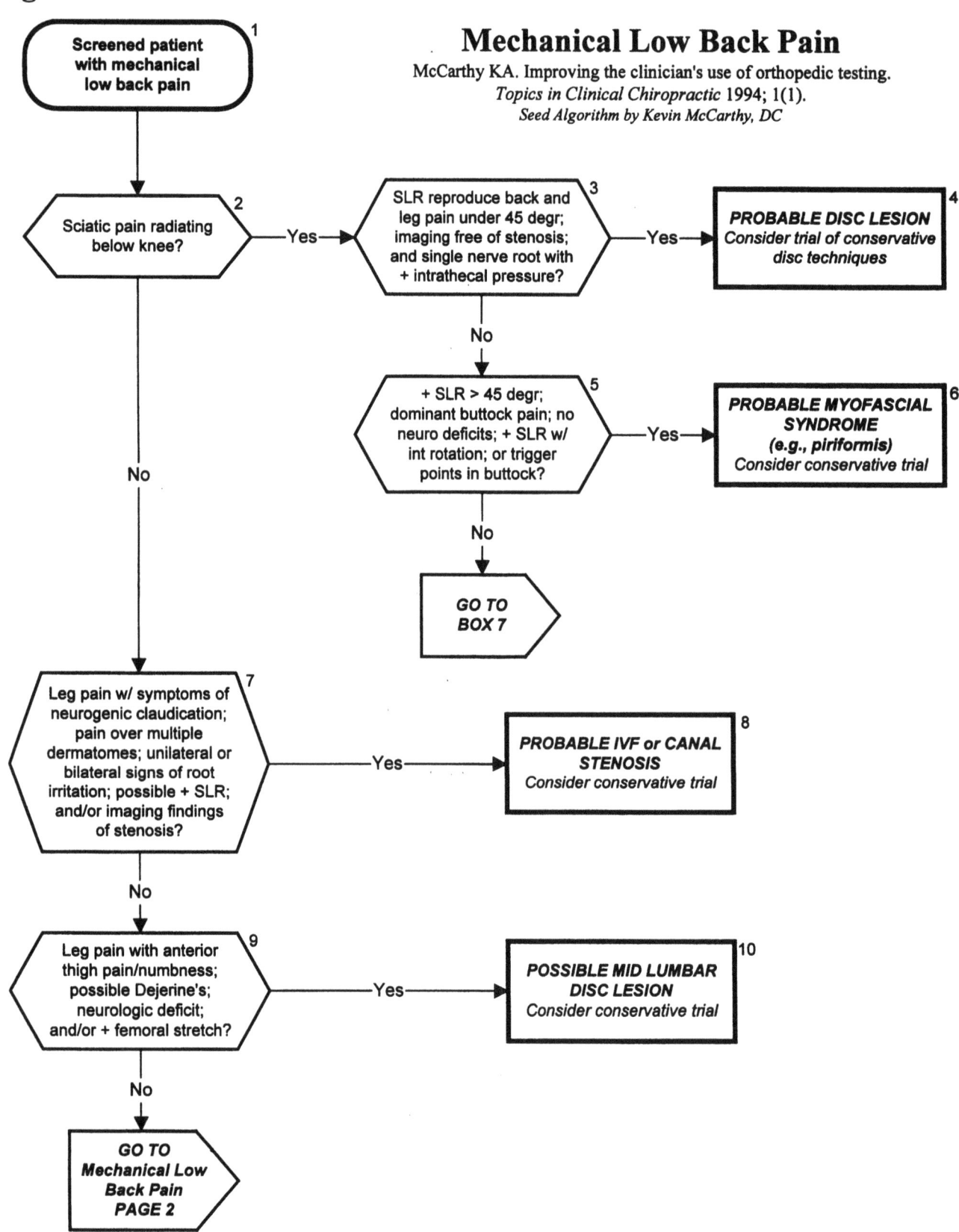

Algorithm 2, continued

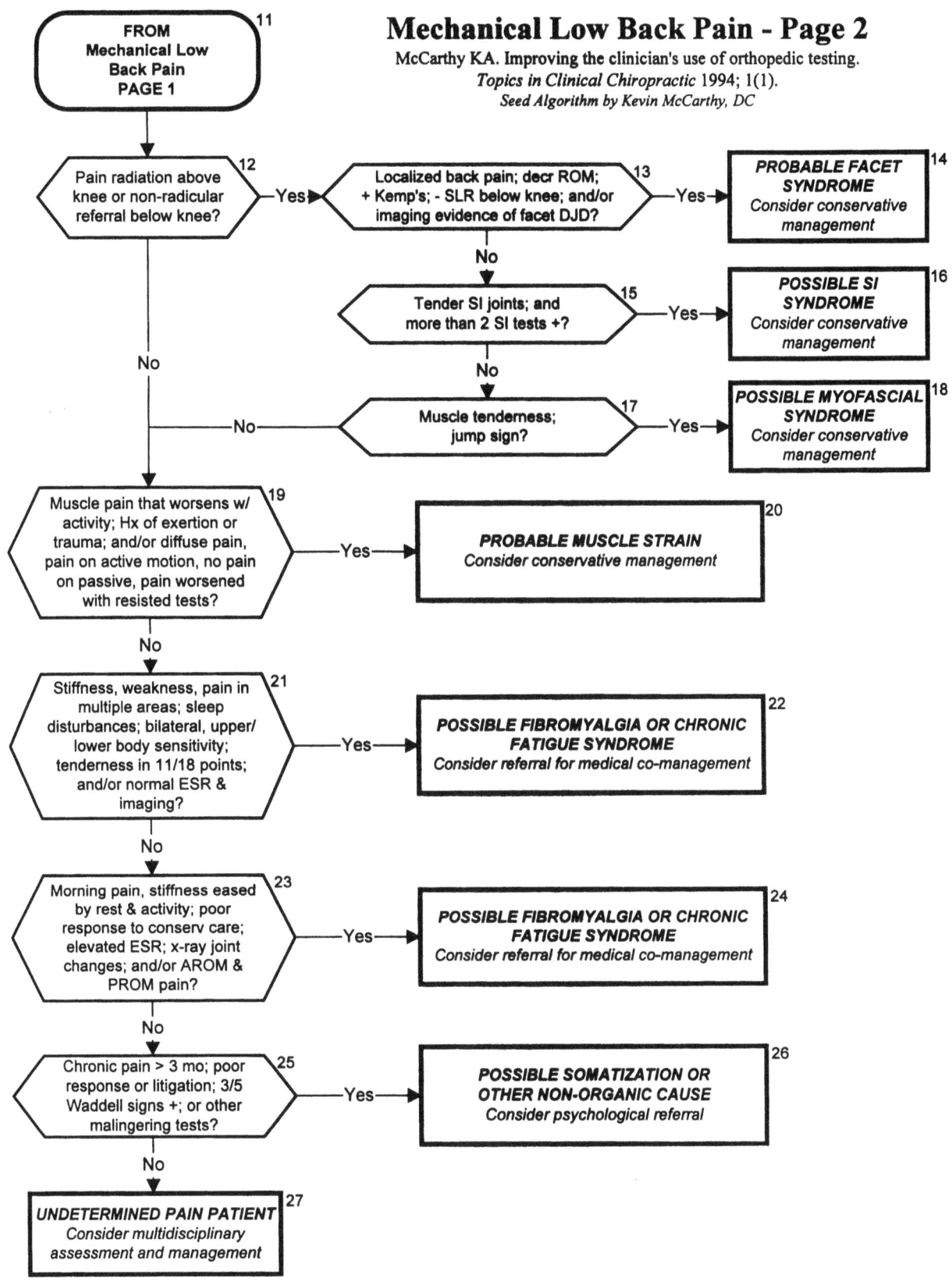

Mechanical Low Back Pain - Page 2
McCarthy KA. Improving the clinician's use of orthopedic testing.
Topics in Clinical Chiropractic 1994; 1(1).
Seed Algorithm by Kevin McCarthy, DC

6
Clinical Considerations in the Mechanical Assessment of the Cervical Spine

Austin D. McMillin

Mechanical lesions of the cervical spine appear to be common etiologies for many presenting complaints in clinical chiropractic settings. Symptoms associated with cervical mechanical dysfunction vary widely and may include local pain, extracervical pain, headache, vertigo, functional limitations, and upper extremity symptoms. Appropriate investigation of cervical complaints requires an awareness of organic pathologic factors that may mimic mechanical symptoms, as well as a thorough history, review of symptoms, and an organized examination. In this way, those patients most appropriately managed through manual methods can be readily identified.

The cervical spine consists of two separate but interrelated functional regions—the upper and lower cervical spine—each of which have unique mechanical characteristics with distinct evaluation implications. Although differing in anatomy and function, these regions are integral in function and relate directly with other areas, including the thoracic outlet, dorsal spine, shoulder complex, and temporomandibular joint (TMJ). Direct examination of these associated areas may therefore be warranted in the context of a cervical examination. Thus, an understanding of anatomic and functional relationships, including the progression of functional motor system dysfunction from the central nervous system to the peripheral neuromuscular junction, and an appreciation of the potential recruitment of adjacent and related peripheral anatomic sites can be valuable in assessing mechanical problems of the cervical spine.[1]

AN APPROACH TO WORK-UP OF THE CERVICAL SPINE PATIENT

Cervical spine evaluation focuses on establishing a sound working diagnosis, constructing a reasonable management course, and identifying relevant outcomes to monitor. The working diagnosis is synthesized from patient history and examination findings after ruling out any possible nonmechanical or significant pathologic etiologies. Key to this process is functional assessment, including determination of any correlation between abnormal functional findings and patient complaints. Provocative testing that identifies which mechanical maneuvers exactly reproduce the patient's complaints assists in establishing this relationship. An overview of some of the etiologies of cervical spine symptoms is provided in Table 1.

Multiple interrelated contributing problems may confound the work-up, warranting the clinician to attempt to systematically prioritize primary and secondary causative factors from those that may have no bearing on the current presentation. Of course, diagnostic and management plans should be developed for any unrelated incidental problems that may be uncovered (eg, hypertension, local extremity complaints), in addition to plans for the main complaint.

Secondary pathomechanics caused by organic lesions may also be a consideration. For example, the patient with ankylosing spondylitis may gain benefit from functional management even though manual therapy has not been shown to correct the processes responsible for the condition. Some cases may require concurrent medical management, in which case follow-up evaluations should also assess the appropriateness and value of further conservative management. A number of medically managed cervical spine conditions may benefit from a course of chiropractic care. Status post-resection of cervical nuclear herniation, postresolution of

Adapted from *Top Clin Chiro* 1995; 2(3): 1–18
© 1995 Aspen Publishers, Inc.

Table 1. Etiologies of cervical complaints

Organic lesions
  Neoplasm
  Infection
  Rheumatologic lesions
    Rheumatoid arthritis, ankylosis spondylitis
    Polymyalgia rheumatica
  Pathologic fracture
Anatomic/structural lesions
  Discopathy
  Central and IVF stances
    Congenital
    Degenerative
      Articular
      Periarticular
        Ligament hypertrophy (flavum)
  Neurologic lesions
    Myelopathy
    Peripheral neuropathy
  Congenital anomaly
    Cervical rib
    Segmentation anomalies
Mechanical lesions
  Subluxation
  Degenerative lesions
  Postural lesions
  Traumatic lesions
    Facet/arthropathy
    Discopathy
    Muscular strain
    Ligamentous sprain
    Instabilities
    Myofascial
      Traumatic
      Adaptive
    Entrapment neuropathy
Combined lesion (eg, anatomic derangement with a mechanical component)
Referral/visceral
Inorganic/psychogenic/symptom augmentation

Table 2. Major mechanical factors in cervical spine myelopathy

Static factors
  Developmentally small central canal
  Osteophytosis
  Disc herniation/sequestration
  PLL (posterior longitudinal ligament) ossification
  Uncovertebral arthrosis/deformation
  Apophyseal joint deformation/inflammation
  Hypotonic/hypertrophied flaval ligament
Dynamic factors
  Motion—normal and abnormal
  Loads—normal and abnormal
  Mechanical properties of spinal cord
  Mechanical properties of spinal column (ie, instability)
  Hypotonic flaval ligament

Source: White AA, Panjabi MM. Biomechanical considerations in the surgical management of cervical spondylotic myelopathy. *Spine.* 1988;13(7):856–860. © copyright 1988, Lippincott Williams & Wilkins.

---

discitis, or 6 months post–cardiac bypass surgery for an assessment and care of cervicothoracic spine and rib cage dysfunction are examples of conditions that may benefit from manual approaches.

With complaints of mechanical origin, identification and classification of the nature, stage, and severity can be useful to assist in the management plans for various conditions and chronicities.[1,2] This also facilitates a more accurate prognosis, which can emphasize functional restoration and full return to precondition status. Table 2 summarizes a number of mechanical pathologies that can have significant clinical implications.[3] During the history and examination, contraindications to mechanical management may also be identified. Algorithm 1 illustrates a sequence for cervical spine assessment.

Mechanical assessment of the cervical spine

A thorough and adequately detailed history should guide the line of investigation and detail required in the examination.[4–9] History taking need not be overly time consuming; however, a cursory interview is likely to miss vital diagnostic clues. The physical examination of the patient with cervical spine complaints should encompass a methodical progression of both the cervical spine and related regions. A wealth of functional information is available to the observant physician that can enhance the development of a suitable management approach and recovery expectations.

In assessing mechanical dysfunction, the possibility of organic pathology must first be ruled out. Central and peripheral neurologic lesions may also be of clinical concern in the cervical spine. Structural pathology (eg, fracture) and serious mechanical pathology (eg, instability, facet dislocation) must be ruled out as well. Viikari-Juntura[10] reported poor standardization of examination methods to be a factor in reliability of examination procedures, suggesting the need for consistency in examination protocol. Subsequent to physical and regional examination, clinical laboratory evaluation, radiography and special imaging, and electrodiagnostic testing may contribute valuable data. Special studies should be carefully selected and coordinated to achieve the greatest diagnostic and therapeutic yield without adding to unnecessary physical and financial strain on the patient.

Chief complaint and history of present condition

Any new patient evaluation, whether of a mechanical focus or not, requires a careful history, beginning first with a review of chief complaints.[4,5,9,11-16] A thorough history may offer more to the overall impression than the physical examination itself.[4,17] History taking should not be rushed, as this may increase the likelihood of diagnostic errors.[5] For example, a history that includes reports of direct head trauma or myelopathic signs may necessitate expediting imaging procedures to rule out fracture, dislocation, or instability.

The earliest clues of a mechanical etiology can often be extracted from details about the onset and behavior of symptoms (Table 3). Red flags also become apparent during the interview that can raise concerns regarding nonmechanical pathology (Table 4). This illustrates the importance of particular attention to a thorough past health history, including familial and socioeconomic histories as well as a sufficiently detailed review of systems.

Patients should be questioned regarding precipitating and relieving factors, location of pain (including radiating patterns), and the presence of neurologic symptoms. Pain and symptom reports, however, should be confirmed by direct observation and localization testing during the examination, as there may be overlap in the symptomatic distribution between different conditions.[18,19] Pain originating from articular and muscular involvement, for example, have similar regional distributions (Fig 1). One of the most commonly reported cervicogenic symptoms, headache, shares a common pain distribution with posterior fossa tumors.[20]

Table 3. Historical clues to mechanical etiology

- History of recent/remote trauma (macro or repetitive micro)
- Onset typically sudden, with specific trauma usually recalled; may be insidious and nontraumatic with certain conditions (eg, degenerative conditions)
- Symptoms increase with motion/activity
- Symptoms typically reproduced with a particular direction/motion
- Symptoms typically improve with rest
- Upper extremity symptoms usually unilateral; symptoms may be cranial, especially with upper cervical dysfunction; scapular, upper quarter, and anterior chest referral more common with lower cervical involvement
- Movement asymmetry/restriction commonly reported
- Locking/catching phenomenon
- Residual subluxation following resolution of severe joint/bony injury or regional surgery.
- Pain of joint etiology typically sharp, intermittent
- Pain of muscular etiology typically diffuse, achy; may refer in identifiable (trigger point) pattern

Table 4. Symptoms raising suspicion of nonmechanical pathology

- Trunk or lower extremity neurologic symptoms, especially long tract signs
- Bilateral upper extremity pain or neurologic subluxation
- Remote symptoms with neck movement (ie, lower extremity)
- Signs of sphincter dysfunction, bowel/bladder dysfunction/incontinence
- Fever, unrelenting nocturnal pain, weight loss, chronic fatigue
- Recent infection/surgery
- Polyarthralgia
- Onset with associated direct head trauma, loss of consciousness[26]
- Sudden onset without trauma/incident
- Dysphagia[20]
- Nuchal flexion/extension rigidity, especially in absence of trauma[20]
- Cranial neurologic deficit/central nervous system symptoms
- Pain related to general exertion (ie, stair climbing)
- Associated gastrointestinal symptoms
- Subluxation pattern inconsistent with that of functional lesion
- Symptoms unchanged or progressive, despite previous functional management

Expanded current and past medical histories

To fully understand the nature of present complaints, records may need to be obtained, including the results of prior diagnostic testing and treatment. This can minimize test duplication and avoid replication of unsuccessful therapy. A review of the past medical history, including familial history and system review,[4,5,9,12,21] typically reveals pertinent findings. A history of past trauma, surgeries, and shoulder complex injuries resulting in subclinical mechanopathology (eg, clavicular fracture or cervical fusion) may result in altered mechanics that can impact management of a current complaint.

A review of medication usage may assist in determining the appropriateness or safety of manual techniques (eg, anticoagulant or long-term corticosteroid use). Many medications commonly have side effects,[22] some of which may mimic mechanical pathology, such as upper extremity paresthesias. Questions relating to current medication use may need to be discussed with the prescribing physician.

A history of cancer, cardiovascular disease, or cerebrovascular disorders is also significant. Smoking history is pertinent due to possible cardiovascular and pulmonary pathology and the relationship to intervertebral discopathy and because it is a risk factor for pharyngeal and bronchiole conditions that can cause symptoms in the cervical region. Con-

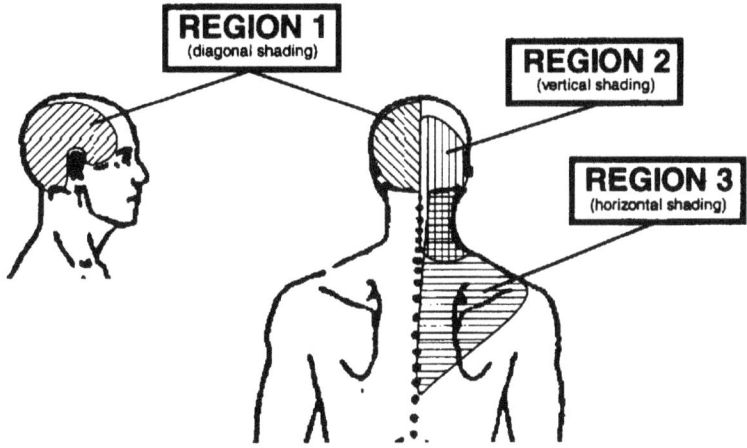

Structures potentially responsible for regional pain patterns:

REGION	Joint origin	Muscular origin

REGION 1 (diagonal pattern)	C2-3	suboccipitals
		cervical erectors
		  - semispinalis cervicis
		  - semispinalis capitis
		  - splenius cervicis
		  - splenius capitis
		upper trapezius
		sternocleidomastoid

REGION 2 (vertical pattern)	C3-4	upper trapezius
		lower trapezius
		levator scapulae
		cervical erectors
		  - semispinalis cervicis
		  - semispinalis capitis
		  - splenius cervicis
		  - splenius capitis
		multifidus

REGION 3 (horizontal pattern)	C4-5	middle trapezius lower trapezius levator scapulae multifidus

Fig 1. Common cervical pain patterns from muscular and joint structures. *Sources:* Travell J, Simons DG. *The Trigger Point Manual.* Baltimore, Md: Williams & Wilkins; 1983. Bogduk N, Marsland A. The cervical zygopophyseal joints as a source of neck pain. *Spine.* 1988;13(6):610–617.

---

ditions such as rheumatoid arthritis and ankylosing spondylitis may involve the cervical spine. Diabetes mellitus may contribute to upper extremity symptomatology (eg, peripheral neuropathy).

Objectifying subjective information

Several methods of data collection can help to substantiate or objectify patient reports and offer simple but useful outcome measures.[1] Pain may be graded using visual analog scales (VASs) and characterized using pain drawings.[3] Such instruments can be useful in identifying intensity and nonorganic pain patterns. Comparing pain drawings with known patterns of pain referral helps to target a probable etiology. Patterns correlating with dermatomal root levels, zygopophyseal pain patterns, discogenic patterns, myofascial referral, and sclerotogenous distributions drawn by patients help localize the source, especially when correlated with all available information. Diagrams with nonanatomic symptom distributions may indicate somatization, overlay, or symptom magnification.[3] Patterns of widely varying and fluctuating distributions, intensities, and subjective functional limitations may help suggest a psychogenic component to the clinical presentation, especially when out of proportion to objective findings.

Functional measures such as the Neck Disability Index have been shown to reliably document the impact of complaints on quality of life.[24] Along with VASs and pain drawings, these types of functional assessment can help to document a relevant clinical outcome and measure the patient's perspective of progress over time. Strategies for monitoring and overseeing active functional restoration programs in the low back have been suggested by Cook and Mootz.[1] A similar approach may be applicable in the cervical spine (Table 5).

Cervical examination

Efficient examination of the cervical spine begins with a synthesis of information gleaned during the history. Depending on the patient presentation and history, a general physical and regional examination may be warranted. Vital signs, including bilateral blood pressures, cranial examination, and nasopharyngeal examination, should be routine in patients with new cervical complaints. This allows assessment of regions where underlying pathology may produce cervical symptoms. For example, esophageal lesions may create sensations of neck tightness, and intracranial lesions may produce radiation patterns similar to those produced by cervicogenic headache. Ideally, cervical examination should uncover the source of the patient's complaints. Suspicion of extracervical causes should direct the clinician toward specific regional or system examination and to special studies that may help differentiate systemic or referred origins.

If intake information suggests that physical examination may be unsafe (as in the case of suspected fracture or dislocation), certain physical maneuvers may be inappropriate, and the patient may have to be referred or special studies obtained prior to continuation of the examination. Mechanical symptoms can usually be reproduced with provocative testing. Sources other than cervical elements should be considered if asymmetry, tenderness, and impaired mobility are absent[21,25] or symptoms are not reproducible. Different musculoskeletal dysfunctions may share common symptoms, regardless of the site. Tenderness, asymmetry, restricted movement, and tissue texture changes are usually present in any soft tissue lesion.[5]

A standard systematic approach to regional cervical spine examination includes observation, palpatory procedures, and functional tests. A work-up of adjacent structures, including the upper thorax, thoracic outlet sites, upper extremities, cranial nerves, eyes, ears, and nasopharynx, is routinely included in the cervical spine work-up.[11] Multisystem examination may also be indicated, including extended neurologic examination, abdominal examination for subdiaphragmatic structures, and chest examination, if the history warrants or suspicion of pain referral from these structures is high.[23,25,26–29] Similarly, many upper extremity complaints warrant investigation in the cervical spine or thorax, even when the neck region appears asymptomatic.[12]

Several cervical functional tests have shown limited reliability in research settings. However, their utility has been widely discussed, and their inclusion remains standard in cervical examination. Limitations in reliability illustrate the need for standardization and consistent application and interpretation, as variability in testing procedure may affect reliability.[10] Clark and Haldeman[31] reported that physicians were poorly skilled at determining disability and impairment, which necessitated the development of standardization criteria for guidelines. Anchoring the end points of a test measurement may help increase reproducibility. Such grading scales allow for more precision in reporting and comparing pre- and postintervention progress. For example, myospasm documented only as "spasm" is difficult to quantify later. Grading systems can involve standard and consistent verbal descriptors such as "absent," "mild," "moderate," and "severe." These can also be converted to a corresponding numeric system (eg, 0/3, 1/3, 2/3, 3/3) for expedient recording.

Vital signs

Vital signs are obtained routinely on intake and are important in evaluating new cervical complaints. Fever raises the index of suspicion for infection. Asymmetric blood pressure suggests unilateral vascular compromise, such as may be present in a thoracic outlet entrapment. Peripheral pulse and vascular changes may also be found with thoracic outlet syndrome and with autonomic involvement from the cervicothoracic chain.[8] Such conditions must be differentiated from peripheral vascular disease. Auscultation for bruits over subclavian and carotid arteries may indicate vascular compromise, which may affect cervical symptomatology or

---

Table 5. Monitoring strategies for functional restoration

Health status questionnaires—baseline, 4 weeks, discharge
Subjective factors indicating improvement—weekly
Visual analog scales—weekly during month 1
Anchored functional scales and activities of daily living information—weekly
Functional status surveys (eg, Roland Morris, Oswestry, etc)—every other week
Range of motion measurements—weekly
Functional performance of stabilization exercises—weekly

Reprinted with permission from Cook RD, Mootz RD. Determining appropriateness of exercise and rehabilitation for chiropractic patients. *Top Clin Chiro*. 1994;1(1):32–41. © copyright 1994, Aspen Publishers, Inc.

raise caution regarding the selection of manual therapies.[30] Height and weight not only serve as benchmarks for longterm health monitoring, recent changes may be indicative of endocrine disorders, neoplasms, or certain skeletal and articular derangements such as osteoporosis and degenerative disc disease.

Observation

Observation actually begins when first greeting the patient during a history and continues throughout the examination. Guarding behavior and antalgia may result from pain, soft tissue damage, spasm, or mechanical dysfunction. Generally, restricted motion without apparent acute pain is consistent with degenerative syndromes and chronic myofascial shortening. Signs of advanced neurologic involvement include fasciculation and atrophy and may suggest more extensive pathology. Overt myospasm and gross asymmetry, as in acute torticollis, should be quantified and recorded. Inflammation of deep tissues is typically not visible on inspection unless extensive; however, redness and asymmetric swelling may result from deeper tissue involvement. Ecchymosis suggests moderate to severe acute injury and raises the suspicion of fracture (see Table 7).[29]

Postural inspection, with particular attention to head, neck, thorax, and shoulders, can provide insight as to the nature and site of the lesion. Deviations from neutral posture are common with regional mechanical conditions and have been associated with an etiology of neck pain and related symptoms[29,32-34] and may be a sign of dislocation or fracture[32] or a congenital skeletal anomaly. Postural abnormalities have been implicated in the onset of lumbar facet syndrome,[35] and it is reasonable to suspect that similar processes may occur in the cervical region. Coronal plane inclinations (tilt) with ipsilateral rotation suggest lower cervical involvement by virtue of coupled motion in this region. Head-on-neck inclinations[36] or purely rotational deviations alone are more probably of upper cervical origin.[4] Sagittal plane postural deviations are typically found as ventral glide of the lower cervical region, often with compensatory upper cervical extension. Postural changes such as these may result in increased regional muscular activity, usually on the antigravity side of the distortion,[14] and contribute to soft tissue repetitive microtrauma, myofascial reaction, and degenerative changes.[14,37] Abnormal muscular function can be detected in part by careful observation of postural distortions. Postural changes should be correlated with regional alterations (ie, shoulder girdle) to identify contributing patterns in related musculature (Table 6).[29]

Gait alterations are often a first sign in myelopathy[38] or central nervous system lesions and are not generally expected to be altered in uncomplicated cervical dysfunction. Broad-based, unsteady, or staggering gait should raise questions regarding possible cervical myelopathy.

Table 6. Common cervical regional muscular patterns

Muscles prone to shortening/tightness
   Levator scapulae
   Upper trapezius
   Pectorals
Muscles prone to weakness
   Deep cervical flexors
   Lower scapular stabilizers

Source: Janda V. Muscles and cervicogenic pain syndromes. In: Grant R, ed. *Physical Therapy of the Cervical and Thoracic Spine.* New York, NY: Churchill Livingstone; 1988.

Palpation

Static palpatory procedures should note sensitivity to superficial and deep pressure. Depending on the nature of a cervical spine problem (eg, as in a patient with painful, acute torticollis), performing deep palpation may be best deferred until after active range of motion has been assessed. Superficial sensitivity is atypical for mechanical conditions and may be a sign of psychologic overlay.[39] Inflammatory signs include temperature and edematous changes, but these may be difficult to assess, given the depth of many structures. Circumferential neck measurements may assist in lending objectivity to regional inflammatory changes.[28]

Deep palpation can be organized into quadrants (right anterior and posterior, left anterior and posterior) to prevent oversight (Table 8). Common static palpatory findings of mechanopathology include pain over musculotendinous, articular, and ligamentous structures and the identification of

Table 7. General signs of acute or severe cervical condition

Stage of early examination	Examination findings
Observation	Marked antalgia
	Marked limitation of general movement
	Diaphoresis
	Battle sign (suboccipital/occipital bruising)
	Bakody's sign (arm held supported/overhead)
Static palpation	Masses
	Lymphadenopathy
	Severe isolated vertebral/spinous pain
Active range of motion	Severe limitation secondary to pain

Table 8. Overview of structures of mechanical importance per quadrant

Quadrant	Structures

Anterior (right mirrors left)	Muscular
	  Strap muscles
	  Scalenes
	  SCM
	  Deep flexors
	  Pectorals
	  Intercostals
	  Masticatory muscles
	Articular
	  Anterior aspect of vertebral joints
	  First rib
	  Sternoclavicular joint
	  Acromioclavicular joint
	  TMJ
	  Sternocostal articulations
	  Intervertebral disc
	Other soft tissues
	  Brachial plexus and nerve roots
	  Anterior intervertebral ligaments
	  Shoulder bursae
	  Subclavian and carotid arteries
	Entrapment sites
	  Central canal
	  IVF
	  Thoracic outlet syndrome
	    Scalene triangle
	    Costoclavicular space
	    Subcoracoid/pectoralis minor fulcrum

Posterior (right mirrors left)	Muscular
	  Suboccipitals
	  Cervical intrinsics
	  Cervicodorsal groups
	  Cervicoscapular groups
	  Scapulothoracic musculature
	  Rotator cuff and scapular stabilizers
	Articular
	  Craniovertebral joints
	  Upper cervical joints, posterior aspect
	  Lower cervical joints, posterior aspect
	  Costovertebral/transverse joints
	  Dorsal spine joints, posterior aspect
	Other soft tissues
	  Occipital nerves
	  Supra- and interspinous ligaments
	  Nuchal ligament
	Entrapment sites
	  Suboccipital triangle
	  Suprascapular notch

myofascial trigger points. Structural tenderness and muscular tone should be assessed.[40] Tenderness may be quantified with pressure algometry, which has been shown to be clinically useful in assessing tissue compliance and pain thresholds.[41] Spasm, trigger points, and muscular rigidity are common components of mechanical lesions and often accompany joint dysfunction. It is often difficult to differentiate between a primary articular and a musculotendinous lesion if both are present, and the two may require separate treatment considerations.[8] Methods for differentiating different forms of hypertonicity ranging from spasm to tightness have been described by Liebenson[40] and are summarized in Table 9. Ligaments painful to palpation should be considered abnormal.[11] Any complaints elicited during palpation should be documented and correlated with the chief complaint.

Active ranges of motion

Active ranges of motion (AROM) should be tested prior to passive or provocative procedures.[12,17] This allows for an estimate of general functional ability to guide further testing and prevents undue exacerbation of discomfort during passive motion.[42] Potentially painful movements should be performed last to avoid accentuating secondary reactions such as myospasm that may alter maneuvers performed later.[12]

Active motion has characteristics that are both quantitative and qualitative; thus, an in-depth description beyond merely the available excursion adds insight to the condition. Noting where discomfort or crepitus arises within the range, attending to fluidity and symmetry of movement, and noting any associated guarding or unusual ancillary muscular recruitment are obvious characteristics that may be of clinical value. Active range is typically measured in degrees in all planes, which allows for one baseline on which to gauge change.

The American Medical Association (AMA) *Guidelines to Physical Impairment*[43] recommends a standardized approach to measuring AROM using a dual inclinometer method, which is simple to perform. This method has also been described and recommended in the chiropractic literature.[9,31] Visual estimation of AROM has shown only fair reliability;[10] therefore, standard anchoring of patient positioning, instrument location, and movement protocols offer the best chance at consistency, objectification, and reproducibility of these kinds of measurements. Although there is variability regarding what may be considered "normal" range of motion, differences among various authors are reasonably close and provide a general guide to AROM evaluation.[4,12,43] Obviously, inaccuracies in measurement methods and anatomic variability limit detailed precision; however, measurements in the cervical spine of differences within a range of

Table 9. Differential diagnosis of abnormal muscular findings

	Examination shows			
Distribution	Is pain expected?	Related findings	Probable source	Additional considerations
Follows distinct muscular anatomic distributions	+	Hx typical for trauma or acute onset; isometric and stretch pain is typical; +/− inflammatory signs	Myospasm (reflex or posttraumatic)	Multiple muscles may be involved and will then show a multiple distribution.
Follows distinct muscular anatomic distributions	−	Hx common for chronicity; ROM loss with firm end feel; region may show pattern of recurrent pain/discomfort	Muscular tightness (noncontractile shortening)	Degenerative or chronic postural components are common; antagonist weakness may be found.
Follows muscular anatomic distributions w/distinct intrinsic foci	+/−	Referral pain with compression over trigger area; stretch irritability; weakness in associated muscle; muscular "jump" with pressure	Myofascial trigger point (MTP)	Possibility of satellite MTPs in related regions. Spontaneous pain is not necessarily present with latent MTPs but will show pain pattern with MTP provocation (eg, palpation).
Follows distinct muscular anatomic distributions	+	Stretching provokes pain; signs vertebral articular involvement expected	Segmental hypertonicity (facilitated segment)	Typically associated with involvement of the vertebral joint. Facilitation/inhibition patterns common in agonist/antagonist groups.
No muscular anatomic distribution; general regional involvement expected	−	Hx may show chronicity; psychologic component likely (stress, chronic pain behavior)	Limbic hypertonicity	Examination may be relatively nonspecific for specific regional mechanical pathology.

Sources: Travell J, Simons DG. *The Trigger Point Manual.* Baltimore, Md: Williams & Wilkins; 1983. Liebenson C. Active muscular relaxation techniques. Part 1: basic principles and methods. *J Manipulative Physiol Ther.* 1989;12(6):446–453.

perhaps 5° to 10° may be meaningful. Table 10 summarizes expected active normal ranges for cervical motion.

Range of motion should be symmetric in the coronal and transverse planes. Mechanical factors affecting AROM include degenerative conditions, discopathy, capsulitis, acute musculotendinous trauma, chronic myofascial shortening and postural syndromes, and joint dysfunction. Again, observations relating to the onset and character of symptoms through the range, as well as general difficulty or apprehension with movement, should be noted. Abnormalities of movement often occur as deviations from the plane of motion or muscular substitution able to be observed as altered muscular contraction patterns throughout the range. Limitations may or may not be significant to the clinical presentation.[42] However, such findings may be useful in assessing functional mechanical abnormalities. Inflammation or involvement of cervical facet capsules and/or synovial membranes can produce capsular patterns of restricted movement that typically manifest as limitations in all ranges, excluding flexion.[44] A typical pattern of capsular restriction involves extension, ipsilateral lateral flexion, and rotation toward the painful side.[17]

Table 10. Cervical active excursion ranges

Activity	Range of excursion
Flexion	80° to 90°
Extension	70°
Lateral flexion	20° to 45°
Rotation	70° to 90°

Significant AROM limitation or severe pain throughout the normal physiologic range suggests a more serious or acute condition. The remainder of the examination must be approached cautiously in these cases.

Reproducible snapping suggests periarticular soft tissue involvement. Fine crepitus is typically articular and degenerative; however, primary joint disease (such as with rheumatoid arthritis) should not be overlooked. Articular pops from cavitation within the active range may be incidental, although they may also suggest hypermobility. Locking phenomenon is generally considered to indicate mechanical pathology of the cervical three-joint complex.[36]

Passive ranges of motion

Gross passive ranges of motion (PROM) may be best conducted in a recumbent position to minimize postural activity of the cervical muscles. The passive examination allows for differentiation of noncontractile tissue involvement, although muscular injury may also show pain at the end range of passive stretch. All planes of motion should be tested, and combined motions are useful in assessing for joint restriction.[8] During passive challenge, palpatory overpressure can be applied to the joint during the physiologic range to help assess quality of motion and at the end range to evaluate end feel. Joint end-feel assessment yields information regarding abnormalities in function relating to such factors as internal derangement, capsular restriction, myospasm, or ligamentous damage.[42]

Overpressure is probably more specific to the evaluation of noncontractile elements. Voluntary resistance is readily apparent during testing and may be the result of apprehension in more severe conditions or may suggest psychologic overlay. Directions of general restriction should be noted for all cardinal planes for an assessment of flexibility. Adaptive myofascial shortening, capsular and periarticular adhesion, acute myospasm, trigger point stretch reactions, and myofibrosis are mechanical lesions that may adversely affect flexibility and PROM. Individual muscular groups may be assessed for flexibility and shortening by passive isolation stretch, although due to the abundant and complex nature of the cervical musculature, collateral and antagonist muscle group recruitment can frequently frustrate these assessment attempts.

Skilled passive intersegmental motion assessment, typically referred to as "motion palpation," is a qualitative rather than a quantitative procedure. Treleaven et al[34] reported passive segmental examination to be more sensitive in detecting joint dysfunction than examination of active motion; but its reliability is in question. However, cervical mechanical assessment has been considered incomplete without a skilled examination of passive articular motion.[4,8,12] All directions of free movement should be assessed for each cervical segmental level, with particular attention paid to symptom behavior and quality of motion. Complicating intersegmental motion assessment are variations in articular symmetry and orientation.[45] Reliability of motion palpation of the cervical spine generally appears to be weak, but some degree of reliability is possible in the lower cervical spine.[45,46] Interpretation of active and passive motion, symptomatic patterns, onset factors extracted from the history, and static palpatory data might best be integrated for a more global perspective of intersegmental restriction in the cervical spine.

Testing muscular function

Resistance tests may be useful in evaluating contractile tissue. Production of pain during an isometric contraction suggests a muscular lesion.[8,12,42] Weakness with pain is consistent with more severe muscular injury. In the complete absence of pain, weakness is more probably neuropathic.[42]

Strength and endurance of cervical musculature may be evaluated using simple, quantifiable maneuvers similar to those available in assessing trunk musculature.[1,12] This can be done from a recumbent position by rating the ability to lift the head in all planes against gravity. Each direction can be graded on a 1 to 4 scale based on time or repetitions (Table 11). Studies indicating that cervical pain has been shown to improve with muscular strengthening over several weeks point to the potential clinical value of assessing strength.[47]

Weakness and faults of neuromuscular patterning can be found by watching for substitution patterns[29] during active movements, observing posture, and thoroughly evaluating relational patterns of strength and weakness (reciprocal inhibition and facilitation). For example, Janda[29] described abnormal flexor patterning and weakness of deep cervical flexors by observing a predominate sternocleidomastoid (SCM) contraction and chin jutting in supine testing of flexion. Weakness of deep cervical flexors is thus implied. Similar patterns can be observed in posterior groups. Forward head posture and deep cervical muscular weakness have been correlated with cervicogenic headache.[33] Cervical deep flexor weakness and low endurance are also identified by a relative inability to hold the chin-tucked head 1 cm from the examination table in a supine position or by observation of shakiness.[34]

Mechanical provocation testing

Maneuvers designed to reproduce symptomatology and differentiate various mechanical lesions are described in Table 12. Table 13 summarizes expected findings in some of the more commonly encountered cervical mechanical conditions.

Neurologic examination

A minimal neurologic examination in an otherwise healthy cervical complaint patient should encompass the cranial nerves and upper extremities. However, a complete neurologic examination is often required. Peripheral findings resulting from pathology in the cervical region might include

Table 11. Functional strength testing of the cervical spine*

Cervical muscle group	Test description	Strength rating (scored 1–4)**	Criteria for rating
Cervical flexors (isometric test focuses primarily on deep neck flexors)	Repetition testing: the patient lifts the head in a chin-tucked fashion from a supine position. Isometric testing: the patient holds the chin-tucked head/neck 1 centimeter from the exam table.	1 = normal strength 2 = mild weakness; functionally fair 3 = moderate weakness; functionally poor 4 = severe weakness; non-functional	1 = able to hold the isometric position for 20–25 seconds w/ no onset of shakiness, or can perform 6–8 repetitions. 2 = able to hold the isometric position for 10–19 seconds, or can perform 3–5 repetitions. 3 = able to hold the isometric test position for 1–9 seconds, or can perform 1–2 repetitions. 4 = unable to hold the isometric position without shakiness, or cannot perform a single repetition.
Cervical extensors	The patient extends the head and neck from a prone position.	As above.	As above. Isometric testing should be conducted in the mid-to-end range of extension.
Cervical lateral flexors (testing to be conducted bilaterally)	The patient lifts the head and neck to the side from a side-lying position.	As above.	As above. Isometric testing should be conducted in the mid-to-end range of lateral flexion.
Cervical rotators (testing to be conducted bilaterally)	The patient lifts the head and neck with predominate rotation to one side.	As above.	As above. Isometric testing should be conducted in the mid-to-end range of rotation.

*This method of testing considers only strength in cardinal planes with no consideration for neuromuscular coordination or substitution patterns.
**The lower the score, the better the strength. The lowest regional score (6; one point each for flexion, extension, and bilateral rotation and lateral flexion) is considered normal.
Source: MaGee DJ. Cervical spine. In: *Orthopedic Physical Assessment*. 2nd ed. Philadelphia, Pa: WB Saunders; 1992.

---

upper motor neuron (UMN) signs in upper and lower extremities, UMN signs in the lower extremities with lower motor neuron (LMN) signs in the upper extremities, or UMN changes in the lower extremities alone.

Neurologic screening routinely includes deep tendon reflexes; sensory appreciation, particularly to pain and light touch; and motor strength. Asymmetry and hyperactivity in deep tendon reflexes are perhaps more clinically meaningful than bilaterally "diminished" ones, which are more likely a normal variant. Given the potential variability from patient to patient along with limited specificity and probable reliability problems in the test itself, gradation of responses may be of only limited usefulness. However, when testing sensitivity, changes can be readily scaled by assigning an anchoring system that patients readily understand. For example, by assigning the normal side a value of $1.00 (=100%) and then having patients value a contralateral deficit, a relative worth of 75¢ translates to a 25% hypesthesia. This can be compared over time to help establish consistent patterns. Equilibrium tests, pathologic reflex testing, and vibration and temperature appreciation can be valuable, especially if central lesions are suspected. Again, emphasis is placed on the importance of consistent anchoring, positioning, and measurement strategies.

Neurologic examination also requires girth measurement, which is an indicator of muscle mass, as an indirect method of examining motor supply. Girth measurement may detect atrophy with greater objectivity than visualization of symmetry and can serve as a baseline for serial monitoring. Atrophy may be observed without measurement in upper extrem-

Table 12. Common cervical mechanical conditions*

Common presenting conditions	Predominant physical examination findings	Keep in mind
Acute musculature	+ Isometric isolation pain or weakness ± Pain at end of range stretch + Palpation likely for myospasm or pain + Probable altered AROM/PROM + Probable multilevel articular restriction	• Palpable defect = sign of more serious injury • High likelihood of associated noncontractile involvement • Imaging and special studies not likely to be significantly contributory
Chronic myofascial dysfunction	+ Probable postural changes + Probable soft tissue imbalances, weakness, and tightness + Multiple restrictions in AROM, PROM + Probable diffuse muscular tenderness ± Isometric pain/provocation + Probable trigger point activity ± Degenerative changes on imaging + Probable multilevel joint dysfunction	• Radiographs may show contributory degenerative changes
Osteoarthritis	+ Probable postural changes + Probable soft tissue imbalances, weakness, and tightness + Probable crepitus + Multiple restrictions in AROM, PROM ± pain, capsular patterns likely + Probable diffuse muscular tenderness + Probable trigger point activity + Degenerative changes on imaging + Probable multilevel joint dysfunction	• Diagnosis confirmed radiographically • Be alert to myelopathic, root entrapment, and vertebrobasilar insufficiency signs • Assess for canal stenosis when posterior osteophytosis is seen
Root syndrome with radiculitis	± Antalgia + Pain in dermatomal distribution, often demonstrated on pain drawing + Probable restricted AROM, PROM + Normal neurologic examination + Axial compression/foraminal compromise tests w/pain reproduced + Ipsilateral quadrant; may see focal facet-type pain + Focal or radicular response with brachial traction test ± Brachial plexus Tinel's sign	• Compression can be by any space-occupying lesion; histology and examination help determine the probable etiology • More common etiologies are disc derangement/nuclear herniation, osteophytosis • Radiographs may show foraminal osteophytosis • Advanced imaging generally not indicated unless treatment fails or condition worsens • Monitor for progressive neurologic deficits
Root syndrome with radiculopathy	• As above, but with demonstrable neurologic deficit + Greater functional impact ± Brachial plexus Tinel's sign	• As above • Root-related weakness is a poor sign • Advanced imaging may be indicated if history suggests or conservative care fails • Consider electrodiagnostic studies • Arm or shoulder pain may be significantly greater than neck pain

continues

Table 12 (continued)

Common presenting conditions	Predominant physical examination findings	Keep in mind

Thoracic outlet entrapment	+ Poor shoulder girdle carriage and shortened anterior musculature
	+ AROM restriction in lateral flexion.
	+ Likely multilevel articular and myofascial restrictions
	+ Pain with percussion in anterior quadrant
	+ Supraclavicular pressure may reproduce symptoms
	+ AER (abduction and external rotation) elevated arm stress test
	+ May see ulnar or lower root neurologic deficits
	± Brachial plexus Tinel's sign
		• Be aware of structural factors such as clavicular fracture callus, cervical rib, fibrous band; radiographs often confirmatory
		• Symptoms often bilateral
		• Severity grading:†
		  Mild = positional paresthesia and numbness w/AER elevated arm test
		  Moderate = above + isolated muscle weakness and pain
		  Severe = constant symptoms w/ pain, numbness, paresthesia, weakness, hand dysfunction

Uncomplicated joint dysfunction	± AROM alteration, typically in posterior quadrant directions + May see pain at end of PROM + Probable focal pain + Referral patterns: cranial, scapular common + Passive restrictions ± Catching/locking ± Postural abnormality	• May be a component of a more extensive problem • May be no history of trauma • Radiographs may show arthridity; static radiographs of little practical value; dynamic radiographs may show hyper/hypomobility

*PROM used to include passive intervertebral assessment
†Liebenson C. Thoracic outlet syndrome: diagnosis and conservative management. *J Manipulative Physiol Ther.* 1988;11(6):493–499.

---

ity musculature with reasonable reliability, particularly in the hand.[10] Weakness may be present but is often difficult to test reliably using manual testing measures.[9] The use of a dynamometer improves accuracy in evaluating forearm strength. Repetitive contraction of muscles may help elicit more subtle weakness by revealing asymmetric fatigability.

Attention to signs of nerve root involvement is important. Typically, root signs first show up with sensory changes rather than motor weakness. Peripheral nerve involvement may display a mixed segmental distribution or distribution along the trajectory of the peripheral nerve. Tinel's sign (pain or symptoms resulting from percussion over a nerve distribution) may be found at multiple cervical and upper extremity sites, implying neurologic involvement. A positive Tinel's sign found over the cervical anterior quadrants may suggest a more proximal lesion of the brachial plexus.[12]

SPECIAL STUDIES

Because neurologic symptoms may be transient and take time to demonstrate abnormalities, electrodiagnostic studies should not be considered a routine part of the initial work-up.[28] However, if the clinical picture strongly suggests root involvement or primary neuropathology, or if there is a worsening or persistence of neurologic symptoms despite intervention, electrodiagnostic studies may be valuable. Nerve conduction velocity (NCV) and electromyography (EMG) studies help to assess integrity of peripheral nerves, while somatosensory evoked potentials (SSEPs) and dermatomal evoked potentials (DEPs) may help evaluate involvement of spinal cord tracts and reflexes. It is important to correlate any positive electrodiagnostic findings with the current clinical presentation.[48] A long-standing condition in an unrelated level or nerve distribution (eg, late-stage C-8 denervation findings) should not justify diagnostic or therapeutic considerations in the work-up of a patient with an acute onset of C-5 radicular pain. Clear signs of radiculopathy may indicate the need for advanced imaging (computed tomography [CT] or magnetic resonance imaging [MRI] studies with or without contrast) to define such structural etiologies as disc herniation or protrusion, osteophytosis, or tumor. Clinical laboratory tests may be warranted to rule out some systemic conditions such as diabetic neuropathy.

Radiographic imaging

Plain film radiography may be indicated to confirm suspicions raised during examination. There is an increasing trend

Table 13. Summary of commonly used cervical mechanical tests

Test	Classic interpretation	Qualitative/functional interpretation
Axial compression[4,8,12,14,31]	± Radicular pain—suggests root entrapment; good reliability[8]	Focal pain—suggests facet involvement; may see arthrogenic scapular referral; lateral flexion and extension positions may accentuate findings
Cervical distraction[4,8,12,14,31]	± Radicular pain relief consistent with root entrapment; good reliability[8]	Regional pain common with cervical muscular and ligament injury
Upper cervical quadrant[17]: Head extension with full ipsilateral rotation, then lateral flexion	See next column	Upper facets in maximum compression; contralateral anterior quadrant muscles stretch/flexibility; perform test bilaterally; look for articular patterns
Lower cervical quadrant[12,15,17]: Full neck extension, lateral flexion, then ipsilateral rotation	See next column	Upper cervical joints in maximum compression; perform test bilaterally; look for articular pain patterns; be aware of CNS signs from vertebrobasilar insufficiency
Cervical vertigo test: Bilateral sitting trunk rotation w/cervical spine and head held neutral	± Reproduction of vertigo; onset suggests cervical vs vestibular origin; has shown early correlation with segmental dysfunction	See preceding column
Adson's maneuver[4,8,12,14,27,31]: Cervical rotation w/ ipsilateral rotation and held deep inspiration	± Reproduction of entrapment symptoms; tests proximal thoracic outlet for compromise; mechanism is assumed to be mechanical compromise of scalene triangle; questionable reliability	Assess relative excursion; limitation may be from degenerative changes, ipsilateral facet dysfunction, contralateral scalene shortening/spasm
AER test w/overhead work[29]: Arm in abduction, external rotation; elbows behind coronal plane; rapidly open and close hand × 3 min	+ Reproduction of thoracic outlet syndrome symptoms; strong pulse at end of tests but w/ symptom onset suggests neurologic vs vascular etiology	See preceding column
Brachial plexus tension test[12]: Glenohumeral abduction and external rotation, elbow extension, and forearm supination; wrist and finger extension added	+ Root/brachial plexus symptom reproduction indicates lesion	See preceding column
Shoulder depression test[4,12]: Manual depression of the shoulder with contralateral cervical side bending	+ Radicular symptoms associated with space-occupying lesion or dural and periarticular adhesion	Assess excursion for relative flexibility of lateral and posterolateral soft tissues
First rib mobility test[14]: Maximum contralateral cervical rotation w/ forward bending in the sagittal plane while first rib palpated for motion	+ Restriction indicative of first rib fixation	May be + in thoracic outlet syndrome Compare bilaterally

to limit imaging to those cases where a significant diagnostic yield from such a study would change a treatment plan that would be indicated in the absence of films.[49,50] While plain film radiography may confirm postural observations seen on inspection or show degenerative changes, the clinical value of radiographs as a routine screening tool has been called into question.[50-55] The degree of radiographically demonstrated degenerative change does not appear to correlate with patient symptomatology.

Positive radiographic findings must be correlated with the rest of the clinical presentation to determine the significance of abnormalities. The judicious use of cervical radiography in the work-up of traumatic and mechanical complaints might include films to rule out fracture and dislocation (eg, prevertebral soft tissue swelling or dysphagia may raise suspicion of occult fracture). Assessment for complicating structural variations, such as cervical ribs, evaluation of the preservation of normal static joint integrity, evaluation for central and IVF (intervertebral foramen) stenosis, and determination of instability and loss of normal motion integrity are examples of clinical considerations that may indicate a need for radiographs. Radiographic studies may also be warranted in patients more than 50 years old or in individuals who have failed to respond to a few weeks of conservative care.

Stress (dynamic, motion) studies may offer clues to ligamentous damage. Flexion integrity of the upper cervical complex is best assessed using motion studies. The atlantodental interval (ADI) increases with rupture of the transverse ligament of C-1. The likelihood of this condition is increased in cervical spine trauma or enthesopathic conditions such as rheumatoid arthritis or ankylosing spondylitis.

A lucent cleft sign (a cleft formed by traumatic avulsion of the annulus) suggests acute disc avulsion (rim lesion).[56] This is distinct from vacuum signs found with degenerative conditions[56,57] and can usually be differentiated by a history of trauma, an anterior rim (versus central disc or central end plate) location, and the absence of degenerative changes. This is often a transient sign, disappearing as granular tissue infiltrates. When present, a lucent cleft may be associated with more extensive damage to related structures, such as facet hemarthrosis and root sheering, which may be difficult to assess in physical examination. Instabilities and loss of ligamentous integrity are demonstrated by disruptions in the posterior vertebral body line[56] and may occur with motion in either direction. White et al's criteria[58] for instability suggest that subluxation greater than 3.5 mm or segmental angular alteration of more than 11° is confirmatory. Radiographic assessments of stability are probably best made in the postacute stage due to the acute effects of muscular guarding and splinting.[28]

Overlay templating of dynamic radiographs has been described as a method for detecting hyper- and hypomobilities[27]; however, normative data using this technique have not yet been presented. Patient malpositioning (eg, rotation) may preclude an accurate templating procedure. Loss of intersegmental integrity assessed using this methodology is a basis for a significant assigned physical impairment, according to the AMA.[43] However, it is unclear how actual rating was calculated.

Recent studies[54,59-61] have determined that the instantaneous axis of rotation (IAR) can be easily and reliably determined for an assessment of motion patterns at individual vertebral levels (Fig 2). Abnormal IAR plots have been correlated with cervical symptoms, although the abnormality has not been identified to correlate with the symptomatic segmental level.[54] Mechanical abnormalities determined by IARs can be demonstrated in up to 72% of cases where radiographs are otherwise assessed as normal. This is done by localizing the IAR based on a ratio to vertebral height to width, with the IAR plotted on a normogram against the expected normal location. These studies reported reliability in measurement, accounted for technical errors to increase the confidence, and established a normal range for each cervical motion segment.[54,59-61] Some studies have cited a relationship with the direction of IAR shift away from the normal location to structural damage causing the shift; posterior axis shifts are associated with a loss of stability anteriorly (ie, disc or ALL avulsion) or structural restriction posteriorly (ie, joint fixation, myospasm, or adhesion). The opposite would be true for anterior axis shifts.[62,63] Abnormal IAR locations should be considered an objective marker for mechanical abnormalities in the cervical region that correlate with symptoms.

Advanced imaging: CT, MRI, and videofluoroscopy

Computed tomography

CT studies are particularly helpful in assessing bony pathology such as osteophytosis and central canal diameter. Discs, spinal cord, and other soft tissues are less clearly imaged. The use of contrast medium allows for improved imaging of the cord and root sleeves and is the preferred method for imaging extradural, intradural, and intramedullary lesions.[64] The need for less contrast material than with plain film myelography increases the safety of this procedure for the patient,[65] and computer reformatting offers multiple visual perspectives. CT studies are static and therefore nonfunctional in nature. They are rarely indicated unless there is failure of conservative management of radicular pain due to suspected bony pathology or central canal pathology is suspected. Degenerative findings on plain radiography increase the likelihood that the CT may be a more appropriate imaging tool than other options. CT is also of value in ruling out occult fracture, as is scintography (bone scan).

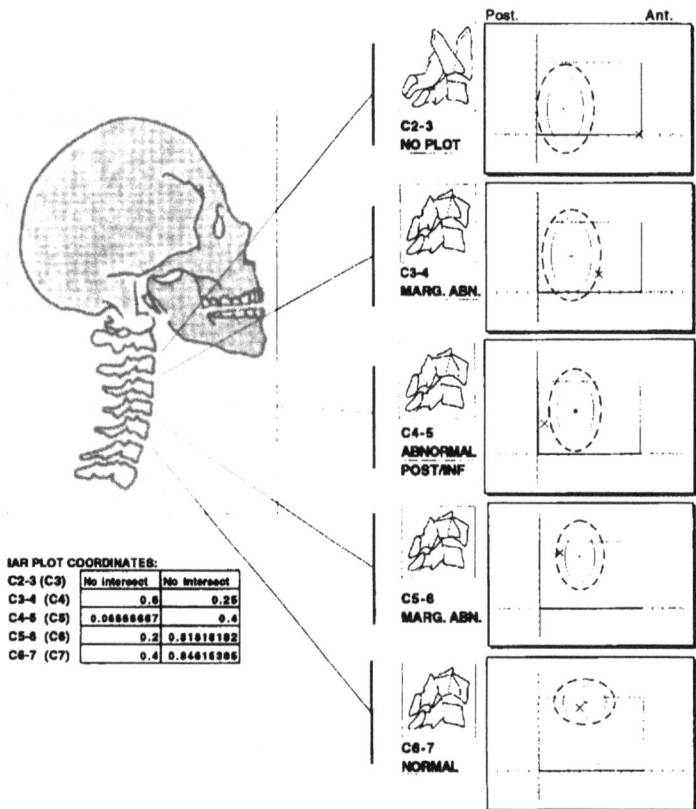

Fig 2. Cervical spine instantaneous axis of rotation (IAR) study. IARs are obtained using flexion/extension radiographs. The end result is a plot called a "normogram" (shown on the right) with the vertebra below superimposed on an XY axis. An IAR plot falling within the solid oval is "normal." An IAR plot between the solid and stippled ovals is "marginally abnormal." An IAR plot outside of the stippled oval is "abnormal." *Sources:* Amevo B, April C, Bogduk, N. Abnormal instantaneous axes of rotation in patients with neck pain. *Spine.* 1992;17(7):748–756. Amevo B, Worth D, Bogduk N. Instantaneous axes of rotation of the typical cervical motion segments: II. Optimization of technical errors. *Clin Biomech.* 1991;6:38–46. Amevo B, MacIntosh JE, Worth D, Bogduk N. Instantaneous axes of rotation of the typical cervical motion segments: I. An empirical study of technical errors. *Clin Biomech.* 1991;6:31–37. Amevo B, Worth D, Bogduk N. Instantaneous axes of rotation of the typical cervical motion segments: a study in normal volunteers. *Clin Biomech.* 1991;6:111–117.

Magnetic resonance imaging

Soft tissue lesions are imaged exceptionally well with MRI, making it the procedure of choice when soft tissue pathology is suspected. Like CT, MRI scans are static and therefore yield no functional mechanical information. Abnormalities demonstrated on MRI must be correlated with all other clinical findings due to established false-positive findings in asymptomatic patients.[66] This is often a more preferred imaging technique when patients have failed conservative management of radicular symptoms, when soft tissue lesions are the suspected etiology, or when further evaluation of myelopathic signs is required.

Videofluoroscopy

Videofluoroscopy (VF) (formerly known as "cineradiography") has been used to help define mechanical lesions, particularly hypermobility and instability. Foreman and Croft reported the results of a sensitivity study in which VF was able to detect abnormalities in 18 of 39 cases where standard radiographs were normal.[28] It is unclear if the standard series included stressed views, or if templating or IAR studies were also abnormal.

Drawbacks to VF typically include high X-ray exposure to the patient (although newer technologies are improving radiation exposure doses) and only fair to moderate interrater agreement in interpretation.[67] VF has been recommended in research settings,[55] but the value of widespread clinical application has been challenged.[68] Therapeutic utility appears lacking unless the plain films had been taken recently, symptoms had persisted or worsened for 6 to 12 months, symptoms were present with a history of cervical spine surgery, and/or upper cervical ligamentous damage is strongly suspected with negative or equivocal plain film studies (including stress views).[68] Furthermore, no objective support for serial studies appears to have been identified.[68]

CONCLUSION

An organized approach to evaluation of mechanical disorders of the cervical spine is likely to yield a database of information that can optimize a treatment approach (see Algorithm 1). Even in cases where obvious mechanical etiologies are correlated with symptom onset, it is prudent to perform a thorough history and review of systems and take a regional approach to examination of the cervical spine and adjacent structures. When complaints cannot be reproduced through mechanical provocation, suspicion of referral from systemic or organic sources should increase, and the scope of the examination should be expanded to include body systems that are known to refer to the cervical region. Special studies, including radiography, should be used judiciously when there is a likelihood of a reasonable diagnostic yield that could impact treatment decisions.

A synthesis of all clinical findings is crucial for the development of an accurate clinical impression. Mechanical and muscular disorders, including joint dysfunction, hypertonicity, myospasm, myofascial trigger points, sprain and strain, and neurologic involvement are readily differentiated with standard assessment protocols. Specificity in assessment methodology offers clinical information that can facilitate an appropriate treatment direction. Uncomplicated mechanical and muscular dysfunction should respond rapidly to chiropractic care. When response is slow or absent, further investigation is essential.

REFERENCES

1. Cook RD, Mootz RD. Determining appropriateness of exercise and rehabilitation for chiropractic patients. *Top Clin Chiro.* 1994;1(1):32–41.
2. Fitz-Ritson D. The chiropractic management and rehabilitation of cervical trauma. *J Manipulative Physiol Ther.* 1990;13(1):17–25.
3. White AA, Panjabi MM. Biomechanical considerations in the surgical management of cervical spondylotic myelopathy. *Spine.* 1988;13(7):856–860.
4. West H. Physical and spinal examination procedures utilized in the practice of chiropractic. In: Haldeman S., ed. *Modern Developments in the Principle and Practice of Chiropractic.* Norwalk, Conn: Appleton-Century-Crofts; 1980.
5. Mennell JM, ed. Clinical examination. In: *The Musculoskeletal System: Differential Diagnosis from Symptoms and Signs.* Gaithersburg, Md: Aspen; 1992.
6. Mennell JM. History taking. In: Mennell JM, ed. *Joint Pain: Diagnosis and Treatment Using Manipulative Techniques.* Boston, Mass: Little, Brown; 1964.
7. Magery ME. Examination and assessment in spinal joint dysfunction. In: Greive G, ed. *Modern Manual Therapy of the Vertebral Column.* New York, NY: Churchill Livingstone; 1986.
8. Magery ME. Examination of the cervical spine. In: Greive G, ed. *Modern Manual Therapy of the Vertebral Column.* New York, NY: Churchill Livingstone; 1986.
9. Haldeman S, Chapman-Smith D, Peterson DM. *Guidelines for Chiropractic Quality Assurance and Practice Parameters.* Gaithersburg, Md: Aspen; 1993.
10. Viikari-Juntura E. Interexaminer reliability of observations in physical examinations of the neck. *Phys Ther.* 1987;67(10):1,526–1,532.
11. Zohn DA, Mennell JM. Clinical examination. In: *Musculoskeletal Pain: Diagnosis and Physical Treatment.* Boston, Mass: Little, Brown; 1976.
12. McGee DJ. Cervical spine. In: *Orthopedic Physical Assessment.* 2nd ed. Philadelphia, Pa: WB Saunders; 1992.
13. Birnbaum JS. The neck and upper back. In: *The Musculoskeletal Manual.* Orlando, Fla: Academic Press; 1982.
14. Buschbacher RM. Head and neck. In: Buschbacher RM, ed. *Musculoskeletal Disorders: A Practical Guide for Diagnosis and Rehabilitation.* Boston, Mass: Andover Medical; 1994.
15. Kenna C, Murtagh J. Examination of the neck: part 1. *Aust Fam Physician.* 1986;15(8):1,015–1,020.
16. Kenna C, Murtagh J. Examination of the neck, part 2. *Aust Fam Physician.* 1986;15(9):1,204–1,212.
17. Corrigan B, Maitland GD. *Practical Orthopedic Medicine.* London, England: Butterworth; 1983.
18. Travell J, Simons DG. *The Trigger Point Manual.* Baltimore, Md: Williams & Wilkins; 1983.
19. Bogduk N, Marsland A. The cervical zygopophyseal joints as a source of neck pain. *Spine.* 1988;13(6):610–617.
20. Meyer JS. Headache: an illustrated practitioner's guide. *Hosp Med.* 1986;October:146–170.
21. Clinical highlights. *Hosp Med* 1982;18(12):95.
22. *Physician's Desk Reference 1993.* Oradell, NJ: Medical Economics; 1993.
23. Heller JG. The syndromes of degenerative cervical disease. *Orthop Clin North Am.* 1992;23(3):381–394.
24. Vernon H, Mior S. The neck disability index: a study of reliability and validity. *J Manipulative Physiol Ther.* 1991;14(7):409.
25. Souza TA. Back to basics: differentiating mechanical pain from visceral pain. *Top Clin Chiro.* 1994;1(1):1–12.
26. Watts C. Trauma to the cervical spine. *Hosp Med.* 1986;April:101–128.
27. Pratt NE. Neurovascular entrapment in the regions of the shoulder and posterior triangle of the neck. *Phys Ther.* 1986;66(12):1,894–1,899.
28. Foreman SM, Croft CC. *Whiplash Injuries: The Cervical Acceleration/Deceleration Syndrome.* Baltimore, Md: Williams & Wilkins; 1988.
29. Janda V. Muscles and cervicogenic pain syndromes. In: Grant R, ed. *Physical Therapy of the Cervical and Thoracic Spine.* New York, NY: Churchill Livingstone; 1988.
30. Clark W, Haldeman S. The development of guideline factors for the evaluation of disability in neck and back injuries. *Spine.* 1993;18(13):1,736–1,745.
31. Evans RC. *Illustrated Essentials in Orthopedic Physical Assessment.* St. Louis, Mo: Mosby; 1994.
32. Cibulka MT. Evaluation and treatment of cervical spine injuries. *Clin Sports Med.* 1989;8(4):691–701.
33. Watson DH, Trott PH. Cervical headache: an investigation of natural head posture and upper cervical flexor muscle performance. *Cephalalgia.* 1991;11(3):155–159.
34. Treleaven J, Jull G, Atkinson L. Cervical musculoskeletal dysfunction in post-concussion headache. *Cephalalgia.* 1994;14:273–279.

35. Hourigan C, Bassett JM. Facet syndrome: clinical signs, symptoms, diagnosis, and treatment. *J Manipulative Physiol Ther.* 1989;12(4):293–297.
36. McNair JFS. Acute locking of the cervical spine. In: Greive G, ed. *Modern Manual Therapy of the Vertebral Column.* New York, NY: Churchill Livingstone; 1986.
37. Sweeney T. Neck school: cervicothoracic stabilization training. *Occup Med.* 1992;7(1):43–54.
38. Clark CR. Cervical spondylotic myelopathy: history and physical findings. *Spine.* 1988;13(7):847–849.
39. Waddell G, McCulloch JA, Kummel E, Venner RM. Non-organic physical signs in low back pain. *Spine.* 1980;5:117–125.
40. Liebenson C. Active muscular relaxation techniques. Part 1: basic principles and methods. *J Manipulative Physiol Ther.* 1989;12(6):446–453.
41. Sanders GE, Lawson DA. Stability of normal soft tissue compliance in normal subjects. *J Manipulative Physiol Ther.* 1992;15(6):361.
42. Henniger R. Back to basics: evaluation of soft tissue pain. *Top Clin Chiro.* 1994;1(2):1–7.
43. American Medical Association. *Guidelines to Physical Impairment.* 4th ed. Chicago, Ill: American Medical Association; 1993.
44. Cyriax JH, Cyriax PJ. *Illustrated Manual of Orthopedic Medicine.* 2nd ed. London, England. Butterworth; 1993.
45. Gottlieb M. Absence of symmetry in superior articular facets on the first cervical vertebra in humans: implications for diagnosis and treatment. *J Manip Physiol Ther.* 1994;17(5): 314–320.
46. Mior SA, King RS, McGregor M, Bernard M. Intra and interexaminer reliability of motion palpation in the cervical spine. *J Can Chiro Assoc.* 1985;29:195–198.
47. Berg HE, Berggren G, Tesch PA. Dynamic neck strength training effect on pain and dysfunction. *Arch Phys Med Rehabil.* 1994;45:661–665.
48. Griggs RC, Bradley WG, Shahani BT. Approach to the patient with neuromuscular disease. In: Braunwald E, Isselbacher KJ, Petersdorf RG, Wilson JD, Martin JB, Fauci AS, eds. *Harrison's Principles of Internal Medicine.* 11th ed. New York, NY; McGraw-Hill; 1987.
49. Deyo R. Lumbar spine films in primary care. *J Gen Intern Med.* 1986;1(1):20.
50. Mootz RD, Meeker WC. Minimizing radiation exposure to patients in chiropractic practice. *J Chiro.* 1989;26(4):65–70.
51. Freidenberg ZB, Miller WT. Degenerative disc diseases of the cervical spine. *J Bone Joint Surg.* 1963;45A:1,171–1,178.
52. Heller CA, Stanley P, Lewis-Jones B, Heller RF. The value of x-ray examinations of the cervical spine. *Br J Med.* 1983;287:1,276–1,279.
53. Gore DR, Sepic SB, Gardner BS. Roentgenographic findings of the cervical spine in asymptomatic people. *Spine.* 1986;11:521–524.
54. Amevo B, April C, Bogduk N. Abnormal instantaneous axes of rotation in patients with neck pain. *Spine.* 1992;17(7):748–756.
55. Breen A, Allen R, Morris A. Spine kinematics: a digital videofluoroscopic technique. *J Biomed Engineering.* 1989;11:224–228.
56. Yochum TR, Rowe LJ. *Essentials of Skeletal Radiology.* Baltimore, Md: Williams & Wilkins; 1987.
57. Taylor JR, Twomey LT. Acute injuries to cervical joints: an autopsy study of neck sprain. *Spine.* 1993;18(9):1,115–1,122.
58. White AA, Southwick WD, Panjabi MM. Clinical instability in the lower cervical spine: a review of past and present concepts. *Spine.* 1976;1:15–27.
59. Amevo B, Worth D, Bogduk N. Instantaneous axes of rotation of the typical cervical motion segments: II. Optimization of technical errors. *Clin Biomech.* 1991;6:38–46.
60. Amevo B, MacIntosh JE, Worth D, Bogduk N. Instantaneous axes of rotation of the typical cervical motion segments: I. An empirical study of technical errors. *Clin Biomech.* 1991;6:31–37.
61. Amevo B, Worth D, Bogduk N. Instantaneous axes of rotation of the typical cervical motion segments: a study in normal volunteers. *Clin Biomech.* 1991;6:111–117.
62. Haler TR, O'Brien M, Felmly WT, et al. The effect of the three columns of the spine on the instantaneous axis of rotation in flexion and extension. *Spine.* 1991;16(8)(suppl):S312–S318.
63. Yoshioka T, Tsuji H, Hirano N, Sainoh S. Motion characteristics of the normal lumbar spine in young adults: instantaneous axis of rotation and vertebral center motion analyses. *J Spinal Disorders.* 1990;3(2):103–113.
64. Garvey TA, Eismont FJ. Diagnosis and treatment of cervical radiculopathy and myelopathy. *Orthop Rev.* 1991;XX(7): 595–603.
65. Alker G. Neuroradiology of cervical spondylotic myelopathy. *Spine.* 1988;13(7):850–853.
66. Boden SD, McCowin PR, Davis DO. Abnormal magnetic imaging scans of the cervical spine in asymptomatic subjects. *J Bone Joint Surg.* 1990;72A:1,178–1,184.
67. Croft AC, Krage JS, Pate D, Young DN. Videofluoroscopy in cervical spine trauma: an interpreter reliability study. *J Manipulative Physiol Ther.* 1994;17(1):20–24.
68. Schultz GD. A literature review of spinal videofluoroscopy. In: Hansen D, Craven S, Vernon H, et al (eds). *Chiropractic Science in Health Policy and Research.* San Jose, Calif: Consortium for Chiropractic Research; 1993.

Clinical Considerations in the Mechanical Assessment of the Cervical Spine 87

Algorithm 1

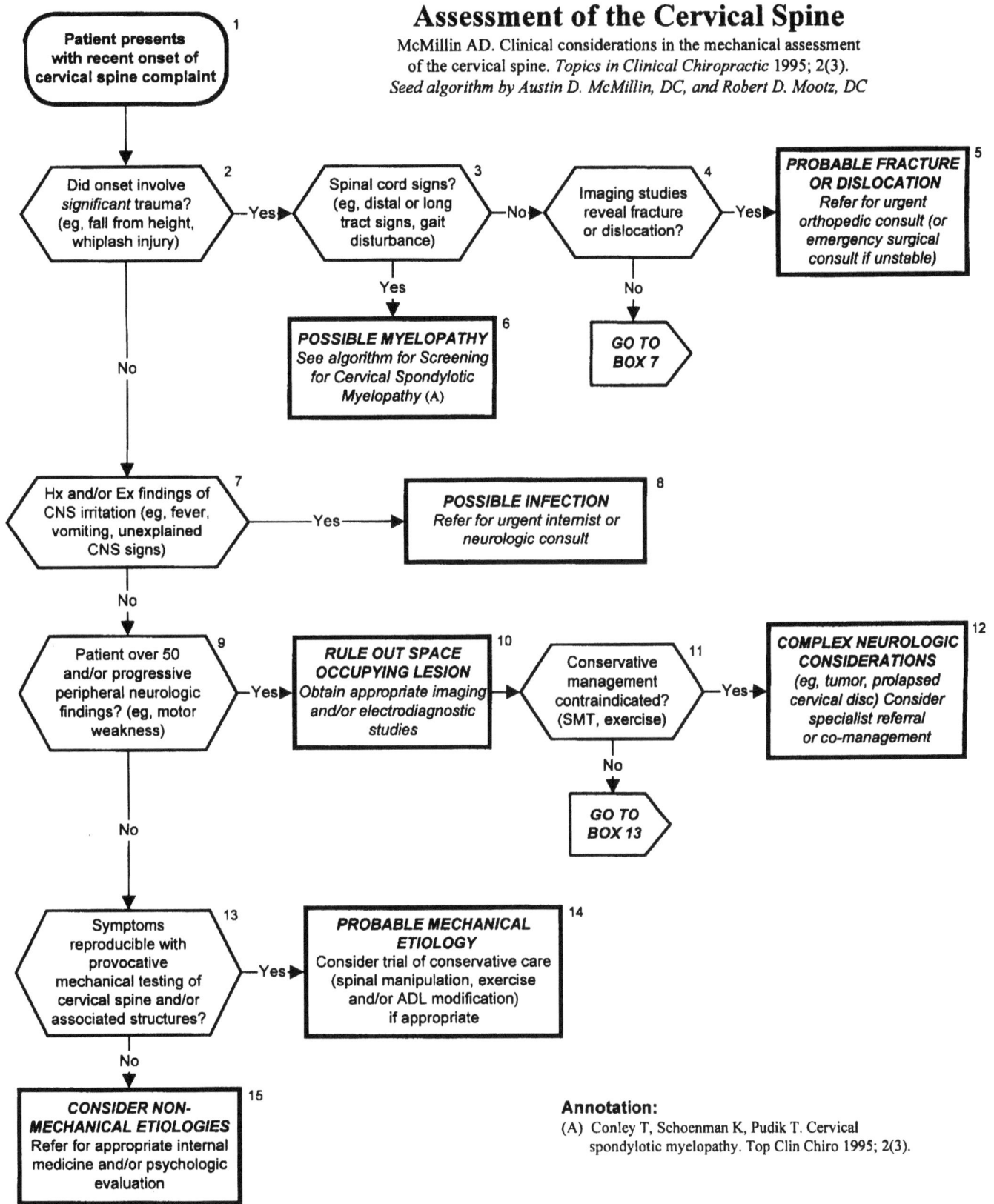

Assessment of the Cervical Spine

McMillin AD. Clinical considerations in the mechanical assessment of the cervical spine. *Topics in Clinical Chiropractic* 1995; 2(3).
Seed algorithm by Austin D. McMillin, DC, and Robert D. Mootz, DC

Annotation:
(A) Conley T, Schoenman K, Pudik T. Cervical spondylotic myelopathy. Top Clin Chiro 1995; 2(3).

7

Is Radiography Appropriate for Detecting Subluxations?

Gary D. Schultz and John M. Bassano

Radiography is considered a central tool for the assessment of back pain, so much so that patients sometimes feel less confident about their physician when it is not employed in the diagnostic phase of the evaluation.[1] In short, radiography is an accepted and often expected modality in the evaluation of back complaints. Patients presenting to chiropractors usually do so because of spine-related pain or complaints that could be attributed to the spine.[2] Out of this widespread expectation has arisen a number of justifications for ordering radiographs. The various rationales can be divided into two categories: clinical and nonclinical.

The clinical rationales for ordering X-rays have been widely discussed.[3–8] These generally assume that conditions to be ruled in or ruled out will have diagnostic or therapeutic significance. Additionally, it is likely that the benefits of the examination in these situations outweigh the cost and potential harm of the test (see Table 1).

Nonclinical reasons include legal mandate, litigious patient, fear, secondary gain on the part of the physician or the patient, habit, and peer pressure.[3,8,9] Most of these reasons are shunned, as they are peripheral to the treatment needs of the patient. Yet the chiropractic profession has been plagued for over two decades with the "nonclinical" administrative mandate to irradiate some patients in order to be reimbursed for the treatment provided.

HISTORICAL SIGNIFICANCE

Consider the following scenario involving a patient covered by Medicare: "Mrs. Jones, although I don't really need them to care for you, in order for your chiropractic treatment to be reimbursed under your Medicare Part B, we have to take some X-rays.... No, I'm sorry, the cost of those films is not covered by Medicare, and neither is the examination I should use to determine the need for the X-rays."

For over 20 years the chiropractic profession has been charged with the responsibility of providing radiological evidence of the chiropractic "lesion" for Medicare reimbursement. The subluxation, as viewed with plain film imaging, could be reported as any one of or a combination of three categories: static subluxation, functional subluxation, and/or regional subluxation.[10] These early "Medicare guidelines" evolved from a politically charged gathering of chiropractic leaders—the so-called Houston Conference in 1972. The implicitly designed X-ray guidelines were widely disseminated throughout the profession using regional seminar programs and mailed audiotapes and notes. The guidelines were tied to the Medicare reimbursement system and quickly found their way into the other federally funded programs (eg, federal workers' compensation). Today, federal benefits such as Medicare are even becoming benchmarks for other regional and private sector payers.

Although the Medicare categories of subluxation as viewed on radiographs never achieved a place in mainstream practice and are no longer reportable, the X-ray policy remains in the Medicare reimbursement system. This requirement has certainly stood the test of time, with no administrative changes made in the past 22 years (except imaging for chronic cases). To the government purchasers and policy people, *the* reason chiropractors take radiographs when treating Medicare patients is to demonstrate the existence of a subluxation.

Now, after 22 years (and the opportunity to study the theories of the chiropractic lesion in more depth), what has emerged that supports the early Medicare action as good or bad? Is there sufficient evidence (and agreement) that the

Table 1. Rationale for ordering radiographs

Clinical rationales
- Need to rule in or rule out conditions
- Possible diagnostic or therapeutic significance of radiographs
- Outweighing of costs and potential harm by benefits
- Contraindications to manipulation

Nonclinical rationales
- Legal or administrative mandate (eg, Medicare policy)
- Need to practice defensive medicine
- Litigious patient
- Fear
- Secondary gain (provider, patient)
- Habit
- Peer pressure

---

subluxation lesion as used by chiropractors is indeed a radiographically identifiable clinical entity?

MALPOSITION VERSUS FUNCTIONAL LESIONS

Subluxation has never been considered a nonclinical reason to order radiographs, but its appropriateness as a clinical indication has been questioned for a long time.[11–13] Part of the controversy is due to the fact that the definition of subluxation continues to be hotly debated within the profession. Definitions and models of subluxation fall into many general categories, including biomechanical, neurophysiological, trophic, kinetic dysfunctional, and psychosocial models.[14] For the sake of simplicity, we will treat the various models as mainly classifiable into two general categories: anatomic malposition and functional lesion hypotheses.

The role of radiography differs depending upon which hypothetical perspective one chooses to take. Following is an assessment of what may or may not be appropriate about the application of radiography from both a mechanical malposition perspective and a functional lesion perspective.

The "malposition" model is the hypothesis that subluxation consists of an abnormal position between vertebral segments. This abnormal position may cause local or far-reaching deleterious somatic and visceral effects.[15] The "functional lesion" hypothesis holds that abnormal joint motion between vertebral segments of the spine characterizes subluxation. The static position of the segments may or may not be related to the function of the segment in this second model.

Because of the complexity and variety of potential models associated with subluxation[14] and the wide variation in opinions about the various perspectives, a multitude of definitions and concepts regarding chiropractic subluxation have evolved.[16] Although few would suggest that spinal subluxation or dysfunction of some sort does not exist, the limited available research on the subject remains largely in the realm of nonchiropractic basic physiology studies theoretically extrapolated to explain clinical observations. However, several responsible attempts have been made within the profession to appraise what is understood and use formal, explicit processes to evaluate the literature and synthesize expert and community-based clinical opinion.[16–18]

In either case, the purpose of chiropractic intervention is to reduce or eliminate the subluxation, which is accomplished by administering the chiropractic adjustment. Although radiographs are considered by some to be an integral component of the documentation of the subluxation, there has not been a cogent delimitation of the ability of radiography to be a scientifically valid, reliable messenger of the information required to establish this diagnosis.

THE APPROPRIATENESS OF RADIOGRAPHY FOR DIAGNOSING SUBLUXATIONS

The practical question from a health policy standpoint is whether radiography is necessary and appropriate for the diagnosis of subluxations of any type or severity. Appropriateness is a complex issue. The performance characteristics of an appropriate test include safety, availability, reliability, and validity. In addition, the condition in question should not be adequately depicted by other means and should be worthy of detection to the degree made available by the test.[19]

In order words, radiographs are justifiable for the detection of subluxations if they are safe, generally available and affordable, capable of reliably and validly differentiating subluxations from other conditions, and can accurately represent the nature of the subluxations so that adjustments can be used to reduce them (see Table 2).

There is little doubt as to the availability of radiography in chiropractic. American Chiropractic Association data indicate that over 83% of chiropractic practices have radiographic units in their offices. Approximately three-quarters of new patients receive an average of 3.4 radiographic views, and 17% of patients receive follow-up studies averaging 2.6 views.[20] The prevalence of radiographic units within practices may partly explain the extensive use of radiographs: they are employed for purposes of diagnosis because they are easily available.[21]

Table 2. Performance characteristics of an appropriate test

- Safety
- Available and affordable
- Capable of reliably and validly detecting and differentiating disease from "normal" and other conditions
- Impacts clinical decision making

The safety of radiography has been questioned because of the potential deleterious somatic and genetic effects of radiation exposure. Using current technology, such as rare-earth cassettes with matched film, high-frequency radiographic equipment, and automatic processing, dosage levels can be kept relatively low. Still, it must be acknowledged that all radiation exposure represents a risk of some type, especially in the case of children and women of child-bearing age.[22,23]

The affordability of radiographs in the clinical setting has come under more scrutiny in recent decades. Regardless of one's impression of what is costly, radiographs contribute significantly to the overall cost of a case of back pain, especially when used in a serial fashion or when large numbers of views are ordered.[24,25] Therefore, radiology for subluxation detection as well as for other diagnostic purposes deserves investigation as to necessity.

The performance characteristics of reliability and validity are difficult to address in subluxation detection by radiography when one considers that two models exist that would necessitate very different applications and interpretations of the technology. Reliability can be measured using intra- and interexaminer methods. Additionally, malpositions can be measured in vitro and the radiographic correlation with their magnitude, direction, and morphology can be tested. The advantage of this method is that estimates of magnitude of error can be established.

Validity is best measured by comparing performance against a gold standard. Since a gold standard for chiropractic subluxation as a whole does not seem to exist, this method cannot be employed. Using symptomatic foci as the locus of the subluxation, at least the location of the lesion can be tested using a test-retest method.

THE MALPOSITION HYPOTHESIS

Radiographs have been used in chiropractic to determine the location of "misplaced" vertebrae almost since their advent.[26] Considerable investigation has been undertaken to evaluate the potential of radiography as it relates to vertebral malposition. Suboptimal radiographic reliability might be due to asymmetry of morphology,[11,27,28] positional and geometric distortion,[11,29-31] or measurement inaccuracy.[29,32,33]

Saraste and coworkers[34] evaluated radiographic measurements of the lumbar spine. They found that measurement errors of radiographic variables stem from poor definition of anatomic measuring points, changes in patient position, and intra- and interobserver variation. They concluded that combined factors may produce an error amounting to 50% of measured values.

Schram and colleagues[35] evaluated errors in Gonstead pelvic radiographic analysis due to positioning. They concluded that small degrees of incorrect positioning may result in significant errors. Each degree of rotational change allowed a 1.87-mm change in the radiographic listing. In another study, Schram and Hosek[31] evaluated error limitations in radiographic kinematics of the spine. They concluded that errors of 0.5 mm were capable of producing apparent rotation in excess of 5°.

Zengel and coworkers[36] evaluated the effects of radiographic projectional distortion on apparent vertebral rotation. They found that vertebrae displayed 1 mm of apparent rotation for every 2–3 cm of lateral off-centering. Apparent rotation will increase as the object-film distance increases, and a larger rate of distortion can be expected.

In literature involving the upper cervical spine, much lower error measurements have been reported than in other literature.[37] Interestingly, the reported threshold of significance is considerably smaller as well, with some authors advocating that less than 1° of rotation represents a therapeutically significant lesion.[38,39] The precise explanation for this lowered threshold is not intuitively obvious. One might hypothesize that the improved reliability may be due to the patient's being clamped in position, reducing positional error, coupled with improved practice and experience in a particular measuring procedure.

In summary, the reliability of static marking of radiographs to detect "bones out of place" remains controversial. Error margins often exceed the actual measured values or the magnitude of change expected to be accomplished with the intervention, rendering the procedure of dubious reliability.[40] However, one must not assume there is no reliability.

The use of static marking systems for predicting symptomatic spinal lesions also remains controversial. The ability of radiography to yield consistently accurate results is dependent upon many variables, and these variables are difficult to control in the clinical setting. Furthermore, precisely what causes the pain or the symptomatic state remains a mystery.

In most clinical circumstances, it is reasonable to assume that measured distances of greater than 2 mm are likely due to real malposition rather than error. Angles measured in the spine should exceed 2° prior to assumption of abnormal under the most rigorous of conditions and 3–5° in less than optimal settings.[41-43] Positional changes pre- and posttreatment less than 3 mm or 4–5° are difficult to attribute to therapy, given the potential effect of cumulative error on multiple measurements.

Even in the upper cervical spine, not all authors agree that small increments of alignment abnormality correlate with clinical signs. Anderson[44] tested the upper cervical chiropractic theory by radiographic analysis. He concluded the data of upper cervical misalignments were not correlated with the presence or absence of symptoms. The results of these investigations should not be generalized to measurement reliability outside the upper cervical spine because of the uniqueness of the positional and projectional parameters.

A corollary of the malposition model is the "perfect posture" hypothesis—the belief that there is an optimum posture that every normal spine should have.[45] This hypothesis has been evaluated in the literature. In the cervical spine, there appears to be a correlation with the symptomatic state and hypolordosis.[12,46] However, other static parameters relating to assumed normal posture cannot be identified with confidence.[47]

The association of symptoms with other static radiographic parameters has not fared well in the literature either. Specifically, lordotic and minor lateral deviations of spinal posture have not been found significantly more frequently in symptomatic populations than in asymptomatic populations.[34,48–51] Another challenge facing radiographic evidence of postural or segmental malpositions involves the relationship of such malpositions to future spinal health or function. For example, is it possible that asymptomatic subluxations as "seen" on radiographs may be predictors of future illness, dysfunction, postural imbalance, or other pathology?

Another assessment of validity relates to the pre- and postmanipulation assessment of vertebral position. An analysis of reduction in symptoms and postadjustment change in position was performed by Plaugher and coworkers.[40] Once again, the magnitude of posttreatment change was well within the range of generally accepted error, invalidating conclusions drawn from this retrospective study.

THE FUNCTIONAL LESION HYPOTHESIS

In order to evaluate the possibility of a functional lesion in the spine radiographically, functional radiographs (usually stress radiographs) need to be employed. Stress radiographs have long been used to evaluate the spine for instability, in particular the cervical spine, where post–motor vehicle accident radiographs often include flexion/extension views.

Many methods of measuring excursion and total movement have been developed. Evaluation of these methods has been done elsewhere, and it appears that, in the case of the cervical spine, templating using acetate overlays of the stress views of the spine is the most reliable, clinically feasible method for comparing vertebral position on separate views.[52,53] However, the same generic limitations encountered in mensuration of static radiographs pertain to this method. This quantitative evaluation of motion serves to document hypomobility as well as hypermobility, assuming they are of sufficient magnitude to exceed error ranges. Difficulties in radiographically demonstrating such gross motion abnormality as orthopaedic instability in the lumbar spine underline the obstacles to imaging functional subluxations.[42,54–59]

Once again, controversy exists as to what constitutes normal motion patterns and whether asymmetry is normal.[42,54,57] The literature comparing radiographic findings on symptomatic and asymptomatic cases suggests that asymmetry may be the rule in low back range of motion. This conclusion is consistent with clinical assessments of this issue.[60] Further, little correlation of radiographically visualized abnormality and level or severity of symptomatology has been demonstrated.[42,54,61]

Videofluoroscopy

Videofluoroscopy (VF) has been employed to a limited degree in the evaluation of motion of the spine, particularly the cervical spine. The uniqueness of VF lies in its qualitative assessment of motion. The concept of aberrant motion is consistent with the functional lesion hypothesis, and there is evidence that aberrant motion exists in the spine. VF would seem to be well suited for the investigation and validation of this hypothesis. However, there are a number of impediments to the application of VF for this purpose.

First, there is the issue of patient safety. Although technical advances have reduced radiation from VF, in many circumstances a considerably higher radiation dosage may be delivered to the patient (and the doctor) than in other forms of imaging.[62] Next, comes the issue of what constitutes normal motion in the spine qualitatively, which has given rise to considerable controversy.[63–66] Even more controversial is the definition of what is abnormal.[62] In other words, while VF has promise as a tool for evaluating the qualitative component of motion, extensive disagreement on what constitutes normal and abnormal motion still exists, and thus there is no specific standard of motion in the spine as viewed fluoroscopically (or even vaguely agreed-upon standard, for that matter). Therefore, very few cogent conclusions can be drawn from fluoroscopic studies.

IMPACT ON CLINICAL DECISION MAKING

The last variable in the appropriateness puzzle is whether a finding of subluxation (even if the condition is perfectly detected and characterized by a radiograph) has any importance in determining the course of treatment or the prognosis of the patient. In other words, are the outcomes of patients treated because of a presumptive diagnosis of subluxation any different from the outcomes of patients with "radiographically proven" subluxations?

A number of studies have evaluated the effectiveness of manipulation for spinal complaints. It is difficult to know if the patients treated in these studies actually had subluxations. Most doctors would accept that the patients had mechanical back complaints, that there were no contraindications to manipulation, and that the conditions were at least similar to subluxations. If one subscribes to the belief that subluxations are being adjusted in the many randomized controlled trials that have been performed comparing chiropractic manipulation to other therapies, then it is clear that the radiograph is not an essential component of the treatment regime except where necessary to confirm the absence of contraindications to manipulation.

Hubka has demonstrated the validity of using palpation of the spine to locate areas of pain. He assumes that the subluxation resides in the region of the painful area. Applying chiropractic adjustments to these areas provided relief of pain in his study population.[67] Based on such information, it again appears that many back complaints (minus any contraindication to manipulation) can and are effectively treated using chiropractic methods in the absence of radiographs. It is entirely possible that many subluxations do not require exact characterization for appropriate and effective chiropractic care to be administered.

CONCLUSION

The two hypotheses (malposition and functional lesion) each are associated with a body of conflicting literature regarding the utility of radiographic imaging. Significantly, the use of radiographs for the detection and characterization of subluxations continues despite lack of substantive evidence supporting its use. Such lack of evidence is not completely attributable to the lack of scientific inquiry into this topic; rather it is a result of the failure of the hypotheses about subluxation to be supported using radiography. Ultimately, the ability of imaging to precisely document subluxations in chiropractic will depend on the development of a concise, cogent, testable definition of the term. Once again, the current state of affairs is an indictment of the hypotheses as much as it is an indictment of radiography (Table 3).

Regarding the malposition hypothesis, the literature has identified several factors that affect reliability: anatomic unpredictability, positional inconsistency, geometric distortion, and measurement error. It suggests that these factors add up to a margin of error of at least 2 mm of distance and at least 3° of angular measurement error. This is likely to be an optimistic assessment. It is reasonable to think that practice conditions do not usually approach the levels of precision existing in a laboratory. However, at least some quantification of the error has been accomplished. It is likely that most of the misalignments proclaimed to be chiropractic subluxations on radiographs are smaller than these error limits, and therefore one cannot rely upon their actual existence radiographically.

One apparent exception to this rule occurs when examiners are trained rigorously in a measurement procedure and patients are "clamped" into a position in a standardized radiographic unit, as in the upper cervical treatment systems. In this instance, there is evidence to suggest that reliability can be considerably improved. However, those advocating upper cervical techniques insist that measurements smaller than 2 mm or 2° are significant. Therefore, they are left with the same reliability issues.

The validity of radiography for the identification of symptomatic, treatable subluxations remains unknown. At best, the literature supporting the relationship between symptomatology and radiographic postural observations is of dubious quality. More methodologically sound studies have very often failed to find even a rudimentary correlation between posture and symptoms.

It is possible that postural changes in the spine potentiate symptomatic states, but this potentiation has yet to be demonstrated. Even if potentiation can be demonstrated, certainly the value of these factors for predicting the development of symptomatic states will be exceedingly difficult to establish given the prevalence of postural aberrations and back pain as individual entities.

The functional lesion hypothesis suffers from nearly the same impediments as the malposition hypothesis. However, there is an added burden—multiple measures are necessary to achieve a conclusion using stress radiographs. The need for multiple measures increases the likelihood of numerous errors per conclusion, and furthermore, their impact cannot be assumed to be linear (the calculation of error thresholds becomes a very cumbersome task, one that is unlikely to render them clinically appealing).

Assessment of the validity of radiographs for predicting symptomatic functional lesions has been performed in well-designed studies. Little or no difference has surfaced between postural measured parameters comparing weight-bearing and recumbent radiographs. Attempts to show a correlation between the location of symptoms in the low back and measured abnormalities have also failed, and comparisons of measured postural findings in symptomatic and asymptomatic populations have not uncovered differences between the populations.

Table 3. Summary of evidence

Misalignment	Functional lesion
Reliability	
Anatomic unpredictability	Same as misalignment
Positional inconsistency	Multiple measures likely
Geometric distortion	compound measurement error
Measurement error	
Validity	
Dubious correlation between radiographic posture observations and symptoms	No difference in measured parameters comparing weightbearing and recumbent radiographs
	No difference in measured findings between symptomatic and asymptomatic populations

On the other hand, the investigations that have been done are too sparse to conclude that no such validity exists. Once again, the quality and quantity of the literature is insufficient to rule out this possibility. Note, however that the evidence there is places a significant burden of doubt upon the assertion that validity is still out there lurking in the numbers.

Dynamic examination of the spine using videofluoroscopy holds exciting promise, but the modality needs more study before it becomes generally acceptable. Principally, there is a lack of understanding of qualitative norms for motion. This all but eliminates any ability to understand what abnormal function of the spine might be or how it relates to what chiropractors adjust on a daily basis.

Given the suboptimal reliability and the lack of demonstrated validity for either model of subluxation, the conclusions derived from radiographs of supposed subluxations are at best system noise except in the case of very large abnormalities. When one compares radiography's performance potential with the proven ability of simple palpatory investigation of spinal tenderness to determine where adjustments should be applied to the spine, there is ample reason to question the appropriateness of radiography as a primary modality for characterizing chiropractic subluxations.

So, is radiography appropriate for detecting subluxations? The short answer appears to be "sometimes." It is widely available, mildly invasive, and more expensive than other methods commonly used. Radiography has not demonstrated adequate reliability or validity for the detection and characterization of subluxations, especially as a screening tool for the subluxations most commonly seen on plain films. Furthermore, it appears that there are less invasive, more accurate methods of characterizing subluxations. This all but obviates the need for radiography as an initial component in the hunt for subluxations.

In a situation where other clinical tests suggest a subluxation of sufficient magnitude to contraindicate or alter a therapeutic intervention (eg, spondylolisthesis or scoliosis), radiography is probably appropriate early in the clinical course. Furthermore, where it is difficult to distinguish subluxation from other conditions that contraindicate chiropractic adjustments, radiography should be employed early in the clinical course to ensure the patient's safety.

FUTURE CHALLENGES

Although practitioners will likely continue to differ in their beliefs regarding the use of radiography for assessing chiropractic subluxations, the questions posed here indicate the kind of research that should be pursued. The margin of error in positioning and measurement will need to be below the magnitude of the subluxations found and the amounts of measurable change expected from chiropractic adjusting. Perhaps of greater importance will be the need to demonstrate that patient management based in part on radiographic information will lead to better patient outcomes than can be achieved without such information. It can be anticipated that as clinical accountability and cost competition increase in the future, chiropractors will experience more pressure to justify the use of radiography for subluxation detection.

REFERENCES

1. Deyo R, Diehl A, Rosenthal M. Reducing roentgenography use: can patient expectations be altered? *Arch Intern Med.* 1987;147:141–145.
2. Shekelle PG, Brook RH. A community-based study on the use of chiropractic services. *Am J Pub Health.* 1991;81:439–442.
3. Deyo R, Diehl A. Lumbar spine films in primary care. *J Gen Intern Med.* 1986;1:20–25.
4. Kelen G, Noji E, Doris P. Guidelines of the use of lumbar spine radiography. *Ann Emerg Med.* 1986;15:245–251.
5. Schultz G, Phillips R, Cooley J, et al. Diagnostic imaging of the spine in chiropractic practice: recommendations for utilisation. *Chiro J Aust.* 1992;22:141–152.
6. Halvorsen JG, Swanson D. Indications of office radiographs. *J Fam Pract.* 1990;31:521–529.
7. Marquart DJ. A review of the cognitive process used to decide which patients require diagnostic imaging. *Council on Diagnostic Imaging.* 1992;7(3):16–20.
8. Taylor JAM, Resnick D. Imaging decisions in the management of low back pain. In: Lawrence D, et al., eds. *Advances in Chiropractic.* Vol. 1. Chicago: Mosby–Year Book; 1994.
9. Wyatt L, Schultz G. The diagnostic efficacy of lumbar spine radiography: a review of the literature. In: Hodgsen M, ed. *Current Topics in Chiropractic.* Sunnyvale, CA: Palmer College of Chiropractic-West; 1987.
10. Swanson HE, Schaefer RC, eds. *Basic Chiropractic Procedural Manual Emphasizing Geriatric Considerations.* Des Moines, IA: American Chiropractic Association; 1977.
11. Howe J. Facts, fallacies and misconceptions in spinography. *J Clin Chiro.* 1972;34:34–45.
12. Meeker W, Mootz R. Evaluating the validity, reliability and clinical role of spinal radiography. In: Coyle B, ed. *Current Topics in Chiropractic.* Sunnyvale, CA: Palmer College of Chiropractic-West; 1985.
13. Hildebrant R. Chiropractic spinography and postural roetgenology, I: clinical basis. *J Manipulative Physiol Ther.* 1980;3:87–92.
14. Gatterman MI, ed. *Foundations of Chiropractic Subluxation.* St. Louis: Mosby–Year Book; 1995.
15. Herbst RW, ed. *Gonstead Chiropractic Science and Art.* Mt. Horeb, WI: Sci-Chi Publications; 1968.
16. Lantz CA. A review of the evolution of chiropractic concepts of subluxation. *Top Clin Chiro.* 1995;2(2):1–10.
17. Gatterman MI, Hansen DT. Development of chiropractic nomenclature through consensus. *J Manipulative Physiol Ther.* 1994;17:302–309.
18. Haldeman S, Chapman-Smith D, Peterson D, eds. *Guidelines for Chiropractic Quality Assurance and Practice Parameters.* Gaithersburg, MD: Aspen Publishers; 1992.

19. Schultz G. Decision analysis: are calculations and clinicians really on a collision course? *Top Clin Chiro.* 1996;3(1):10–19.
20. Goertz C. Summary of the 1995 ACA annual statistical survey on chiropractic practice. *J Am Chiro Assoc.* 1996;33:35–41.
21. Hillman B. Self-referral for diagnostic imaging. *Radiology.* 1992;185:633–634. Editorial.
22. Curry T, Dowdey J, Murry R. *Christensen's Physics of Diagnostic Radiology.* 4th ed. Malvern, PA: Lea & Febiger; 1990.
23. Krain LS. Some thought about the importance of X-ray exposure histories for patients. *Med Hypotheses.* 1992;37:225–231.
24. Hillman B, Olson G, Griffith P, et al. Physician's utilization and charges for outpatient diagnostic imaging in a Medicare population. *JAMA.* 1992;268:2050–2054.
25. Royal HD. Technology assessment: scientific challenges. *AJR.* 1994;163:503–507.
26. Hildebrant R. Chiropractic spinography and postural roetgenology, II: clinical basis. *J Manipulative Physiol Ther.* 1981;4:191–201.
27. Rupert R. Anatomical measures of standard chiropractic skeletal references (a preliminary report). In: *Proceedings of the Biomechanical Conference of the Spine.* Boulder, CO: Palmer College of Chiropractic, 1980.
28. Nash C, Moe R. A study of vertebral rotation. *J Bone Joint Surg.* 1969;51A:223–229.
29. Phillips R. An evaluation of the graphic analysis of the pelvis on the A-P full-spine radiograph. *J Am Chiro Assoc.* 1975;9:139–148.
30. Davis B, Rozeboom D. A model to test the radiographically determined pelvic subluxation. In: *Proceedings of the Advances in Conservative Health Sciences.* Lombard, IL: National College of Chiropractic Academic press; 1983.
31. Schram S, Hosek R. Error limitations in X-ray kinematics of the spine. *J Manipulative Physiol Ther.* 1982;5:5–10.
32. Rozeboom D. Reliability of full-spine X-ray analysis. In: *Proceedings of the Advances in Conservative Health Sciences.* Lombard, IL: National College of Chiropractic Academic Press; 1983.
33. Sigler D, Howe J. Intra- and interexaminer reliability of the upper cervical marking system. *J Manipulative Physiol Ther.* 1985;8:75–80.
34. Saraste H, Brostrom L, Aparisi T, et al. Radiographic measurement of the lumbar spine: a clinical and experimental study in man. *Spine.* 1985;10:236–241.
35. Schram S, Hosek R, Silverman H. Spinographic positioning errors in Gonstead pelvic X-ray analysis. *J Manipulative Physiol Ther.* 1981;4:179–181.
36. Zengel F, Davis B, Rozeboom D. Lack of effect of projectional distortion on Gonstead vertebral endplate lines. In: *Proceedings of Advances in Conservative Health Sciences.* St. Louis, MO: Academic Press; 1982.
37. Owens E. Line drawing analyses of static cervical X-ray used in chiropractic. *J Manipulative Physiol Ther.* 1992;15:442–449.
38. Messer A, Salsman W, Parker B. The cervical subluxation: its correction and effect upon the body. *J Clin Chiro.* 1972;2:122–135.
39. Grostic J. Grostic procedure seminar notes, Ann Arbor, MI, 1944.
40. Plaugher G, Cremata E, Phillips R. A retrospective consecutive case analysis of pretreatment and comparative static radiological parameters following chiropractic adjustments. *J Manipulative Physiol Ther.* 1990;13:498–506.
41. Keessen W, During J, Beeker T, et al. Recordings of the movements at the intervertebral segments L5-S1: a technique for the determination of the movement in the L5-S1 spinal segment by using three specified postural positions. *Spine.* 1984;9:83–90.
42. Hass M, Nyiedo J. Interrater reliability of roentengenological evaluation of the lumbar spine in lateral bending. *J Manipulative Physiol Ther.* 1990;13:179–189.
43. Coyle B. Errors in X-ray analysis in digitization. *Proceedings from the Conference on Chiropractic Research.* Sunnyvale, CA: Conference on Chiropractic Research, 1987.
44. Anderson R. A radiographic test of upper cervical chiropractic theory. *J Manipulative Physiol Ther.* 1981;4:129–133.
45. Aragona R. *Basic Standard of Practice Procedural Manual Addressing Common Technical ASBE Questions: Standards of Care.* ASBE white paper; 1991.
46. Gay RE. The curve of the cervical spine: variations and significance. *J Manipulative Physiol Ther.* 1993;16:591–594.
47. Mick T. The use of functional radiographs in diagnosis: a literature review. Presented at the Conference on Chiropractic Research and Education, 1992, Palm Springs, CA.
48. Hanssen T, Bigos S, Beecher P, et al. The lumbar lordosis in acute and chronic low back pain. *Spine.* 1985;10:154–155.
49. Frymoyer J, Newberg A, Pope M, et al. Spine radiographs in patients with low back pain. *J Bone Joint Surg.* 1984;66A:1048–1055.
50. Bryner P, Mousalli ME. Lumbar spine lordosis in low back pain: an analysis of radiographs. *Chiro J Aust.* 1992;22:42–46.
51. Jackson RP, McManus AC. Radiographic analysis of sagittal plane alignment and balance in standing volunteers and patients with low back pain matched for age, sex and size: a prospective controlled clinical study. *Spine.* 1994;19:1611–1618.
52. Henderson D, Dorman T. Functional roentgenometric evaluation of the cervical spine in the sagittal plane. *J Manipulative Physiol Ther.* 1985;2:5–15.
53. Prantl K. Examination and functional analysis of the cervical spine. *Manual Med.* 1985;8:219–227.
54. Phillips R, Howe J, Bustin G, et al. Stress X-rays and the low back pain patient. *J Manipulative Physiol Ther.* 1990;13:127–133.
55. Panjabi M, Chang D, Dvorak J. An analysis of errors in kinematic parameters associated with in vivo functional radiographs. *Spine.* 1992;17:200–205.
56. Dvorak J, Panjabi M, Novotny J, et al. Functional radiographic diagnosis of the lumbar spine: flexion-extension and lateral bending. *Spine.* 1991;16:562–571.
57. Boden SD, Weisel SW. Lumbosacral segmental motion in normal individuals: have we been measuring instability properly? *Spine.* 1990;15:571–576.
58. Hayes MA, Howard TC, Gruel CR, et al. Roentgenographic evaluation of lumbar spine flexion-extension in asymptomatic individuals. *Spine.* 1989;14:327–331.
59. Haas M, Nyiendo J, Peterson C, et al. Lumbar motion trends and correlation with low back pain, I: a roentgenological evaluation of coupled lumbar motion in lateral bending. *J Manipulative Physiol Ther.* 1992;15:145–158.
60. Gomez T. Symmetry of lumbar rotation and lateral flexion range of motion and isometric strength in subjects with and without low back pain. *J Orthop Sports Phys Ther.* 1994;19:42–48.
61. Dvorak J, Panjabi M, Novotny J, et al. Clinical validation of functional flexion-extension roentgenograms of the lumbar spine. *Spine.* 1991;16:943–950.
62. Schultz G. A literature review of spinal videofluoroscopy. In: *Proceedings of the Conference on Research and Education for the Consortium for Chiropractic Research,* Monterey, CA: Conference on Research and Education for the Consortium for Chiropractic Research, 1993.

63. Howe J. Cineradiographic evaluation of normal and abnormal cervical spine function. *J Clin Chiro.* 1972;2:76–88.
64. Fielding J. Cineroentgenography of the normal cervical spine. *J Bone Joint Surg.* 1957;59A:1280–1288.
65. Jones M. Cineradiographic studies of the normal cervical spine. *California Med.* 1960;93:293–296.
66. Robinson K. Interpretation of videofluoroscopic joint motion studies in the cervical spine: C2–C7. *Digest Chiro Econ.* 1985;12:126–128.
67. Hubka M. Palpation for spinal tenderness: a reliable and accurate method for determining the target of spinal manipulation. *J Chiro Technique.* 1994;6:5–8.

8
Diagnostic Imaging of the Cervical Spine following Whiplash-Induced Injury

John S. Miller and M. Maggie Craw

Whiplash-induced injuries of the cervical spine are among the most common injuries seen in the chiropractic office today. It has been estimated that up to 1 million such injuries occur each year in the United States,[1,2] most of them the result of rear-end automobile collisions.[2-5] It has been suggested that the mandatory use of seat belts, along with the increased use of shoulder-lap belts, has caused an increase in the incidence of this type of injury,[6,7] although a concomitant decrease in the mortality rate has resulted from their use. In addition, several studies have shown a poor correlation between the use of headrests and a decrease in the severity of posttraumatic symptoms,[8,9] with improper positioning implicated as the cause. When headrests are positioned too low, they may act as a fulcrum for the neck, thereby potentially increasing the severity of injury.[2,5,9]

Many clinical efficacy studies have been conducted regarding the use of diagnostic imaging in the evaluation of neck injuries. These studies have primarily been conducted at emergency care facilities.[7,8,10-18] The main criterion for diagnostic yield in these studies was the detection of fractures, dislocations, and/or gross instability of the spine. Extrapolation to the diagnostic needs of a chiropractor presents a significant challenge. Studies regarding prognostic indicators as well as long-term follow-up studies of whiplash patients are helpful in meeting this challenge. An algorithmic approach to the diagnostic imaging of patients, with the intention of maximizing diagnostic yield while minimizing both patient exposure to ionizing radiation and the cost of evaluation, is presented. A seed algorithm for making decisions about the diagnostic imaging of whiplash-induced injuries was developed by the authors and is presented in Algorithm 1.

DIAGNOSTIC GOALS

The primary goal of diagnostic imaging is to rule out serious injuries such as fracture, dislocation, or gross ligamentous instability, whether in a chiropractic office or a trauma center. The secondary goal of diagnostic imaging is to detect findings that may indicate a need to alter the treatment approach or affect the patient prognosis. A partial list of such conditions includes damage to the intervertebral disc; preexisting pathology, including degenerative changes; congenital anomalies; significant alteration of spinal kinematics; acute kyphotic angulation of the cervical curve; and possibly lesser degrees of cervical kyphosis or severe cervical hypolordosis.

INITIAL DIAGNOSTIC WORK-UP

A thorough history and physical examination are prerequisites for determining clinical indications for diagnostic imaging. The history should include the mechanism of injury, location of pain, type and severity of pain or other symptoms, as well as preaccident factors. The physical examination should ascertain whether palpable tenderness, positive orthopaedic and neurologic findings, or gross biomechanical abnormalities are present. In many cases it is prudent to rule out fracture and dislocation utilizing initial radiographs prior to completing the physical examination. It is also important to note that onset of symptoms often occurs 12 or more hours after the time of accident.[7,8]

The authors thank James Borrow, MD, and Joan Davis, DC, for their assistance in the literature search and grammatical revision respectively.

Adapted from *Top Clin Chiro* 1997; 4(1): 26–33
© 1997 Aspen Publishers, Inc.

SELECTION OF PATIENTS FOR PLAIN FILM RADIOGRAPHY

Although some authors advocate the use of cervical spine radiography on every patient who has sustained a whiplash-induced injury,[12,19,20] we feel that selective criteria can be applied. In prospective studies of 1,000 trauma patients at UCLA[11] and 860 trauma patients at another emergency care facility,[13] there were no fractures found in patients who were alert and asymptomatic at the time of examination. In a prospective study of 408 patients who sustained blunt trauma to the neck, results indicate that routine radiography of the cervical spine may not be efficacious, suggesting that greater reliance should be placed on history and physical examination findings.[14] Other studies show similar results.[10,16,17,21,22] In cases of delayed instability[23] or occult cervical spine injuries,[24] pain and muscle spasm are invariably present at the time of initial evaluation. In reported cases of trauma in the absence of neck symptoms at initial examination, there were usually other significant injuries present,[18,25–27] or mental alertness was altered by intoxication[18,25,28] or other factors.[13,14]

RECOMMENDATIONS FOR PLAIN FILM RADIOGRAPHY

At minimum, a three-view cervical spine radiological survey, consisting of APOM (anteroposterior open mouth), AP lower cervical, and neutral lateral views, is indicated for patients with a whiplash-induced trauma presenting with any of the signs or symptoms noted in Table 1.[29–31] The swimmer's lateral view may be valuable in patients in which C-7 is difficult to evaluate on the neutral lateral view.[32] Additionally, left and right oblique views of the cervical spine are indicated when patients present with the signs and symptoms listed in Table 1. These radiographs should be evaluated prior to obtaining flexion and extension views.

Additionally, if flexion or extension motion of the cervical spine is severely limited, it is recommended that flexion and extension views be postponed until muscle spasm decreases. Failure to do so may result in the inability to detect signs of instability.[24,33]

Stress radiography studies are commonly employed in the evaluation of whiplash-induced traumas. Flexion and extension views are indicated for patients whose three-view or five-view cervical spine studies demonstrate the features listed in Table 2. These stress views are also indicated in patients presenting with any of the history or examination findings listed in Table 2[34–36] irrespective of other imaging findings.

Pillar views are used to visualize the articular columns of the cervical spine and may be appropriate when there is an indication of significant lateral hyperflexion/extension injury or clinical suspicion based on other findings, such as those noted in Table 3.

Table 1. Indications for initial imaging of whiplash-induced trauma

Three-view cervical spine examination (APOM, AP lower cervical, neutral lateral)
- Neck pain
- Palpable cervical spine tenderness
- Palpable paravertebral muscle spasm
- Moderately limited cervical spine range of motion

Oblique views (left and right)
- History of head impact during the trauma
- Severe neck pain
- Severe palpable neck tenderness
- Severely limited cervical spine range of motion
- Altered alertness of any etiology, including intoxication and mental deficit
- Painful injuries elsewhere in the body that may mask cervical spine symptoms
- Radiating pain to the upper extremity
- Numbness or paresthesia
- Loss of muscle strength
- Decreased deep tendon reflex

RADIOGRAPHIC INTERPRETATION

The accuracy of radiographic interpretation is dependent upon radiographs of adequate technical quality.[37] Accuracy in radiographic interpretation in any situation has also been shown to be directly related to the training and experience of the interpreter.[38–40] It is highly recommended that the treating doctor seek the expert opinion of a chiropractic or medical radiologist when the possibility of significant injury is suggested by either clinical or radiographic findings. Finally, it is critically important that improper patient positioning is ruled out as a cause of apparent cervical hypolordosis or kyphosis[41] or other biomechanical alteration. The neutral lateral projection must be obtained when the patient is in a true neutral position (ie, the head is positioned in such a way that the hard palate lies on the horizontal plane).[42]

Accuracy in radiological interpretation requires that a search pattern be utilized. The search pattern noted in Table 4 is recommended when plain film studies are being reviewed because of a history of trauma. The pattern commences with an examination of vertebral alignment following the anterior and posterior body margin lines for evidence of anterolisthesis, retrolisthesis, or acute kyphotic angulation.[43] It also traces the spinous-lamina line; atlanto-dental interval;[44] paraodontoid spaces; C1-2 lateral mass-facet alignment; spinous process alignment on the AP view; and articular pillar alignment on lateral, oblique, or pillar views. The alignment and motion on flexion-extension views may provide other clues, such as intradiscal clefts that may be present on the extension view only,[34,45] retrolisthesis or anterolisthesis manifesting during or increased with flexion

Table 2. Indications for flexion-extension lateral views

Pertinent three-view or five-view cervical spine study findings
- Increased atlanto-dental interval (ADI) (greater than 3 mm in adults and 5 mm in children)
- Anterolisthesis or retrolisthesis of 1 mm or greater
- Acute kyphotic angulation between two adjacent cervical vertebrae
- Intradiscal radiolucency (vacuum or cleft sign)[34]
- Widened interspinous distance (fanning of spinous processes)[35]
- Loss of parallelism of opposing facet surfaces
- Prevertebral soft tissue swelling in the absence of fracture
- Degenerative change
- Spinal anomaly potentially affecting intersegmental range of motion (eg, block vertebra, os odontoideum, spondylolysis, incomplete posterior arch of C-1)
- Surgical or osteomyelitic fusion of two cervical vertebrae

Pertinent history or examination findings
- History of moderate to severe hyperextension injury
- History of a condition with a potential for adversely affecting spinal ligaments (Down's syndrome, inflammatory arthritides, spinal infection)
- Symptoms manifesting during or exacerbated by cervical flexion or extension
- Neurological signs manifesting during or exacerbated by cervical flexion or extension[36]
- Orthopaedic findings manifesting during or exacerbated by cervical flexion or extension

Table 3. Indications for pillar views (articular columns)

- History of significant lateral hyperflexion with extension injury
- Clinical suspicion of fracture not demonstrated on other views
- Questionable appearance of articular pillar on other cervical views
- Widened facet joint space
- Widened uncovertebral joint space

---

or extension, and increased ADI manifesting during or further increased with flexion. Template range of motion evaluation based on flexion lateral and extension films has been advocated by some authors.[46–48]

As the search continues, the doctor looks for alteration in bone, joint spacing, or soft tissue. The doctor should note whether the articular pillar height varies by more than 2 mm compared bilaterally at the same level on pillar views.[49] He or she should also check bony matrix and density, intervertebral disc space height and density, interspinous and interlaminar distances on lateral view, uncovertebral joints on AP and oblique views, and prevertebral soft tissue (retropharyngeal and retrotracheal spaces).[44,50]

SUBACUTE OR DELAYED INSTABILITY

Herkowitz and Rothman define subacute instability as "the development of radiographic evidence of cervical instability within 3 weeks of a cervical spine injury when initial adequate roentgenograms show no body or soft tissue abnormality."[23(p348)] If the initial vertebral displacement is within the elastic range of the tissue, the bone may return to its normal position even when overstretching and damage has occurred. As the tissues continue to stretch after the injury, vertebral displacement may progress to the plastic range of deformation, which is not self-reducing. Radiographs taken at this time should show positive signs of instability. The term *instability* is often misunderstood because of historical misuse and overuse. Instability in this context is defined as a condition with the potential for further soft tissue and possibly neurological damage to occur under conditions that would otherwise be considered normal physiologic loading.[23,51,52] The patient may have initially been assessed as having no signs of instability because of inadequate radiographic evaluation, radiographs of substandard technical quality, protective muscle spasm limiting the range of motion on the flexion-extension films, or a confusing clinical situation masking physical signs of significant damage. A partial list of the radiographic signs of instability includes interspinous distance widening (fanning), facet joint widening, and prevertebral soft tissue swelling.[23,24,35,50,51,53] Excessive vertebral translation (greater than 1–2 mm)[33,53] and focal kyphotic angulation (11° or more than adjacent segments)[52] are also important signs. In patients with neck pain or radicular signs and symptoms that are responding unsatisfactorily to conservative care within a 3- to 4-week period of time or in patients with increasing symptomatology or developing neurologic signs, a radiographic reevaluation to rule out instability may be indicated.[23,54]

PROGNOSTIC SIGNIFICANCE OF RADIOLOGICAL FINDINGS

Preexisting degenerative changes have been found to be associated with a poor prognosis following a whiplash-type trauma. Miles and coworkers found that "degenerative changes are associated with a poor prognosis."[55(p493)] Norris and Watt's conclusion was that "pre-existing degenerative changes in the cervical spine, no matter how slight, do appear to affect the prognosis adversely."[15(p611)] Watkinson and coworkers also

Table 4. Recommended search pattern for radiological interpretation

Alignment of vertebrae
1. Anterior body margin line
2. Posterior body margin line (anterolisthesis, retrolisthesis, or acute kyphotic angulation)[43]
3. Spinous-lamina line
4. Atlanto-dental interval[44]
5. Paraodontoid spaces
6. C1-2 lateral mass-facet alignment
7. Spinous process alignment on AP view
8. Articular pillar alignment on lateral, oblique, or pillar views
9. Alignment and motion on flexion-extension views
   - intradiscal clefts may be present on extension view only[34,45]
   - retrolisthesis or anterolisthesis manifesting during or increased with flexion or extension (excluding evenly distributed stairstepping)
   - increased ADI manifesting during or further increased with flexion
   - template range of motion evaluation as demonstrated on lateral flexion and extension films relative to neutral has been advocated by some authors.[46–48]

Alteration in bone, joint spacing, or soft tissue
1. Articular pillar height should not vary by more than 2 mm compared bilaterally at the same level on pillar views[49]
2. Bony matrix and density
3. Intervertebral disc space height and density
4. Interspinous and interlaminar distances on lateral view
5. Uncovertebral joints on AP and oblique views
6. Prevertebral soft tissue (retropharyngeal and retrotracheal spaces)[44,50]

---

found that "patients with degenerative changes initially have more symptoms after 2 years than those with normal radiographs at the time of injury."[56(p308)] Similar findings were reported by Radanov and coworkers[57] and Maimaris and coworkers.[8] Conversely, Hildingsson and Toolanen[58] did not find degenerative change to be prognostically unfavorable. Additionally, Greenfield and Ilfeld[59] found that degenerative changes in the older patient did not affect recovery; however, this may imply that all other patients were affected. On a related topic, a higher incidence of preexisting degenerative findings was present in patients who had demonstrated delayed instability. It is thought that degenerative changes may weaken the ligament, causing delayed plastic deformation following initial elastic deformation.[23]

Acute or focal kyphotic angulation of the cervical curve is well accepted as an indicator of potential ligamentous damage.[24,44] In a 5- to 7-year follow-up study of whiplash cases, Hohl[60] found a higher incidence of degenerative changes in patients who demonstrated a sharp reversal of the cervical curve upon initial evaluation. Hohl also noted that patients with restricted motion at one intervertebral level, as demonstrated using flexion-extension films, tended to have poorer symptomatic recovery and increased incidence of degenerative changes. The significance of lesser degrees of cervical kyphosis or hypolordosis remain controversial. Norris and Watt[15] concluded that patients with altered cervical curves remained symptomatic longer. Conversely, Greenfield and Ilfeld[59] reported no relationship between subjective recovery percentage and cervical hypolordosis or kyphosis. Hildingsson and Toolanen[58] also found no significant relationship between cervical hypolordosis or kyphosis and the development of persistent symptoms in a cervical trauma series. More specific to kyphosis, Maimaris and coworkers[8] reported no association between cervical kyphosis and prolonged disability. Surprisingly, Miles and coworkers[55] found kyphotic angulation to be associated with a good prognosis, although this finding is possibly related to age, as the kyphotic patients in their study were generally younger.

COMPUTERIZED TOMOGRAPHY

Computerized tomography (CT) is well accepted as a valuable imaging technique in the evaluation of cervical spine trauma. Examples of the use of CT in spinal trauma in the literature are numerous.[61–65] CT has good spatial and contrast resolution, providing better soft tissue than either plain film radiography or conventional tomography. While the soft tissue contrast of CT is inferior to that of magnetic resonance imaging (MRI), its ability to demonstrate osseous detail remains superior. An additional advantage of CT is that it provides direct axial imaging, multiplanar reconstruction, and three-dimensional reconstruction without necessitating changes in patient position. In addition, both examination time and patient radiation dose are decreased relative to conventional tomography.[62]

The sensitivity of CT in the detection of fractures has been found to be between 78% and 100%.[63,66–69] The sensitivity levels have generally been established through axial imaging alone. The use of thin section CT (1.5 mm), in conjunction with coronal and sagittal reformatted images, most likely places the true sensitivity of CT toward the higher end of this range.[54]

There are inherent limitations in the use of CT in the evaluation of cervical spine trauma. Dislocations, spondylolisthesis, and subtle alignment abnormalities suggesting ligamentous injury may be more difficult to recognize on sequential axial images than on plain film or conventional tomographic images. Horizontally oriented fractures may also be difficult to detect on axial images,[64,70] although the use of multiplanar and three-dimensional reconstruction appears to improve CT sensitivity in detecting these abnormalities.[62,63,66,67,71,72] In addition, the spinal cord and contiguous soft tissue structures are sometimes poorly demonstrated without benefit of intrathecal enhancement, resulting in a failure to demonstrate lesions such as cord transection or contusion, dural tears, nerve root avulsions, and herniated discs.[65]

Indications for ordering CT for patients with whiplash-induced injuries are listed in Table 5. CT has been found to help in detecting fractures demonstrated or suggested on standard radiographs[63,66] or for evaluating patients where there is a high degree of clinical suspicion of bony injury.[54,63,73] CT is also appropriate for examining areas not well visualized on plain films (typically the craniovertebral junction and cervicothoracic junction)[14,74,75] and in cases in which craniovertebral junction fracture or dislocation is suspected.

CT MYELOGRAPHY

CT myelography has generally been replaced by MRI for the evaluation of the spinal canal and related soft tissue structures.[71] Although both techniques may show discogenic disease and quantify thecal sac and cord compromise, MRI is uniquely able to evaluate internal cord architecture and detect subtle cord contusions. While CT myelography is valuable in the evaluation of nerve root avulsion and dural tears,[71,76,77] it is used primarily when MRI is not available or cannot be performed.[76]

MAGNETIC RESONANCE IMAGING

Although the applications of MRI continue to evolve, its role as an adjunctive procedure in the radiological evaluation of patients with cervical spine trauma is well established. The primary advantages of MRI are its soft tissue resolution and its ability to directly obtain sagittal images.[78,79] Many studies have been done to determine when MRI is most valuable.[62,80–86] The consensus is that it is clearly superior to other imaging modalities in the evaluation of soft tissue. As a result, it is emerging as the modality of choice following plain film radiography in the evaluation of the spinal cord, intervertebral discs, and spinal ligaments and of patients with neurologic deficit.[54,76,87] The tomographic capability of MRI is also helpful in visualizing the cervicothoracic junction and in surveying long segments of the spine.[82]

MRI is the only imaging modality capable of directly demonstrating evidence of intrinsic spinal cord injury.[54,78,87] A spectrum of spinal cord injuries ranging from mild edema to complete cord transection and including delayed sequelae of spinal trauma such as atrophy and syringomyelia can be detected.[54,88–90] Intramedullary hematomas (acute cord hemorrhage) and intramedullary edema (nonhemorrhagic cord contusion) can be recognized and differentiated.[54,63,81,86,88–92] The differentiation of spinal cord hemorrhage from edema has important clinical implications. Patients with acute hematoma typically have no neurologic function below the level of hemorrhage, with an associated poor prognosis for motor recovery,[54,81,85,87,89,90] while patients with intramedullary edema often demonstrate significant neurologic improvement.[81,84,85,87,89] In addition, the prognosis for motor recovery in patients with localized cord edema is better than for patients with extensive cord edema.[63,81–83,88–90,92]

MRI permits noninvasive evaluation of intervertebral discs and as a result plays an important role in the detection of traumatic disc herniation. The current recognition of the frequent association of unstable spinal injuries with acute disc herniation is a result of increased use of MRI in patients with spinal injury.[80,82]

A role is also emerging for MRI in the detection of isolated ligamentous injuries. Although these injuries are usually discovered as a result of the investigation of other abnormalities, injuries of the anterior longitudinal ligament, posterior longitudinal ligament, ligamentum flavum, and interspinous ligaments may be evident on MRI images.[76,78,81,87,93] The early detection of these injuries is critical in identifying patients at risk for delayed instability.[79,82,93]

However, MRI is not without disadvantages. Its resolution of osseous structures is inferior to that of CT.[76] While most fractures and dislocations are demonstrated using MRI, its ability to depict vertebral arch fractures is limited.[83,86] MRI examination times are relatively long. This creates difficulties for the acutely injured patient and leads to increased motion artifact. In addition, patients with magnetic resonance–incompatible life-support systems and orthopaedic traction devices cannot be scanned. Advances in the development of magnetic resonance–compatible equipment are diminishing this problem.[71,94]

In most cases, the contraindication for MRI is related to magnetic field effects, such as cochlear implants, metallic foreign bodies in the eye, ferromagnetic heart valves, intracranial aneurysm clips, intrauterine devices with metallic loops, permanent TENS units, and some cardiac pacemakers. Additionally, because of the relatively small bore size,

Table 5. Indications for CT following whiplash-induced injury

- Further evaluation of fractures demonstrated or suggested on standard radiographs[63,66]
- Further evaluation of equivocal plain film findings
- Further evaluation of patients who have normal plain films but for whom there is a high degree of clinical suspicion of bony injury[54,63,73]
- For completion of radiographic evaluation in areas not well visualized on plain films (typically the craniovertebral junction and cervicothoracic junction)[14,74,75]
- In cases of suspected craniovertebral junction fracture or dislocation

patients with claustrophobia and obese patients are not good candidates for examination in high field scanners. It is generally recommended that pregnant women not undergo MRI unless absolutely necessary because of the uncertainty of its effects on the fetus. Most orthopaedic implants do not constitute a contraindication, but they do contribute to image degradation.

Clinical indications for ordering MRI for patients with whiplash-induced injuries are listed in Table 6. The test is indicated as a follow-up for patients with fractures or dislocations that have a potential for direct cord injury or canal compromise or as a mean of evaluating patients whose plain film or clinical findings suggest severe ligamentous injury.[76,83] MRI should be considered for patients demonstrating neurologic deficit not explained by plain film or CT findings,[71,76,83] those who develop delayed or progressive neurologic deficit, or those who present with signs of myelopathy.

MYELOGRAPHY

The use of myelography for purposes of diagnosis has become very limited since the advent of CT and MRI. Myelography is an invasive procedure that necessitates the subarachnoid injection of contrast material. Hypersensitivity reactions, infection, and bleeding are known complications. In most instances, myelography is the modality of choice only when CT or MRI is unavailable.

CONVENTIONAL TOMOGRAPHY

Conventional tomography plays a limited role as an adjunct to plain film radiography. It is useful in the demonstration of axially oriented fractures such as odontoid and lateral mass fractures,[62,69,71,76,79,95] facet fractures,[69,76] some vertebral body fractures,[69] and some laminar fractures.[76] Conventional tomography may also be of value in imaging multilevel trauma.[76,79,95] However, CT or MRI is recommended over conventional tomography in the evaluation of the posttraumatic cervical spine.

Table 6. Indications for MRI following whiplash-induced injury

- Follow-up of patients with fractures or dislocations with a potential for direct cord injury or canal compromise
- Assessment of patients whose plain film or clinical findings suggest severe ligamentous injury[76,83]
- Evaluation of patients demonstrating neurologic deficit not explained by plain film or CT findings[71,76,83]
- Evaluation of patients who develop delayed or progressive neurologic deficit
- Evaluation of patients with signs of myelopathy
- Evaluation of patients with signs of radiculopathy not satisfactorily responding to conservative care

CONCLUSION

Plain film radiography remains the imaging modality of choice for the initial evaluation of patients with whiplash-induced cervical spine injuries. The number and type of radiographs needed should be determined by the clinical indicators for each patient. CT follow-up is recommended when plain films demonstrate or suggest a fracture or dislocation or when findings on a comprehensive plain film study are equivocal. CT is especially valuable in the evaluation of axially oriented fractures and fractures and dislocations of the craniovertebral junction. MRI is emerging as the examination of choice for demonstrating the spinal cord, intervertebral discs, and spinal ligaments and for trauma patients manifesting neurological symptoms. The roles of myelography and conventional tomography are limited. In situations where plain film findings are equivocal, clinical findings suggest occult injury, or advanced imaging is being considered, consultation with a chiropractic or medical radiologist is recommended.

REFERENCES

1. Evans RW. Some observations on whiplash injuries. *Neurol Clin.* 1992;10:975–996.
2. O'Neil B, Haddon W Jr, Kelley AB, et al. Automobile head restraints: frequency of neck injury claims in relation to the presence of head restraints. *Am J Public Health.* 1972;62:399–406.
3. Deans GT, McGalliard JN, Rutherford WH. Incidence and duration of neck pain amoung patients injured in car accidents. *Br Med J.* 1986;292:94–95.
4. Galasko CS, Murray PM, Pitcher M, et al. Neck sprains after road accidents: a modern epidemic. *Injury.* 1993;24:155–157.
5. Porter KM. Neck sprains after car accidents: a common cause of long-term disability. *Br Med J.* 1989;298:973–974.
6. Bourbeau R, Desjardins D, Maag U, et al. Neck injuries among belted and unbelted occupants of the front seat of cars. *J Trauma.* 1993;35:794–799.
7. Deans GT, Magalliard JN, Kerr M, et al. Neck sprain: a major cause of disability following car accidents. *Injury.* 1987;18:10–12.
8. Maimaris C, Barnes MR, Allen MJ. "Whiplash injuries" of the neck: a retrospective study. *Injury.* 1988;19:393–396.
9. Olney DB, Marsden AK. The effect of head restraints and seat belts on the incidence of neck injury in car accidents. *Injury.* 1986;17:365–367.
10. Fischer RP. Cervical radiographic evaluation of alert patients following blunt trauma. *Ann Emerg Med.* 1984;13:905–907.

11. Hoffman JR, Schriger DL, Mower W, et al. Low-risk criteria for cervical-spine radiography in blunt trauma: a prospective study. *Ann Emerg Med.* 1992;21:1454–1460.
12. Jacobs LM, Schwartz R. Prospective analysis of acute cervical spine injury: a methodology to predict injury. *Ann Emerg Med.* 1986;15:44–49.
13. Kreipke DL, Gillespie KR, McCarthy MC, et al. Reliability of indications for cervical spine films in trauma patients. *J Trauma.* 1989;29:1438–1439.
14. Mirvis SE, Diaconis JN, Chirico PA, et al. Protocol-driven radiologic evaluation of suspected cervical spine injury: efficacy study. *Radiology.* 1989;170:831–834.
15. Norris SH, Watt I. The prognosis of neck injuries resulting from rear-end vehicle collisions. *J Bone Joint Surg.* 1983;65B:608–611.
16. Ringenberg BJ, Fisher AK, Urdaneta LF, et al. Rational ordering of cervical spine radiographs following trauma. *Ann Emerg Med.* 1988;17:792–796.
17. Roberge RJ, Wears RC, Kelly M, et al. Selective application of cervical spine radiography in alert victims of blunt trauma: a prospective study. *J Trauma.* 1988;28:784–788.
18. Walter J, Doris PE, Shaffer MA. Clinical presentation of patients with acute cervical spine injury. *Ann Emerg Med.* 1984;13:512–515.
19. Gebhard JS, Donaldson DH, Brown CW. Soft-tissue injuries of the cervical spine. *Orthop Rev.* May 1994 (suppl):9–17.
20. Woodring JH, Lee C. Limitations of cervical radiography in the evaluation of acute cervical trauma. *J Trauma.* 1993;34:32–39.
21. Bachulis BL, Long WB, Hynes GD, et al. Clinical indications for cervical spine radiographs in the traumatized patient. *Am J Surg.* 1987;153:473–478.
22. Cadoux CG, White JD, Hedberg MC. High-yield roentgenographic criteria for cervical spine injuries. *Ann Emerg Med.* 1987;16:738–742.
23. Herkowitz HN, Rothman RH. Subacute instability of the cervical spine. *Spine.* 1984;9:348–357.
24. Webb JK, Broughton BK, McSweeney T, et al. Hidden flexion injury of the cervical spine. *J Bone Joint Surg.* 1976;58B:322–367.
25. Bresler MJ, Rich GH. Occult cervical spine fracture in an ambulatory patient. *Ann Emerg Med.* 1982;11:440–442.
26. Maull KI, Sachatello CR. Avoiding a pitfall in resuscitation: the painless cervical fracture. *South Med J.* 1977;70:477–478.
27. Nash CL. Acute cervical soft-tissue injury and late deformity. *J Bone Joint Surg.* 1979;61A:305–307.
28. Thambyrajah K. Fractures of the cervical spine with minimal or no symptoms. *Med J Malaysia.* 1972;26:244–249.
29. Davis JW, Phreaner DL, Hoyt DB, et al. The etiology of missed cervical spine injuries. *J Trauma.* 1993;34:342–346.
30. Spitzer WO, Skovron ML, Salmi LR, et al. Scientific monograph of the Quebec Task Force on Whiplash-associated Disorders: redefining "whiplash" and its management. *Spine.* 1995;20(suppl):1S–73S.
31. Wales LR, Knopp RK, Morishima MS. Recommendations for evaluation of the acutely injured cervical spine: a clinical radiologic algorithm. *Ann Emerg Med.* 1980;9:422–428.
32. MacDonald RL, Schwartz ML, Mirch D, et al. Diagnosis of cervical spine injury in motor vehicle crash victims: how many X-rays are enough. *J Trauma.* 1990;30:392–397.
33. Scher AT. Anterior cervical subluxation: an unstable position. *AJR.* 1979;133:275–280.
34. Reymond RD, Wheeler PS, Perovic M, et al. The lucent cleft, a new radiographic sign of cervical disk injury or disease. *Clin Radiol.* 1972;23:188–192.
35. Griffiths HJ, Olson PN, Everson LI, et al. Hyperextension strain or "whiplash" injuries to the cervical spine. *Skeletal Radiol.* 1995;24:263–266.
36. Harris WH, Hamblen DL, Ojemann RG. Traumatic disruption of cervical intervertebral disk from hyperextension injury. *Clin Orthop.* 1968;60:163–167.
37. Gerrelts BD, Petersen EU, Mabry J, et al. Delayed diagnosis of cervical spine injuries. *J Trauma.* 1991;31:1622–1626.
38. Annis JA, Finlay DB, Allen MJ, et al. A review of cervical-spine radiographs in casualty patients. *Br J Radiol.* 1987;60:1059–1061.
39. Mayhue FE, Rust DD, Aldag JC, et al. Accuracy of interpretations of emergency department radiographs: effect of confidence levels. *Ann Emerg Med.* 1989;18:826–830.
40. Taylor JA, Clopton P, Bosch E, et al. Interpretation of abnormal lumbosacral spine radiographs. *Spine.* 1995;20:1147–1154.
41. Juhl JH, Miller SM, Roberts GW. Roentgenographic variations in the normal cervical spine. *Radiology.* 1962;78:591–597.
42. Borden AG, Rechtman AM, Gershon-Cohen J. The normal cervical lordosis. *Radiology.* 1960;74:806–809.
43. Bohrer SP, Chen YM, Sayers DG. Cervical spine flexion patterns. *Skeletal Radiol.* 1990;19:521–525.
44. Clark WM, Gehweiler JA, Laib R. Twelve significant signs of cervical spine trauma. *Skeletal Radiol.* 1979;3:201–205.
45. Taylor JR, Twomey LT. Acute injuries to cervical joints. *Spine.* 1993;18:1115–1122.
46. Dvorak J, Froehlick D, Penning L, et al. Functional radiograph diagnosis of the cervical spine: flexion/extension. *Spine.* 1988;13:748–755.
47. Henderson DJ, Dorman TM. Functional roentgenometric evaluation of the cervical spine in the sagittal plane. *J Manipulative Physiol Ther.* 1985;8:219–227.
48. Penning L. Normal movements of the cervical spine. *AJR.* 1978;130:317–326.
49. Vines FS. The significance of "occult" fractures of the cervical spine. *AJR.* 1969;107:493–504.
50. Penning L. Prevertebral hematoma in cervical spine injury: incidence and etiologic significance. *AJR.* 1981;136:553–561.
51. Daffner RH, Deeb ZL, Goldberg AL, et al. The radiologic assessment of post-traumatic vertebral stability. *Skeletal Radiol.* 1990;19:103–108.
52. White AA, Johnson RM, Panjabi MM, et al. Biomechanical analysis of clinical stability in the cervical spine. *Clin Orthop.* 1975;109:85–96.
53. Green JD, Harle TS, Harris JH. Anterior subluxation of the cervical spine: hyperflexion sprain. *AJNR.* 1981;2:243–250.
54. Cornelius RS, Leach JL. Imaging evaluation of cervical spine trauma. *Neuroimaging Clin N Am.* 1995;5:451–463.
55. Miles KA, Maimaris C, Finaly D, et al. The incidence and prognostic significance of radiological abnormalities in soft tissue injuries of the cervical spine. *Skeletal Radiol.* 1988;17:493–496.
56. Watkinson A, Gargan MF, Bannister GC. Prognostic factors in soft tissue injuries of the cervical spine. *Injury.* 1991;22:307–309.
57. Radanov BP, Sturzenegger M, Di Stefano G. Long-term outcome after whiplash injury. *Medicine.* 1995;74:281–297.
58. Hildingsson C, Toolanen G. Outcome after soft-tissue injury of the cervical spine. *Acta Orthop Scand.* 1990;61:357–359.
59. Greenfield J, Ilfeld FW. Acute cervical strain, evaluation and short-term prognostic factors. *Clin Orthop.* 1977;122:196–200.
60. Hohl M. Soft-tissue injuries of the neck in automobile accidents. *J Bone Joint Surg.* 1974;56A:1675–1682.
61. Clark CR, Igram CM, El-Khoury GY, et al. Radiographic evaluation of cervical spine injuries. *Spine.* 1988;13:742–747.

62. Harris JH. Radiologic evaluation of spinal trauma. *Orthop Clin N Am.* 1986;17:75–86.
63. Kaye JJ, Nance EP Jr. Cervical spine trauma. *Orthop Clin N Am.* 1990;21:449–462.
64. Post MJ, Green BA, Quencer RM. The value of computed tomography in spinal trauma. *Spine.* 1982;7:417–431.
65. Post MJ, Green BA. The use of computed tomography in spinal trauma. *Radiol Clin N Am.* 1983;21:327–374.
66. Acheson MB, Livingston RR, Richardson ML, et al. High resolution CT scanning in the evaluation of cervical spine fractures: comparison with plain film examinations. *AJR.* 1987;148:1179–1185.
67. Borock EC, Gabram SG, Jacobs LM, et al. A prospective analysis of a two-year experience using computed tomography as an adjunct for cervical spine clearance. *J Trauma.* 1991;31:1001–1006.
68. Schleehauf K, Ross SE, Civil ID, et al. Computed tomography in the initial evaluation of the cervical spine. *Ann Emerg Med.* 1989;18:815–817.
69. Woodring JH, Lee C. The role and limitations of computed tomographic scanning in the evaluation of cervical trauma. *J Trauma.* 1992;33:698–708.
70. Lynch D, McManus F, Ennis JT. Computed tomography in spinal trauma. *Clin Radiol.* 1986;37:71–76.
71. Pathria MN, Petersilge CA. Spinal trauma. *Radiol Clin N Am.* 1991;29:847–865.
72. Wojcik WG, Eideken-Monroe BS, Harris JE. Three-dimensional computed tomography in acute cervical spine: a preliminary report. *Skeletal Radiol.* 1987;16:261–269.
73. Bachulis BL, Long WB, Hynes GD, et al. Clinical indications for cervical spine radiographs in the traumatized patient. *Am J Surg.* 1987;153:473–477.
74. Maravilla KR, Cooper PR, Sklar FH. The influence of thin-section tomography in the treatment of cervical spine injuries. *Radiology.* 1978;127:131–139.
75. Tehranzadeh J, Kerr R, Amster J. Magnetic resonance imaging of tendon and ligament abnormalities: spine and upper extremities. *Skeletal Radiol.* 1992;21:1–9.
76. Murphey MD, Batnitzky S, Bramble JM. Diagnostic imaging of spinal trauma. *Radiol Clin N Am.* 1989;27:855–872.
77. Volle E, Assheuer J, Hedde JP, et al. Radicular avulsion resulting from spinal injury: assessment of diagnostic modalities. *Neuroradiology.* 1992;34:235–240.
78. Hall AJ, Wagle VG, Raycroft J, et al. Magnetic resonance imaging in cervical spine trauma. *J Trauma.* 1993;34:21–26.
79. Tehranzadeh J, Palmer S. Imaging of cervical spine trauma. *Seminars in Ultrasound, CT and MRI.* 1996;17:93–104.
80. Davis SJ, Teresi LM, Bradley WG, et al. Cervical spine hyperextension injuries: MR findings. *Radiology.* 1991;180:245–251.
81. Flanders AE, Schaefer DM, Doan HT, et al. Acute cervical spine trauma: correlation of MR imaging findings with degree of neurologic deficit. *Radiology.* 1990;177:25–33.
82. Goldberg AL, Rothfus WE, Deeb ZL, et al. The impact of magnetic resonance on the diagnostic evaluation of acute cervicothoracic spinal trauma. *Skeletal Radiol.* 1988;17:89–95.
83. Goldberg AL, Rothfus WE, Deeb ZL, et al. Hyperextension injuries of the cervical spine: magnetic resonance findings. *Skeletal Radiol.* 1989;18:283–288.
84. Kulkarni MV, McArdre CB, Ropanicky D, et al. Acute spinal cord injury: MR imaging at 1.5 T. *Radiology.* 1987;164:837–843.
85. Mirvis SE, Geisler FH, Jelinek JJ, et al. Acute cervical spine trauma: evaluation with 1.5-T MR imaging. *Radiology.* 1988;166:807–816.
86. Silberstein M, Tress BM, Hennessy O. A comparison between MRI and CT in acute spinal trauma. *Australas Radiol.* 1992;36:192–197.
87. El-Khoury GY, Kathol MH, Daniel WW. Imaging of acute injuries of the cervical spine: value of plain radiography, CT, and MR imaging. *AJR.* 1995;164:43–49.
88. Beers GJ, Raque GH, Wagner GG, et al. MR imaging in acute cervical spine trauma. *J Comput Assist Tomogr.* 1988;12:755–761.
89. Schaefer DM, Flanders A, Northrup BE, et al. Magnetic resonance imaging of acute cervical spine trauma: correlation with severity of neurologic injury. *Spine.* 1989;14:1090–1095.
90. Schaefer DM, Flanders AE, Osterholm JI, et al. Prognostic significance of magnet resonance imaging in the acute phase of cervical spine injury. *J Neurosurg.* 1982;76:218–223.
91. Goldberg L, Daffner RH, Schapiro RL. Imaging of acute spinal trauma: an evolving multi-modality approach. *Clin Imaging.* 1990;14:11–16.
92. Tarr RW, Drolshagen LF, Kerner TC, et al. MR imaging of recent spinal trauma. *J Comput Assist Tomogr.* 1987;11:412–417.
93. Silberstein M, Tress BM, Hennessy O. Prevertebral swelling in cervical spine injury: identification of ligament injury with magnetic resonance imaging. *Clin Radiol.* 1992;46:318–323.
94. Beale SM, Pathria MN, Masaryk TJ. Magnetic resonance imaging of spinal trauma. *Top Magn Reson Imaging.* 1988;1:53–62.
95. Binet EF, Moro JJ, Marangola JP. Cervical spine tomography in trauma. *Spine.* 1977;2:163–172.

Algorithm 1

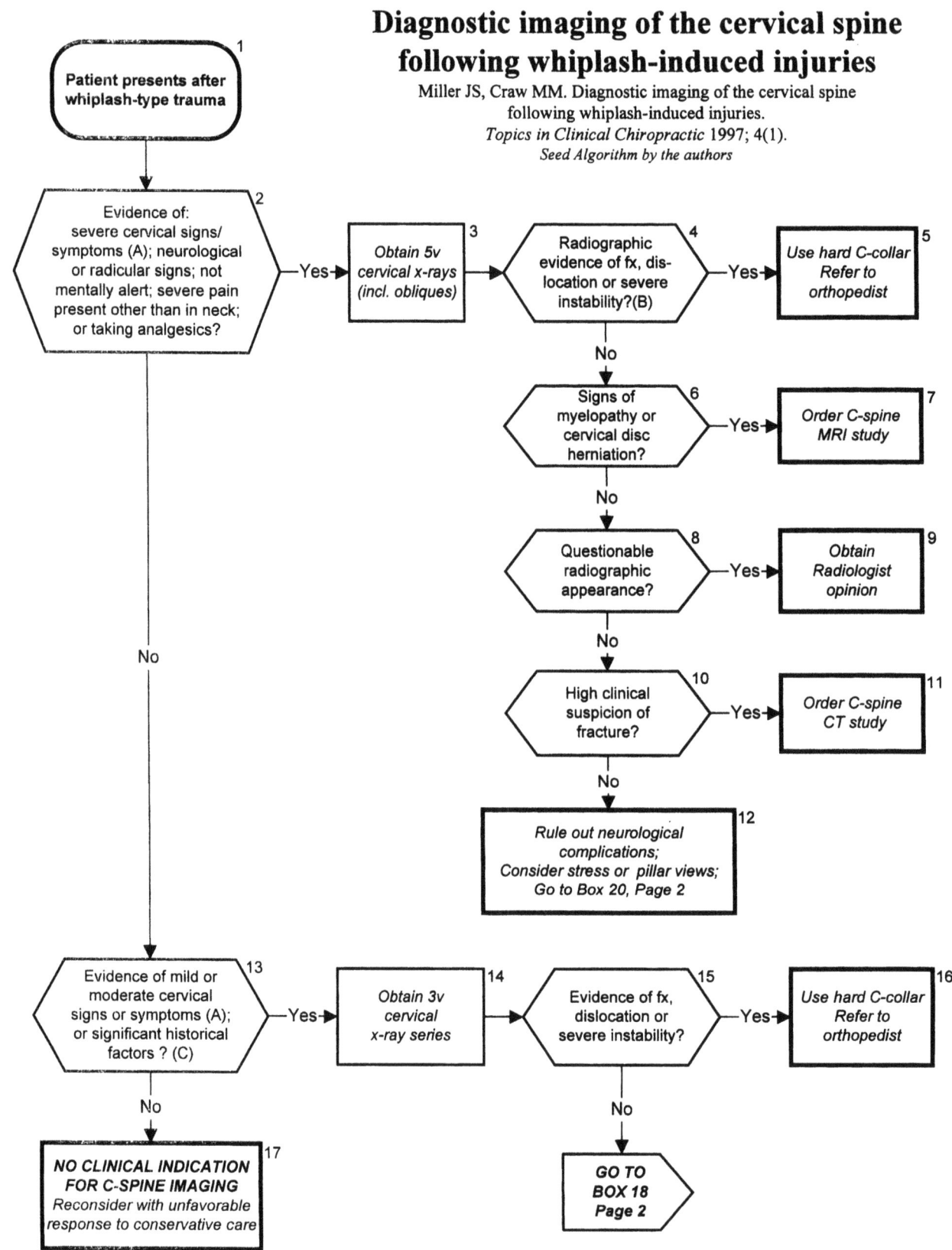

Algorithm 1, continued

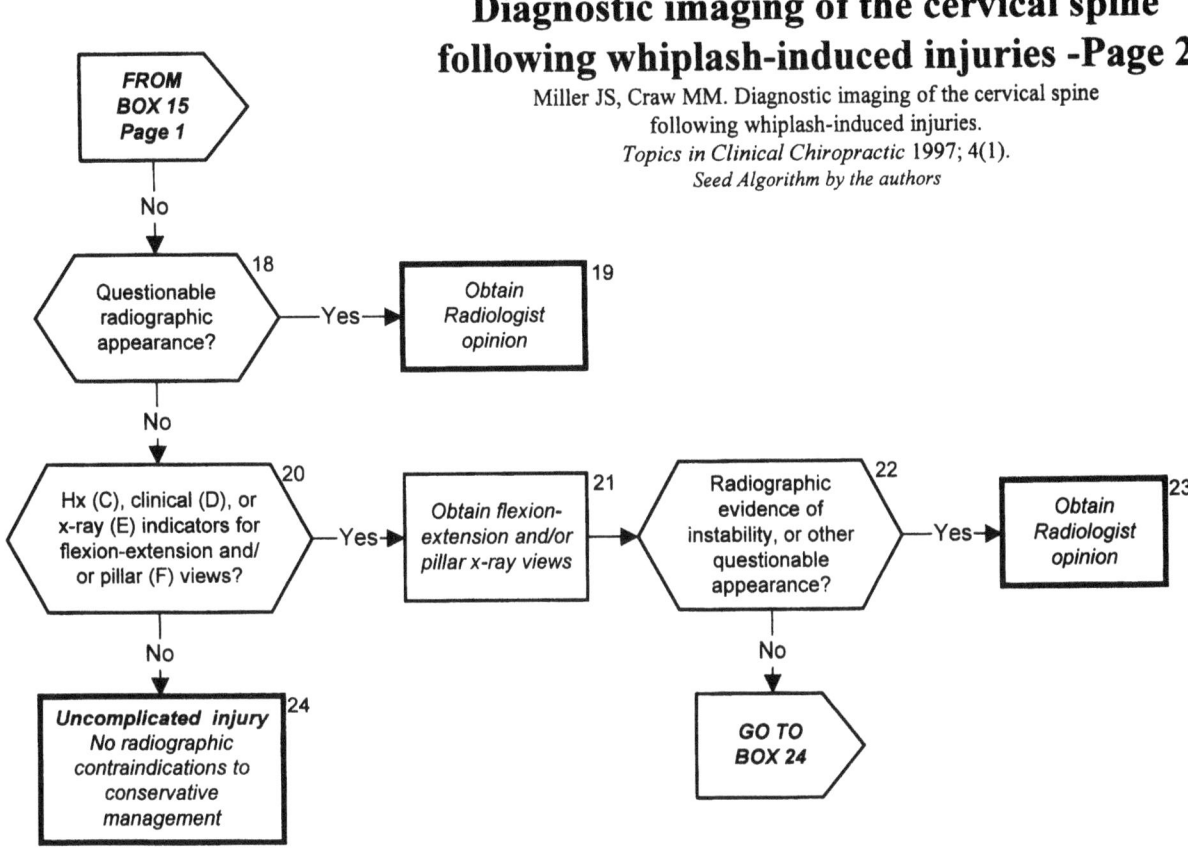

Diagnostic imaging of the cervical spine following whiplash-induced injuries -Page 2

Miller JS, Craw MM. Diagnostic imaging of the cervical spine following whiplash-induced injuries.
Topics in Clinical Chiropractic 1997; 4(1).
Seed Algorithm by the authors

Annotations:
(A) Significant cervical spine physical signs: palpable tenderness; decreased active range of motion; painful range of motion; palpable paraspinal muscle spasm.
(B) Radiographic signs of severe cervical spine instability without fracture or dislocation: anterolisthesis or retrolisthesis greater than 3.5mm; kyphotic angulation between any two vertebrae that is 11 degrees greater than the angulation between the other adjacent vertebrae; perching of articular facets (almost dislocated); atlantodental interval of 1 cm or greater.
(C) Significant history indicating need for flexion/extension views may include: moderate/severe whiplash trauma; inflammatory arthritis; previous c-spine disc herniation, surgery, or infection; Down's syndrome.
(D) Clinical findings indicating need for flexion-extension views: symptoms or orthopedic findings manifesting during or increased by cervical flexion or extension; neurological signs manifesting during or increased by cervical flexion or extension; severe neck spasm. Flexion/extension films need to be delayed until reduction of neck spasm allows sufficient ROM to adequately accomplish the study. Neck immobilization may temporarily be needed if suspicion of instability exists.
(E) Radiographic findings indicating need for flexion/extension views: increased atlantodental interval (ADI>3mm in adults or 5mm in children); anterolisthesis or retrolisthesis of at least 1mm; acute kyphotic angulation between any two cervical vertebrae; intradiscal radiolucency (vacuum or lucent cleft sign); fanning of spinous processes (increased interspinous distance); loss of parallelism of opposing facet surfaces; soft tissue swelling in the absence of fracture; degenerative findings; or cervical spine anomalies which may affect ROM (e.g., os odontoideum, incomplete posterior arch of C1, block vertebra, spondylolysis); acquired intervertebral fusion.
(F) Clinical indicators for pillar views: Hx of significant lateral hyperflexion with extension injury; clinical suspicion of fracture not demonstrated on other views; questionable appearance of articular pillar, widened facet joint space, or widened uncovertebral joint space see on other views.

9

Imaging Modalities for the Lumbar Spine

Sandra M. O'Connor, William S.W. Hsu, and Constance Columbus

It has been reported that 80% to 90% of the population will experience low back pain at one time or another. In fact, this disorder accounts for 40% of all absences from work.[1,2] The diagnosis and management of low back pain are complicated by the difficulty posed in identifying the cause of the pain precisely and isolating it to a specific anatomic site.[3] Fortunately, most acute low back pain results from mechanical problems and is self-limiting in nature.[3] Further investigation is warranted when the condition does not respond to conservative measures in the expected time frame.

The primary role of diagnostic imaging is to gain additional clinical information that can be used in conjunction with the history and physical examination to enable the clinician to formulate a diagnosis and recommend a plan of management. The biggest challenge to the clinician is deciding if imaging is necessary and which imaging modality will provide the most relevant information quickly, inexpensively, and least invasively.[4]

The standard methods of imaging used in the evaluation of lumbar disorders include plain film radiography, myelography, computed tomography (CT), CT-myelography, magnetic resonance imaging (MRI), and radionuclide bone imaging. This chapter provides a brief overview of these imaging modalities and discusses their roles in the assessment of various disorders of the lumbar spine.

PLAIN FILM RADIOGRAPHY

Plain film radiography is often the first imaging procedure performed in the assessment of low back disorders. It is convenient for both the clinician and the patient in that it is readily accessible in both large and small communities and is relatively inexpensive.[5,6] Plain film radiographs of the spine provide valuable diagnostic information relative to the structural and biomechanical integrity of the spine as well as the presence of underlying pathology. Deyo and Diehl[7] report a 90% sensitivity in the ability to detect degenerative and inflammatory diseases, fractures, infections, and neoplasms using plain film radiography in high-risk groups presenting with low back pain. Pain referred to the low back from visceral origin, such as urolithiasis, cholelithiasis, or abdominal aortic aneurysm (Fig 1) can also be detected on plain film radiographs.

Plain film radiography is not without its limitations and potential risks, however. Routine views of the lumbar spine are relatively insensitive in detecting disorders such as spinal stenosis, disc herniations, spinal cord abnormalities, and early bone destruction. A standard five-view series of the lumbar spine can deliver a 2 to 2.5 rad exposure to the skin and is one of the highest doses of any radiologic examination to the gonads.[8,9] Therefore, careful consideration should be given to the necessity of these examinations and whether the information provided will affect the treatment outcome of that patient.

In a recent review article, Simmons and colleagues[10] suggest that radiographs are not necessary for a first episode of low back pain present for less than 7 weeks in low-risk population groups. Table 1 outlines a list of exceptions to this general guideline.

In the initial assessment of low back disorders, a minimum plain film examination of the lumbar spine consists of frontal and lateral views.[11] If indicated, these views can be followed by supplementary films such as oblique views for assessment of the neural arches, an angulated frontal spot view (Hibbs' view) to view the sacroiliac joints, or motion studies to determine the presence of biomechanical abnormalities.

Reprinted from *Top Clin Chiro* 1996; 3(3): 32–44
© 1996 Aspen Publishers, Inc.

Table 1. Indications for lumbar radiography

Atypical history
- Age over 65
- High risk for osteoporosis
- Symptoms of urinary tract dysfunction
- Persisting sensory deficit
- Worsening pain despite adequate treatment
- Intense pain at rest
- Worsening pain at night
- Fever, chills
- Unexplained weight loss
- History of injury or repetitive injury to cause acute or stress fracture
- Recurrent back pain with no radiographs in the past 2 years
- Previous lumbar surgery or fracture
- History of radiographic abnormality reported to patient but no films or report available
- History of finding from another diagnostic study (eg, bone scan) that requires radiograph for correlation
- Patient unable to give a reliable history

Atypical physical findings
- Significant motor deficit
- Unexplained deformity

Psychologic or social circumstances
- Crippling cancerphobia focused on back pain
- Inability to secure another evaluation within 7 weeks from the onset of pain
- Need for immediate decision about career or athletic future
- High risk for violent injury
- Need for legal evaluation

Source: Adapted with permission from Simmons ED, Guyer RD, Graham-Smith A, Herzog R. Contemporary concepts in spine care: radiographic assessment for patients with low back pain. *Spine.* 1995;20:1839–1841. © 1995, Lippincott Williams & Wilkins.

MYELOGRAPHY

Myelography is an invasive procedure involving the injection of radiopaque contrast material into the subarachnoid space. This injection allows the thecal sac and nerve roots to be visualized on plain film radiographs or under fluoroscopy. Any compression on the thecal sac or nerve roots due to osteophytes, bulging discs, hypertrophied ligaments, or adjacent osseous pathology will appear as a focal indentation on the column of contrast. Myelography has, for the most part, been replaced by CT-myelography and MRI.[12] It is still used in those centers where CT and MRI are not available or in those patients who are unable to undergo MRI due to claustrophobia or obesity.[13]

COMPUTED TOMOGRAPHY

CT uses the differential absorption of X-rays as they pass through the body to form digital matrices, which a computer then converts into a cross-sectional image.[14] Scans are usually obtained directly in the axial plane and can be reformatted to produce images in the sagittal, coronal, and oblique planes. With additional software, complex three-dimensional pictures of the spine can be generated from the axial images.

High-resolution CT scans are ideal for imaging the bony and soft tissue structures of the spine and provide direct visualization of the facet joints, intervertebral foramen, neural arches, discs, ligaments, and muscles. The thecal sac is best evaluated after the injection of a radiopaque contrast material into the subarachnoid space (CT-myelography). CT in the axial plane provides excellent information about the dimension and shape of the spinal canal. Any narrowing of the canal due to posterior osteophytes or hypertrophied facet joints and ligaments can be visualized in detail. CT is also useful in the assessment of pathology such as traumas, infections, neoplasms, and metabolic disorders. The only major disadvantage of CT is the radiation exposure to the patient, which is approximately 3 to 5 rad.[8]

MAGNETIC RESONANCE IMAGING

MRI detects the energy released by hydrogen atoms within the body when they are subjected to strong magnetic fields.[14] Generally, structures that are rich in fat and hydrogen, such as bone marrow, hemorrhage, and edema, produce a high MR signal whereas cortical bone and ligaments, having low concentrations of hydrogen, produce a very low MR signal. By using different pulse sequences, specific anatomic structures can be assessed. For example, T1-weighted images enhance fat allowing better visualization of the bone marrow. The brightest signal demonstrated on the T2-weighted images is water, as is seen in the cerebrospinal fluid (CSF) and intervertebral discs. Paramagnetic MR contrast agents, such as gadolinium-diethylenetriamine pentacetic acid (Gd-DTPA) can be used to differentiate postoperative fibrosis from recurrent disc herniation.[15-17]

The major advantage of MRI in the lumbar spine is the ability to visualize the soft tissue structures directly and to differentiate between various tissues within the spinal canal. MRI is capable of detecting such disorders as disc herniation, infection, inflammation, and neoplasms. MRI is also useful in the assessment of syrinx, tumor, infarct, and contusion involving the spinal cord.

MRI has an advantage over CT and plain film radiography because it can reveal the thecal sac, subarachnoid space, and nerve roots in multiple planes without contrast enhancement

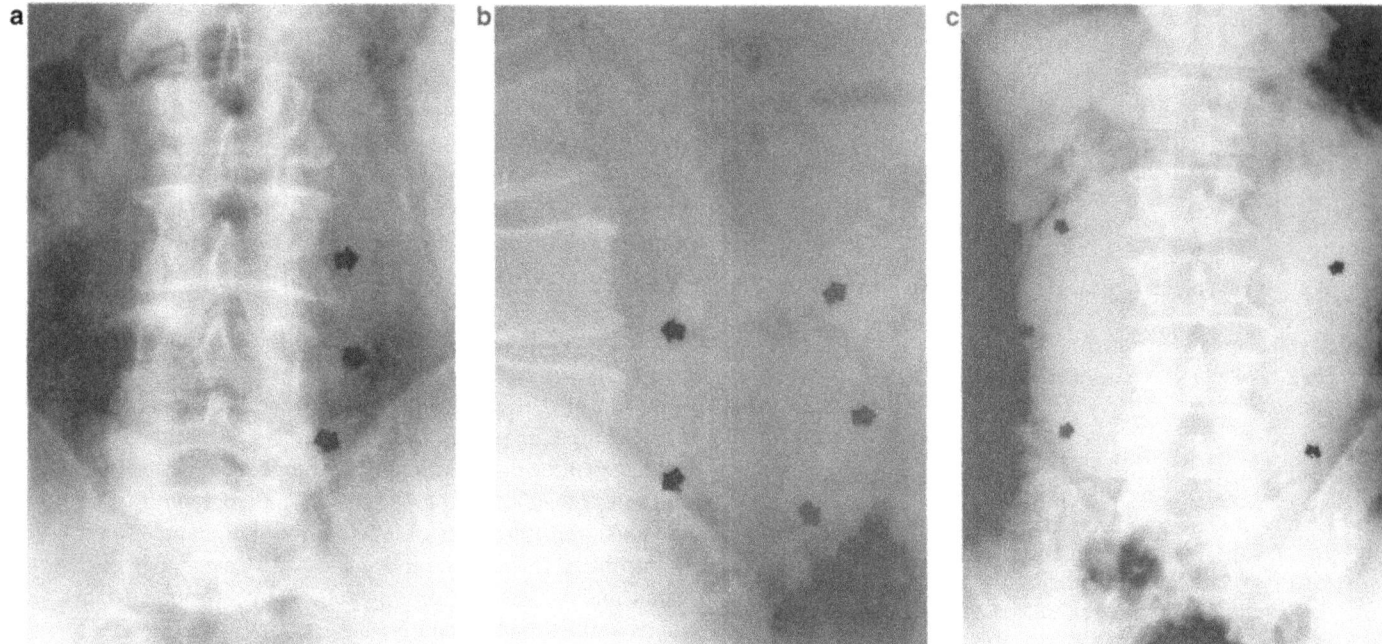

Fig 1. Abdominal aortic aneurysm. Anteroposterior lumbar radiograph of a 68-year-old male demonstrates **(a)** curvilinear calcification in the peripheral wall of the terminal aorta to the left of L-3–L-5. On the lateral view **(b)** an 8-cm abdominal aortic aneurysm is noted anterior to L-4 (arrows). This anteroposterior view of another patient **(c)** shows a 19-cm abdominal aortic aneurysm that has no calcification (arrows). It is important to review all soft tissue structures adjacent to the spine. Courtesy of S.A. Maskall, DC, DACBR, FCCR(C), Grand Forks, British Columbia, Canada.

---

or exposure to ionizing radiation.[18] However, hypertrophic bony and ligamentous changes are better seen on CT as little to no MR signal is generated from these structures.

MRI remains a relatively expensive procedure and is not readily available in smaller communities. Another disadvantage is that claustrophobic patients may find it difficult to remain in the MRI unit for the time required to obtain the images. The presence of ferromagnetic clips in the body or a pacemaker are contraindications to this type of study.

RADIONUCLIDE IMAGING

Nuclear imaging is considered to be the most sensitive technique for detecting early signs of neoplastic or inflammatory disease.[19] Radionuclide imaging can detect as little as 4% to 7% bone loss whereas 30% to 50% loss must occur before it can be detected on plain film radiography.[20,21] Technetium-99m-labeled polyphosphates are the most widely used of the bone-seeking radiotracers.[21,22] After injection, the radionuclides accumulate near areas of abnormal metabolic bone activity such as tumors, infection, fracture, inflammatory disease, and metabolic disease.

Single photon emission computed tomography (SPECT) is basically a bone scan with tomography. SPECT images are considered to be more specific than routine planar scanning because the spine can be visualized in the coronal, axial, or sagittal planes.[14] However, both planar and SPECT images are nonspecific in that they will not provide information regarding the specific cause of the alteration in bone activity. A positive bone scan would require further imaging to determine the exact nature of the pathologic process.

THE ROLE OF RADIOLOGY IN IMAGING LUMBAR SPINE DISORDERS

The following section provides a brief overview of the more common pathologies that can affect the lumbar spine and the imaging modalities used to assess these disorders. This discussion is not a comprehensive review of these disorders. The reader is referred elsewhere for additional information.[11,23]

Congenital abnormalities

Congenital anomalies in the lumbar spine have been categorized by Howard and Rowe[4] into those involving maldevelopment of the vertebral body (Fig 2), neural arch abnormalities (Fig 3), and transitional segments. These ab-

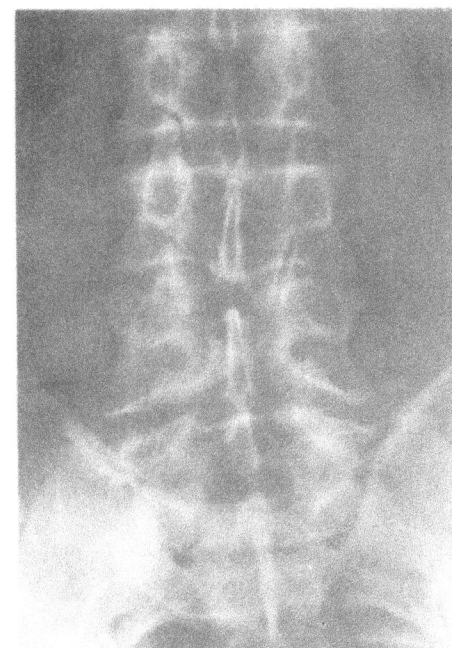
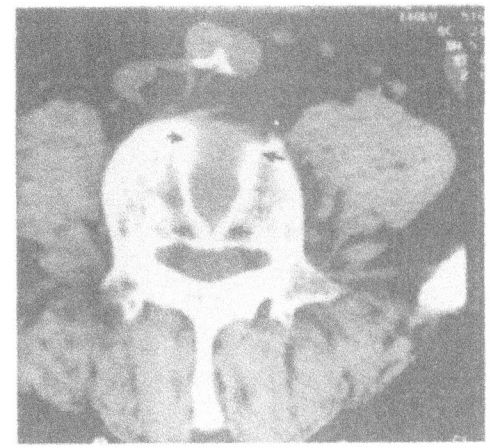

Fig 2. Butterfly vertebra. Characteristic findings of a butterfly vertebra are seen in the anteroposterior view of the lumbar spine (**a**). These findings include a sagittal cleft in the L-4 vertebral body with widening of the vertebral body and interpediculate distance. Also note the deformity of the L-3 and L-5 end plates. The axial CT image with soft tissue contrast (**b**) reveals the central lucency that is isointense with that of disc material. A butterfly vertebra represents failure of midline fusion (dysraphism) of the vertebral body (small arrows). Disc material is usually present within the sagittal cleft. Narrowing of the spinal canal and calcification of the iliac arteries (large arrows) are also noted in this patient who presented with clinical signs of claudication.

---

normalities are readily detected using plain film radiography. Advanced imaging such as CT or MRI adds valuable information as to how these anomalies affect the spinal canal and associated soft tissue structures.

Arthritides

Degenerative changes in the lumbar spine affect the apophyseal articulations and the intervertebral discs. Plain film radiographs demonstrate narrowing of the joint spaces, sclerosis, osteophytes, and the presence of antero- or retrolisthesis. The apophyseal joints are best assessed on the anteroposterior and oblique views; the lateral view clearly demonstrates the disc spaces.

Disc bulges and herniations are best visualized on axial CT or MRI as central or posterolateral soft tissue masses projecting into the spinal canal that may compress the thecal sac or nerve roots. CT will demonstrate if calcification is present within the disc fragment (Fig 4). MRI can also be obtained directly in the sagittal plane allowing for assessment of multiple disc levels simultaneously (Fig 5). Both CT and MRI are more accurate than plain film radiography in evaluating the spinal canal for stenotic narrowing as a result of congenital or acquired changes.[11]

Inflammatory arthritides of the lumbar spine are typically of the seronegative type, the hallmark of which is ankylosing spondylitis (AS). This disorder typically presents in young males and initially starts in the sacroiliac joints. The plain film findings of AS are characteristic, and advanced imaging is usually not warranted (Fig 6) unless complications, such as spinal trauma, occur.

Trauma

Compression fractures are the most common fractures of the lumbar spine. These fractures typically occur in the upper lumbar spine as a result of a combination of flexion and axial loading (Fig 7a,b).[11] Plain film radiography is the primary imaging modality utilized for the assessment of spinal trauma. It provides an overall view of the lumbar spine from which the integrity and alignment of the vertebral bodies can be assessed. With compression fractures, plain film radiographs will demonstrate a loss of anterior vertebral body height and possibly a step defect at the anterior superior margin. Retropulsion of bony frag-

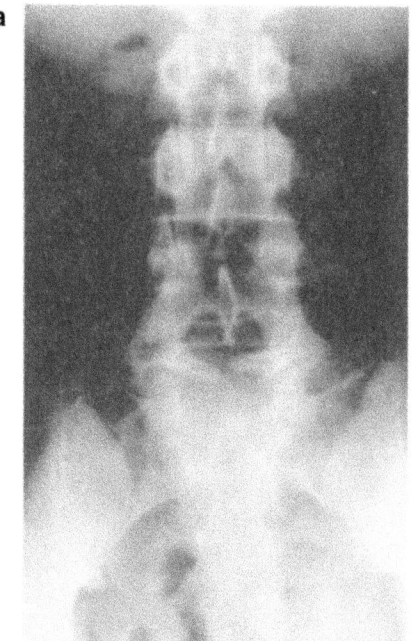 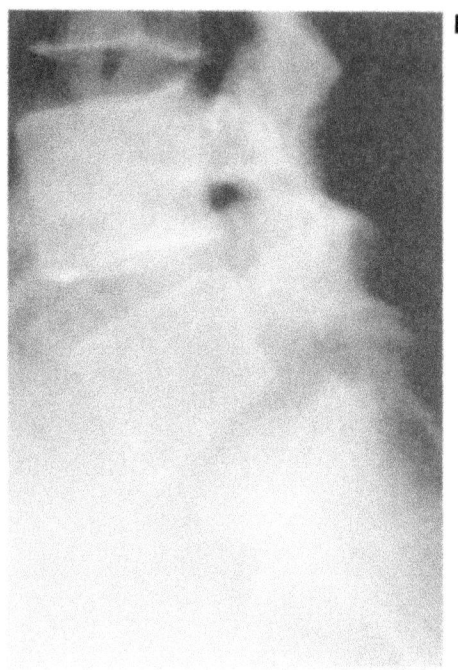

Fig 3. Dysplastic spondylolisthesis. The L-5 neural arch is hypoplastic with nonunion of the posterior elements (a) and (b). A grade 1 anterolisthesis of L-5 on S-1 is noted along with elongation of the pars interarticularis.

---

ments into the spinal canal is best seen on axial CT or MRI (Fig 7c). MRI also provides information regarding the extent of damage to the underlying neural elements.

The presence of an intervertebral vacuum phenomenon in a patient with previous spinal trauma should alert the clinician to the presence of Kümmel's disease (Fig 8). Theoretically, it represents avascular necrosis of the vertebral body.[11] When seen, the clinician should rule out corticosteroid use or thromboembolic disease as contributing factors.

Posterior limbic bones represent separation of the posterior vertebral body ring apophysis. They are most commonly seen at the L-4–L-5 and L-5–S-1 levels; they are thought to occur as a result of trauma.[11] Although difficult to visualize with plain film radiographs, close examination of the posterior margin of the vertebral body may reveal a thin calcification extending into the spinal canal (Fig 9). Posterior limbic bones are best visualized on axial and reformatted CT images.

Infectious disease

Staphylococcus aureus is responsible for approximately 90% of bone and joint infections. The organism usually spreads hematogenously from foci in the skin or the gastrointestinal, genitourinary, or upper respiratory tracts. Spinal infections typically begin in the anterior subchondral region of the vertebrae and spread to the disc and adjacent vertebral end plate. This feature produces the characteristic radiographic appearance of disc space narrowing with adjacent end plate destruction (Fig 10). It is important to keep in mind, however, that conventional radiographs may not demonstrate the destructive changes associated with infection for 2 to 8 weeks.[24]

In the presence of clinical symptoms of infection and negative radiographs, advanced imaging is warranted. Bone scans, using gallium tracers, and MRI scans are highly sensitive in detecting the presence of infection. MRI can further isolate the anatomic location of the infection in the spine and its effect on the adjacent neural structures. This capability makes MRI the diagnostic procedure of choice in the evaluation of spinal infection.[24]

Neoplasms

Spinal neoplasms may be divided into primary lesions, arising directly from the bone, or secondary lesions that arise in a distant site and metastasize to bone. Hemangiomas are common benign lesions that are usually detected incidentally on plain film radiographs or MRIs.

Multiple myeloma commonly involves the spine and is generally seen in patients beyond middle age.[25] It may present radiographically as nonspecific osteopenia or "punched out" lytic lesions. Multiple myeloma can often produce false negative bone scans if little bone reaction is present. MRI is the most sensitive technique in detecting plasma cell infiltration of the spine.[11]

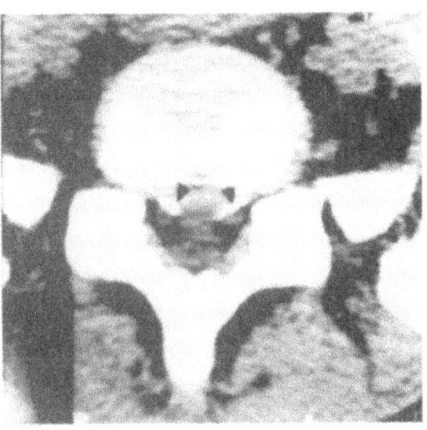

Fig 4. Discal herniation with calcific rim. The axial CT image demonstrates two calcific densities (arrow heads) at the periphery of a large central disc herniation.

Tumors of the spine are most commonly metastatic. Metastases usually arise from melanomas or carcinomas of the thyroid, breast, bronchus, kidney, prostate, or colon.[26] Up to 80% of metastatic lesions are lytic in nature and are detected radiographically by loss of cortical margins or pedicles (Fig 11a,b). A 30% to 50% loss of bone density is required before

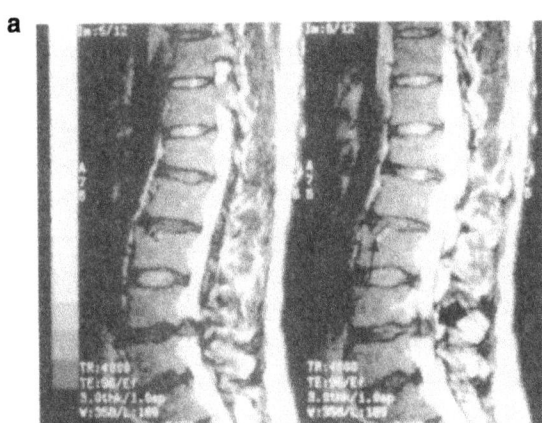
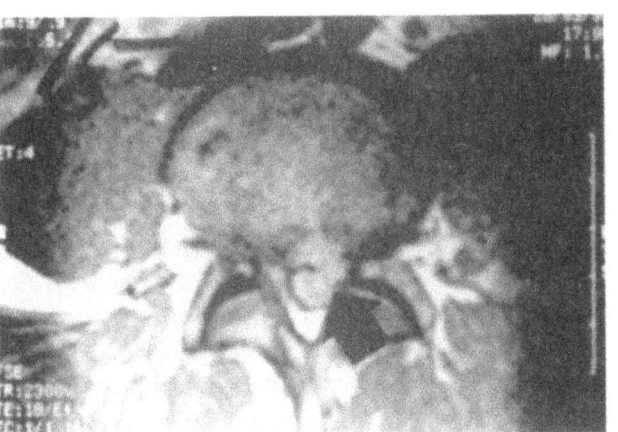

Fig 5. Herniated nucleus pulposus. Sagittal T2 (a) and axial proton-weighted MR (b) images. A large left paramedian disc herniation is noted at L4-5, which is displacing the adjacent nerve roots and occupying a large portion of the spinal canal (arrow). A smaller bulge is seen at L1-2. Note also the large Schmorl's nodule is at the superior end plate of L-3 (small arrow).

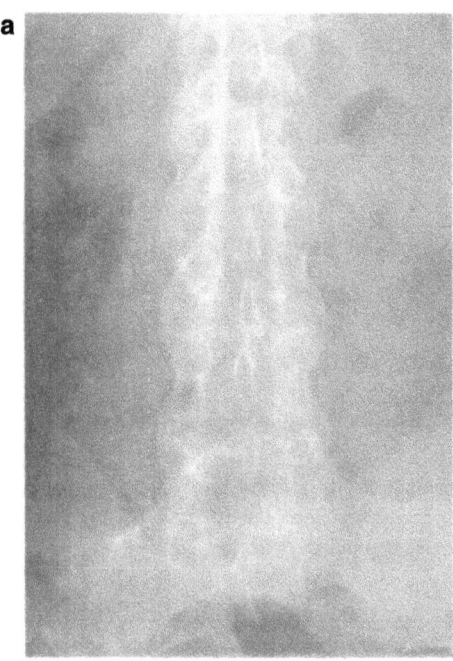
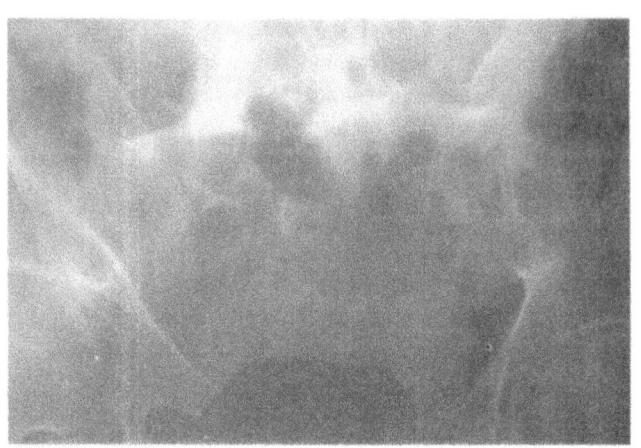
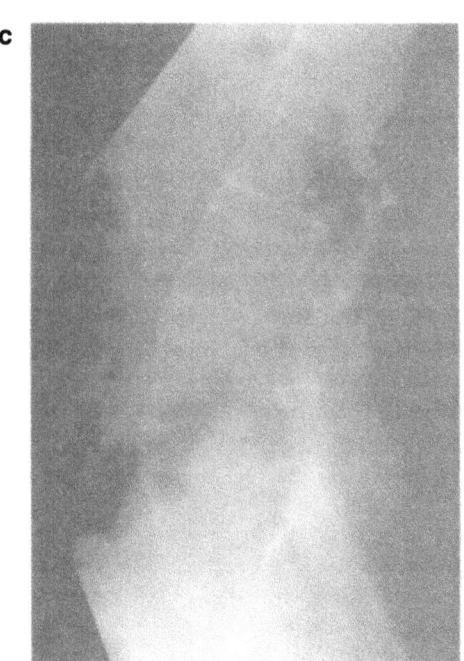

Fig 6. Ankylosing spondylitis. Anteroposterior (**a**) and Hibbs' (**b**) views of a 45-year-old male with known ankylosing spondylitis and low back pain demonstrate end-stage bony ankylosis and obliteration of the sacroiliac joints as well as symmetric, marginal syndesmophytes in the lumbar spine. The lateral lumbar view (**c**) reveals squaring of the vertebral bodies, marginal syndesmophytes and bony ankylosis of the facet joints, which are characteristic radiographic findings of ankylosing spondylitis. Courtesy of Lori S. Ramos, DC, DACBR, WSCC, Berlin, New Hampshire.

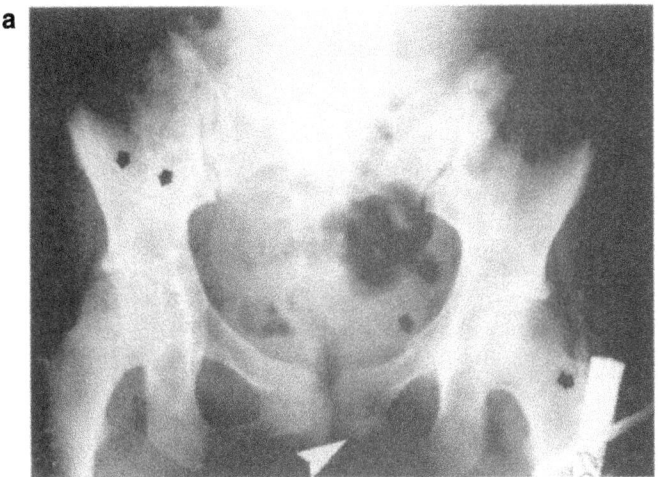
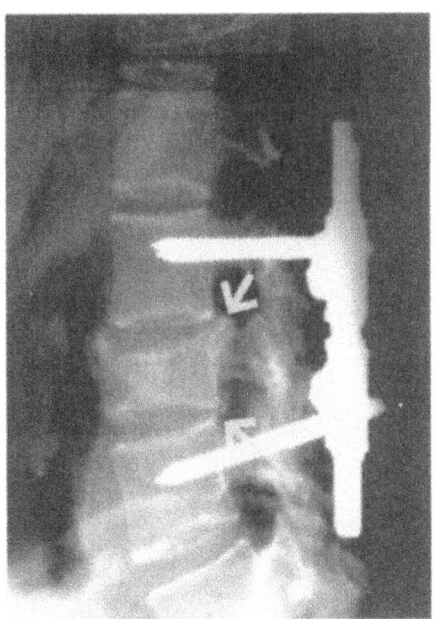
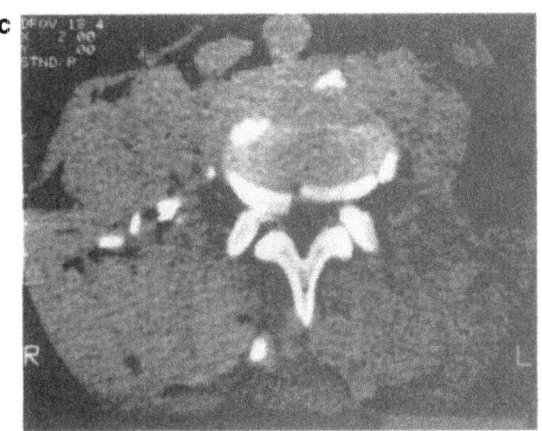

Fig 7. Traumatic compression fracture of L-3 with surgical intervention. **(a)** Anteroposterior pelvic view shows a skeletally immature female, with a Risser's sign of four, who sustained fractures to the right ilium, left superior and inferior pubic rami, left femur, and the L-3 vertebral body (arrows) as a result of a tobogganing accident. The lateral lumbar view **(b)** reveals approximately 30% loss of anterior vertebral body height of L-3 with slight posterior displacement of the vertebral body (arrows). This unstable compression fracture was stabilized with interpedicular screws and rods extending from L-2 to L-4. The axial CT **(c)** was used to assess the degree of fragmentation and retropulsion of bony fragments into the spinal canal.

---

a lesion can be detected with plain film radiographs, whereas bone scans may be positive with only a 4% to 7% bone loss.[21] MRI will detect the replacement of normal fatty marrow in the vertebral bodies by the highly cellular metastatic process, which appears as a low signal intensity area on the T1-weighted images (Fig 11c).

Paget's disease is a tumor-like process of bone typically seen in the axial spine, pelvis, and lower extremities in the older population.[11] Plain film radiographs demonstrate the characteristic features of bony enlargement, coarsened trabecular markings, and thickening of the cortical margins (Fig 12a,b). Scintigraphy can be helpful in demonstrating additional sites of involvement (Fig 12c).

MRI is the diagnostic procedure of choice in the evaluation of spinal cord tumors.[25] Occasionally, indirect signs of intraspinal tumors can be seen on plain film radiographs.

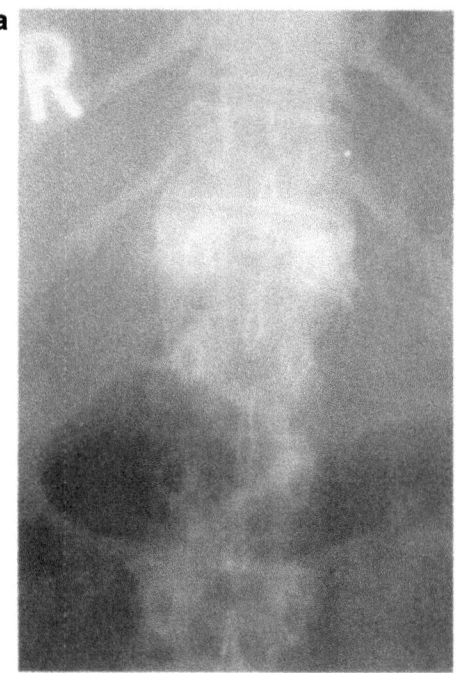
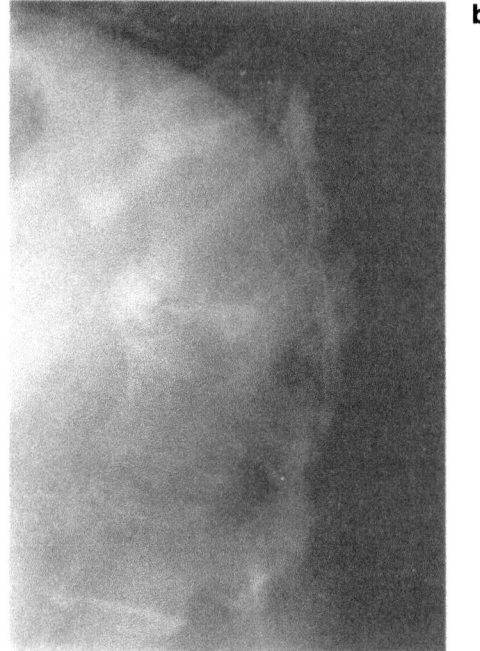
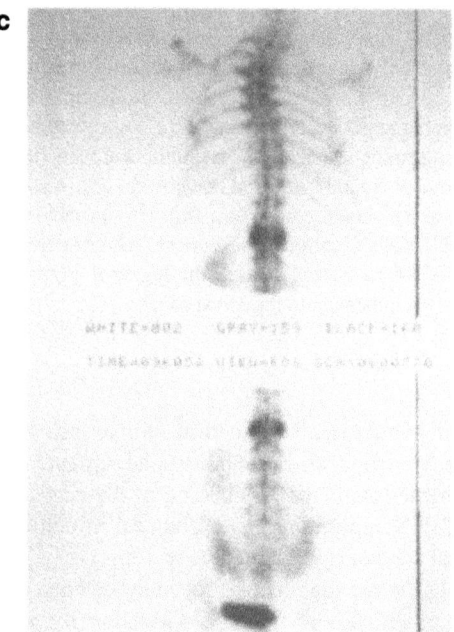

Fig 8. Kummel's disease. Anteroposterior (**a**) and lateral (**b**) views of the lumbar spine. Collapse of the anterior vertebral body with an intravertebral vacuum cleft suggests ischemic necrosis of the vertebral body, often associated with corticosteroid or thromboembolic disease and previous trauma. Increased radionuclide activity is seen at the corresponding vertebra (**c**) indicating nonspecific increased metabolic activity.

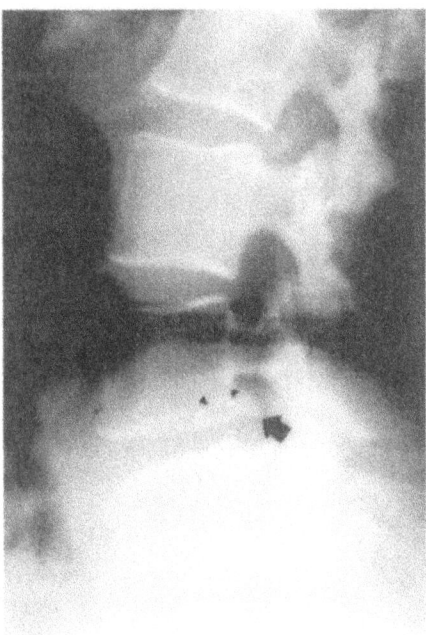

Fig 9. Posterior limbus bone. The spur-like bony projection (arrow) extending from the posteroinferior corner of the L-4 vertebral body on this lateral lumbar view represents avulsion of the posterior ring apophysis. This finding is usually the result of herniation of nuclear material between the ring apophysis and the vertebral end plate prior to skeletal maturity. Courtesy of T.J. Mick, DC, DACBR, Bloomington, Minnesota.

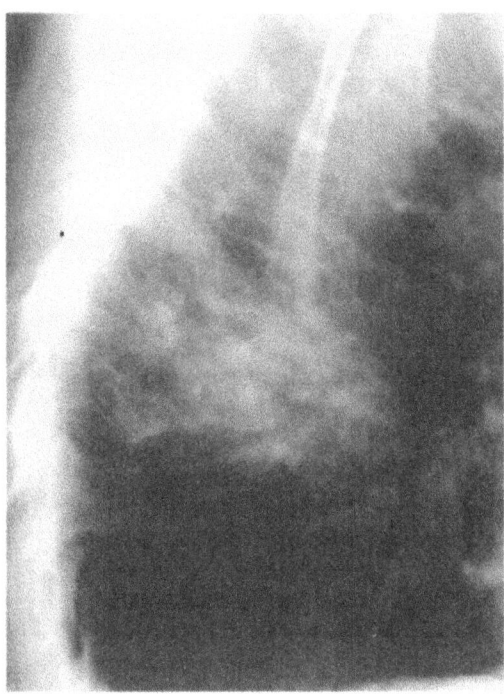

Fig 10. Spondylodiscitis. Lateral view of the lumbar spine showing end plate destruction with bony sclerosis at the anterior corner of the L-3 and L-4 discovertebral junctions (small arrows) in a 39-year-old patient with diabetes. The anteriorly displaced calcified abdominal aorta (large arrow) suggests a prevertebral abscess. These findings are characteristic of infectious discitis and osteomyelitis of the spine.

These signs include scalloping of the posterior vertebral margins, erosion of the medial aspects of the pedicles, and enlargement of the intervertebral foramen. Tumors of the spinal cord are usually classified into intradural extramedullary, intradural intramedullary, and extradural lesions. Intradural extramedullary tumors account for approximately 60% of spinal cord tumors of which meningiomas and neurofibromas (Fig 13) are the most common.[11,25]

SUMMARY

High-quality plain film radiographs continue to be the most commonly used imaging modality due to cost-effectiveness, ready availability, and ability to rule out gross pathology. Advanced imaging procedures such as nuclear imaging, CT, and MRI provide additional information that is not often visible on conventional radiographs. In general, nuclear imaging and MRI are highly sensitive in the detection of bone pathology. MRI produces images demonstrating excellent soft tissue detail and offers direct visualization of the spinal canal and its contents. The trabecular markings and cortical margins of bone are best visualized with CT scans, making this modality valuable in the assessment of arthritic disorders and trauma to the spine.

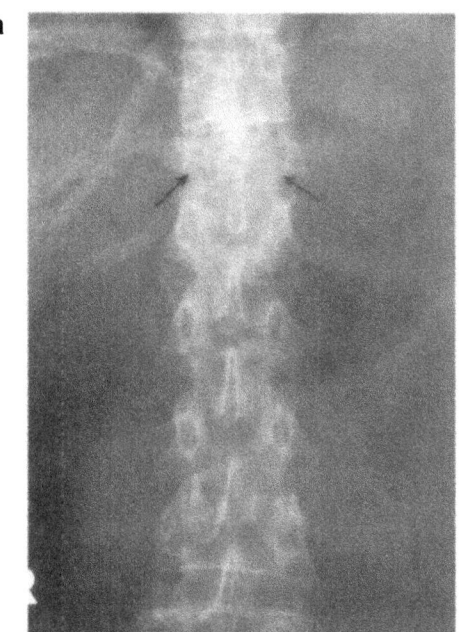
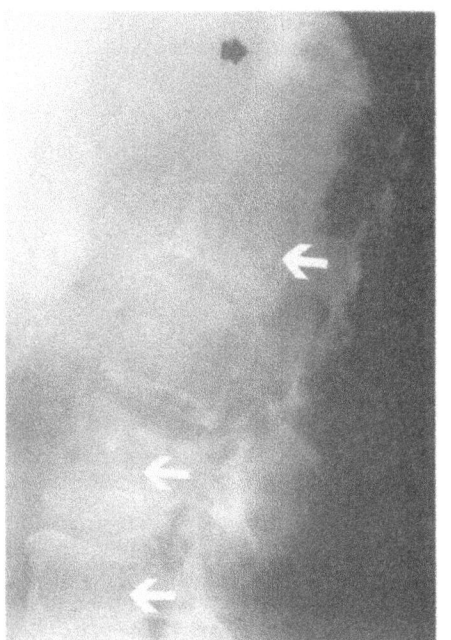
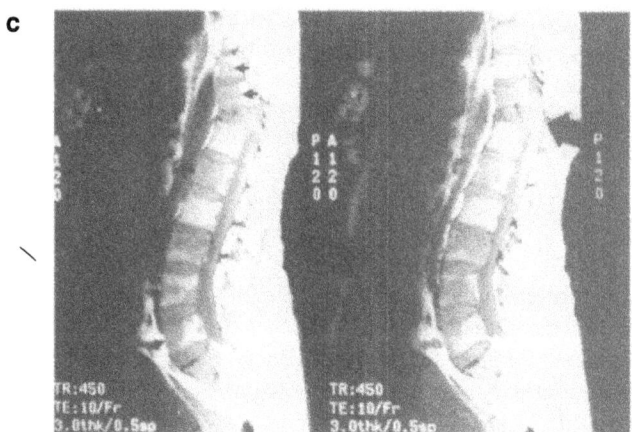

Fig 11. Lytic metastasis from breast carcinoma. The anteroposterior lumbar view (**a**) reveals absence of the pedicles at T-11 (small arrows) consistent with lytic destruction. The lateral view (**b**) reveals a pathologic compression fracture of T-11 and acute kyphotic angulation (black arrow) of the lumbar spine. A second compression fracture is noted at L-1 (white arrow). Mottled lucencies are noted in the vertebral bodies of L-1, L-3, and L-4 (white arrows). T1-weighted MRI in the sagittal plane (**c**) shows the compression of T-11, with collapse and posterior extension into the spinal canal (large black arrow). Lytic metastasis has replaced the normal bright-signal fatty marrow in the T-9, T-10, L-1, and L-3–L-5 vertebral bodies (small black arrows).

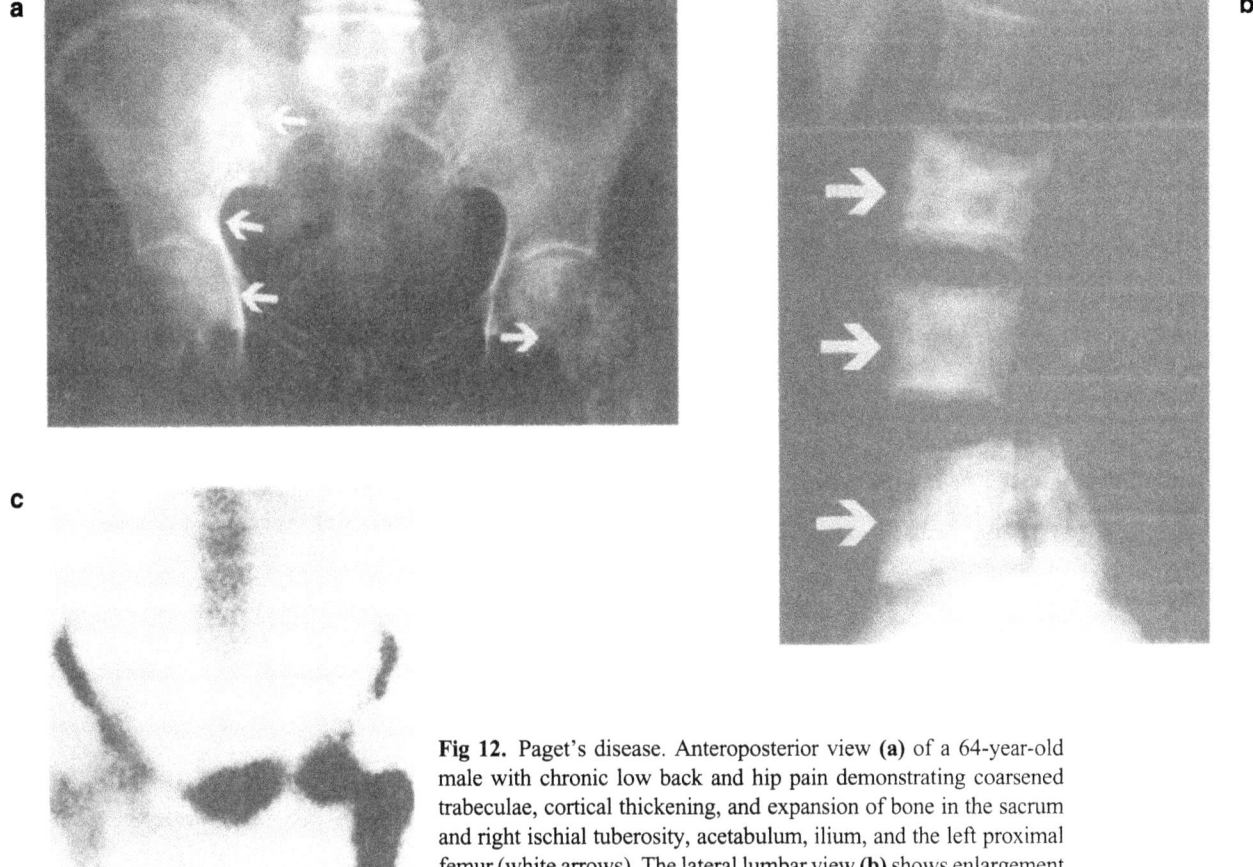

Fig 12. Paget's disease. Anteroposterior view **(a)** of a 64-year-old male with chronic low back and hip pain demonstrating coarsened trabeculae, cortical thickening, and expansion of bone in the sacrum and right ischial tuberosity, acetabulum, ilium, and the left proximal femur (white arrows). The lateral lumbar view **(b)** shows enlargement and cortical thickening of the L-2, L-3, and L-4 vertebral bodies (white arrows) compared with the normal L-1 vertebral body. Increased uptake of radiotracer is noted on the bone scan **(c)** in the corresponding areas seen on the plain film radiographs.

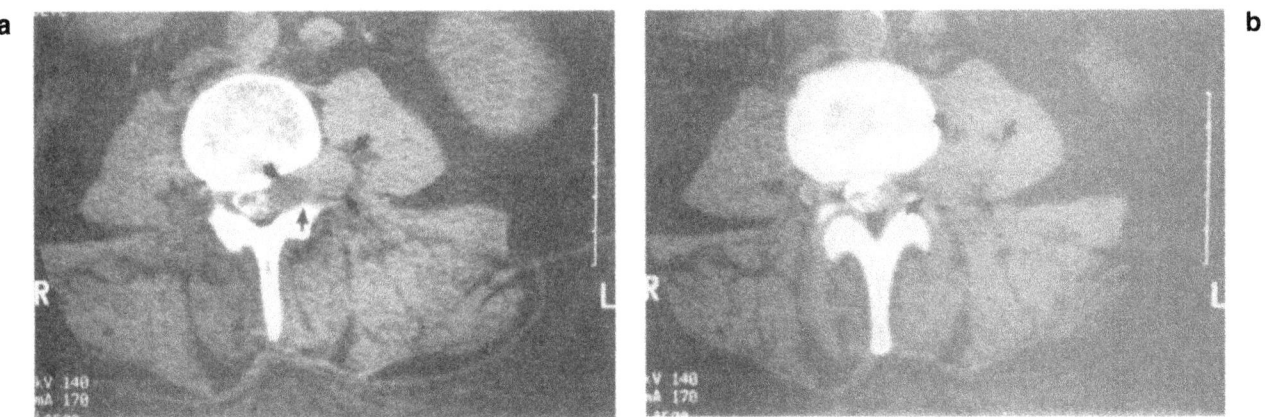

Fig 13. Neurofibroma. Axial CT-myelography, **(a)** and **(b)**, shows a focal soft tissue mass contiguous with the left L-2 nerve root extending through the lateral recess into the paraspinal region (arrows). There is enlargement of the intervertebral foramen and lateral recess and asymmetry of the psoas muscles.

REFERENCES

1. Hall FM. Back pain and the radiologist. *Radiology*. 1980;137:861–865.
2. Gehweiler JA, Daffner RH. Low back pain: the controversy of radiologic evaluation. *Am J Roentgenol*. 1983;140:109–112.
3. Quebec Task Force on Spinal Disorders. Scientific approach to the assessment and management of activity related spinal disorders: a monograph for clinicians. *Spine*. 1987;12:S1–S59.
4. Howard BA, Rowe LJ. Spinal X-rays. In: Haldeman S, ed. *Principles and Practice of Chiropractic*. 2nd ed. Norwalk, Conn: Appleton & Lange; 1992.
5. Whitehouse GH. New imaging techniques in rheumatology. *Br J Rheumatol*. 1986;25:217–222.
6. Sherman R. Chiropractic X-ray rationale. *J Can Chiro Assoc*. 1986;30:33–36.
7. Deyo PA, Diehl AK. Lumbar spine films in primary care: current use and effects of selective ordering criteria. *J Gen Intern Med*. 1986;1:20–25.
8. Taylor JAM, Resnick D. Imaging decisions in the management of low back pain. *Adv Chiro*. 1994;1:1–28.
9. Polz DM, Haddad RG. Radiologic investigation of low back pain. *Can Med Assoc J*. 1989;140:287–295.
10. Simmons ED, Guyer RD, Graham-Smith A, Herzog R. Contemporary concepts in spine care: radiographic assessment for patients with low back pain. *Spine*. 1995;20:1839–1841.
11. Yochum TR, Rowe LJ. *Essentials of Skeletal Radiology*. Baltimore, Md: Williams & Wilkins; 1995.
12. Hashimoto K, Akahori O, Kitano K, et al. Magnetic resonance imaging of lumbar disc herniations: comparison with myelography. *Spine*. 1990;16:1166–1169.
13. Haldeman S, Chapman-Smith D, Petersen DM Jr. Diagnostic imaging. In: Haldeman S, Chapman-Smith D, Petersen DM Jr, eds. *Guidelines for Chiropractic Quality Assurance and Practice Parameters*. Gaithersburg, Md: Aspen Publishers; 1993.
14. Howe J, Foreman SM, Glenn WV. Advanced imaging modalities. In: Haldeman S, ed. *Principles and Practice of Chiropractic*. 2nd ed. Norwalk, Conn: Appleton & Lange; 1992.
15. Thornbury JR, et al. Disk-caused nerve compression in patients with acute low back pain: diagnosis with MR, CT myelography and plain CT. *Radiology*. 1993;186:731–738.
16. Steinberg PM, Hueffle MG, Modic MT, et al. Lumbar spine: postoperative MR imaging with Gd-DTPA. *Radiology*. 1988;167:817–827.
17. Kormano M. Imaging methods in examining the anatomy and function of the lumbar spine. *Ann Intern Med*. 1989;21:335–340.
18. Modic MT, Masaryk TJ, Boumphrey F, et al. Lumbar herniated disc disease and canal stenosis: prospective evaluation by surface coil MR, CT and myelography. *Am J Roentgenol*. 1986;147:757–765.
19. Patton DD, Woolfender J. Radionuclide bone scanning in disorders of the spine. *Radiol Clin North Am*. 1977;2:177–202.
20. Frank JA. Detection of malignant bone tumors: MR imaging vs scintigraphy. *Am J Roentgenol*. 1990;155:1043–1048.
21. Mandell G. Radionuclide imaging. In: Kricun ME, ed. *Imaging Modalities in Spinal Disorders*. Philadelphia, Pa: W.B. Saunders; 1988.
22. Alazraki N. Radionuclide techniques. In: Resnick D, Niwayama G, eds. *Diagnosis of Bone and Joint Disorders*. 3rd ed. Philadelphia, Pa: W.B. Saunders; 1994.
23. Resnick D, Niwayama G, eds. *Diagnosis of Bone and Joint Disorders*. 3rd ed. Philadelphia, Pa: W.B. Saunders; 1994.
24. Reddy S, Leite CC, Jinkins JR. Imaging of infectious diseases of the spine. In: Lee RR, ed. *State of the Art Reviews*. Philadelphia, Pa: Hanley-Belfus; 1995;9.
25. Lee RR. Spinal tumors. In: Lee RR, ed. *State of the Art Reviews*. Philadelphia, Pa: Hanley-Belfus; 1995;9.
26. Vider M, Manyana Y, Navarez R. Significance of the vertebral venous (Batson's) plexus in metastatic carcinoma. *Cancer*. 1977;40:67–71.

10

Advanced Diagnostic Imaging of Adults with Neck or Low Back Pain: A Seed Algorithm

Michael Perillo, Mark Hannan, and David Lemberg

The ordering of an imaging test in the 1990s should be more cognitive than Pavlovian, and our logic more scholastic than lunar.[1(p1765)]

Imaging of the spine through computed tomography (CT) and magnetic resonance imaging (MRI) has existed for approximately three decades. The use of MRI to evaluate the musculoskeletal system was introduced in the early 1980s but was preceded by CT scanning. Although controversy and methodological questions surround both CT and MRI (especially MRI),[2] they both have been studied extensively and been found to be accurate in defining structural abnormalities, particularly of the intervertebral disc, spinal canal, spinal cord, central nervous system, and facet joints. The investigations usually involved comparison of the results of spinal imaging to findings at the time of surgery, the accepted "gold standard" of the day. The strength of CT lies in its ability to define osseous abnormalities, whereas MRI is superior in detecting soft tissue abnormalities. Comprehensive reviews of the technical efficacy of and indications for CT and MRI use may be found in the Mercy Guidelines,[3] and the Agency for Health Care Policy and Research Guidelines for Acute Low Back Problems in Adults.[4] The purpose of this article is to examine issues relating to the appropriate utilization of these modalities in the typical chiropractic care office setting.

Neck and/or low back pain, with or without extremity involvement, is a common patient presentation in chiropractic practice.[5–7] In the clinical setting, a doctor is confronted by a patient with a complaint. The doctor believes the complaint is the result of "something" but does not know exactly what that something is. Rather, the doctor has a probabilistic impression and list of differentials, based upon the information gathered. In other words, the doctor is dealing only with probabilities, not certainties.

Contemporary clinical practice parameters suggest the use of a history and physical examination, perhaps supplemented by plain film radiographs, to develop an initial diagnostic impression, followed by a monitoring of changes in subjective complaints and objective findings to guide the therapeutic process. How should clinical information be used to determine when or if advanced diagnostic imaging should be performed?

APPROPRIATENESS AND GOALS OF SPINAL IMAGING

In the clinical setting, the goal of CT or MRI scanning may be to confirm a diagnostic impression or to investigate or describe the anatomy of the area in question. According to Herzog, the main goal is "to provide precise morphologic data as a means to establish a comprehensive pathoanatomic diagnosis or detect and characterize pathophysiologic changes that may explain the patient's symptomatology."[8(p2486)] In other words, a CT or MRI test should provide new meaningful information regarding the patient's condition and not be merely used to demonstrate a structural abnormality.

Vosburg and coworkers[9] evaluated 71 patient charts that included 90 MRIs of the spine and extremities. They suggested the following questions be answered as a means of judging the appropriateness of a diagnostic study:

1. Are the history and physical examination adequately documented? Is the differential diagnosis supported?
2. Does the diagnostic study provide discriminatory or confirmatory information regarding the differential di-

Adapted from *Top Clin Chiro* 1997; 4(1): 9–14
© 1997 Aspen Publishers, Inc.

agnosis and is it required prior to initial therapeutic intervention?
3. Are the results of the diagnostic study reviewed and do these results direct the therapeutic course?

Additionally, the test results should provide information that helps to guide and possibly change the management of the case.

WHY NOT JUST RELY ON THE RESULTS OF THE TEST?

Should patients with neck or low back pain be evaluated or screened using CT or MRI at the earliest possible time after their presentation? Wouldn't this be the most prudent method for rapidly establishing a "definitive diagnosis?"

A variety of health care policy issues and several important concepts of screening and technology assessment warrant consideration in answering these questions. First, the ability of the proposed test to accurately distinguish between patients who *have* a given disease, condition, or abnormality from those patients who *do not* must be looked at.

Table 1 compares the possible test results from either an MRI or CT scan on a patient with a suspected herniated lumbar disc to the "truth." This model shows that the possible results for a patient who has the test:

(A) The patient has a positive test and has the disease.
(B) The patient has a positive test but does not have the disease.
(C) The patient has a negative test but has the disease.
(D) The patient has a negative test and does not have the disease.

The *sensitivity* of the test is its ability to correctly identify disease in a patient who has the disease (positive in disease, or PID); this is represented by the equation $A/(A+C)$.

The *specificity* of the test is its ability to correctly identify as negative or normal a patient who does not have the disease (normal in health, or NIH); the equation for this is $D/(D+B)$.

A test's sensitivity and specificity represent the test's ability to detect "abnormality." They are theoretical characteristics of the test itself and are not dependent on the prevalence of the disease or condition in any given patient population. (The prevalence is determined by the number of those with the abnormality, both newly developed and previously present.)

Perhaps of greater importance to the clinician is the concept of predictive value. That is, if a patient has a positive test result, how likely is it that the test is "truly positive" (the A cell)? Alternatively, how certain can the clinician be that the patient truly does not have the disease or condition of interest? For instance, in the example under consideration, how certain can the doctor be that the disc abnormality visualized is really the cause of a patient's symptoms and signs, as opposed to something else. The positive predictive value (PPV) = $A/(A+B)$ and the negative predictive value (NPV) = $D/(C+D)$.

Unlike sensitivity and specificity, the predictive values of the test are dependent on the prevalence of the condition in the population upon whom the test is performed. Since the clinician selects the patients to be tested, to a great degree the clinician determines the composition of the test population. Thus, patient selection is crucial.

The importance of patient selection can be demonstrated by means of the following example constructed by Deyo and coworkers.[10] They describe utilizing MRI testing in two patient populations of equal size: a population of patients having sciatica in which 60% truly have a herniated disc (prevalence 60%) and a population of patients with nonspecific low back pain in which 3% truly have a herniated disc (prevalence 3%). In this example, a patient in the low back pain–only population with a positive MRI has a probability of only about 0.12 that any abnormality visualized on the MRI is in fact responsible for causing his or her complaint. In contrast, a patient in the sciatica population has an equivalent probability of about 0.90. Using these concepts, an examination of the literature of live studies follows.

Numerous studies have investigated the diagnostic efficacy (sensitivity, specificity, and predictive value) of CT or MRI scans in the tested populations. Table 2 compares several of these studies.[11–18] False positive rates range from a low of about 9% for disc bulges to a high of about 95% for disc degeneration. Keep in mind that in all of these studies the population evaluated was *asymptomatic!*

Fraser and colleagues[19] reported on a 10-year follow-up study of a group of patients who had lumbar disc herniation and had been treated with saline injection, chymopapain, or laminectomy. They found, after follow-up scanning, that 37% of the patients in each of the treatment groups had persistent disc herniation unrelated to their clinical state. The authors concluded that the presence or absence of herniation on the follow-up scan had no significant bearing on whether the outcome was a successful one.

Brightbill and coworkers[20] describe a series of patients ranging in age from 22 to 46 years old. Each patient had ab-

Table 1. Four outcomes of a diagnostic test

Diagnostic test results	Patient has disease (herniated disc)	Patient does not have the disease	
Positive	True positive (A)	False positive (B)	A + B
Negative	False negative (C)	True negative (D)	C + D
	A + C	B + D	A + B + C + D

Table 2. Summary of studies of diagnostic efficacy of CT and MRI scans

Authors	Test type	Spinal area	Age range	Abnormality noted	False positive			False negative
Jensen et al.	MRI	L/S	20–80	B,P,E	64% 38%*			N/A
Weisel et al.	CT	L/S	<40	H	13–20%			N/A
			>40	H	30–82%			
Boden et al.	MRI	L/S			B	H	D	N/A
			20–39	B,H,D	56%	21%	34%	
			40–59		50%	22%	59%	
			>60		79%	36%	93%	
Weinreb et al.	MRI	L/S	20–39	B,H	9%	44%		N/A
			19–40		10%	44%		
Powell	MRI	L/S	21–30	D,B		34%		N/A
			31–40			60%		
			<70			95%		
Boden et al.	MRI	C/S	<40	H,B,S	14%			NA
			>40		28%			
Schellhas et al.	MRI	C/S	28–41	B,H	50%			NA
Boos et al.	MRI	L/S	20–50	B,H,D	51%	76%	85%	NA

Note: For citations of the studies listed, see references 11–18 at the end of the article.
Key: B = bulge; P = protrusion; E = extrusion; D = degeneration; H = herniation; S = stenosis
*More than one level

normalities demonstrated by lumbar discography and internal disc disruption found at surgery but had *negative MRI* studies of the lumbar spine. Schellhas and colleagues[21] demonstrated similar findings in their study, which compared the results of MRI and discographic examination of cervical discs in an attempt to identify the source(s) of cervical discogenic pain. They report that 27 of 31 cervical discs that appeared to be normal on MRI were shown by discography to have annular tears of varying types and degrees. The results suggest that, depending on the symptomatology, a negative MRI may not imply the absence of an abnormality of the spinal disc. Furthermore, in cases of chemically mediated back or extremity involvement[22] or where diabetic radiculopathy is a possibility,[23] negative study result is likely.

The above-mentioned studies each examined different variables in different patient populations and used different testing instruments and different test protocols. Thus, results cannot be easily combined to generate a single numeric representation of the false positive or false negative rate in CT or MRI testing. The study differences, however, are precisely why the information is important. The wide range of false positive rates, the nonconcordance with other diagnostic tests, and the lack of correlation with patients' current clinical states clearly indicate that the generation of a positive (or negative) test result cannot reliably be accepted as the sole basis for diagnosis.

In cases where there is a suspicion of cervical spondylitic myelopathy[24] or cauda equina syndrome,[25] when manipulative care may be contraindicated, advanced imaging is the diagnostic tool of choice, and the clinician may have to rely upon the test outcome. It should be noted that MRI or CT scanning was not considered to be indicated for the evaluation of suspected segmental instability of the cervical spine.[26]

There are mechanisms to increase the clinician's confidence in the appropriate and productive utilization of MRI and CT scanning. Several authors have studied the estimated accuracy of the medical history detecting conditions such as cancer and a herniated lumbar disc. Deyo and Diehl[27] reported sensitivities of 77% for age greater than 50; more than 90% for bed rest offering no relief; and 100% for a combination of age, prior history of cancer, and unexplained weight loss. Deyo and Tsui-Wu[28] and Spangfort[29] reported a sensitivity of 95% for herniated disc in patients who report a history of sciatica. Analogously, several authors have studied the estimated accuracy of physical examination findings for the diagnosis of herniated nucleus pulposus (HNP) in patients with sciatica. The level of accuracy ranged from a sensitivity of 80% to 99% for a positive ipsilateral straight leg–raising test[30–33] to a specificity of 90% for a positive well leg–raising test. Van den Hoogen and coworkers[34] performed a criteria-based literature review regarding the accuracy of physical examination findings. They expressed confidence only in the accuracy of straight leg– and well leg–raising tests. They also suggested combining positive and negative test results to increase accuracy. Furthermore, they point out that history and physical examination findings that are reproducible over time are more likely to be valid and accurate (chance findings will not be reproducible upon reevaluation).

Unfortunately, few studies have addressed these issues for conditions of the cervical spine. Uchihara and colleagues[35] describe a study comparing the findings of orthopaedic testing of the cervical spine with the results of MRI scans in patients thought to have a brachial plexus lesion. They found positive orthopaedic tests in few (range 0–5) of the patients with negative scans, indicating a high degree of specificity. They found at least one positive test in 28% of patients with positive scans, indicating a generally low sensitivity for most of the classical tests. However, the brachial plexus compression test was positive in 69% of those patients with positive study and negative in 83% of those patients with a negative study. Although this is encouraging, not many other articles that deal with the sensitivity and specificity of orthopaedic tests in the cervical spine could be found. Thus, at this time, there is no analogous "straight leg–raising test" for the cervical spine to help guide decision making by the clinician.

Based on the above information, it seems that the patient's history and physical examination findings (both positive and negative test results) provide the clinician with the best information on which to base an initial diagnosis. Coupling the first examination with successive examinations over time should help to drop out chance findings, further increasing accuracy.

THE ALGORITHM

The authors have constructed an algorithm (or care pathway) intended to help guide the use of CT or MRI testing in the evaluation of neck or lower back pain, with or without extremity involvement (see Algorithm 1). A Medline search of the literature was performed, using search words such as *magnetic resonance imaging, cervical spine, lumbar spine, cervical disc herniation,* and *lumbar disc herniation.* A variety of articles and textbook passages were evaluated. The overwhelming majority of the information dealt with the lumbar spine. Although many authors addressed the issue of appropriate use of these tests, few formally presented flow charts.[4,36–38] The article by Hansen and Mootz[39] was used as a reference for actual algorithm construction.

For the purpose of this presentation, the origin of the patient's complaints is not assumed to be mechanical. Furthermore, as outlined by the Mercy Guidelines, "If diagnostic imaging is to be performed, conventional (plain film) radiography is the initial procedure of choice."[3(p23)] The suggested time frame for performing conventional radiographic evaluation varies from 4 to 7 weeks, depending on the specifics of the patient's characteristics and presenting complaints.[40] Although not an absolute requirement, if the patient is considered a candidate for advanced imaging, most likely plain film radiographic evaluation has already been performed.

It should be noted that referral to a specialist physician is done most often for the purpose of seeking a second opinion and does not necessarily signal the end of chiropractic care. It suggests that in lieu of performing an imaging test at that time, a second opinion, perhaps supplemented with additional pain control, may be helpful and may obviate the need for further testing.

The algorithm presented is untested with respect to its reliability and validity in the clinical setting. Prior to adoption, it should be subjected to a consensus review by a group of "end users," such as a group of practicing chiropractors and representative specialists. As a second step, these end users should take several hypothetical patients through the algorithm to see if the panel doctors each reach similar conclusions. Testing of this algorithm might also involve a retrospective review of real cases (the method used in the Vosberg study),[9] including a comparison of the results of applying the algorithm and the known outcomes.

DISCUSSION

The algorithm may be thought of as a practice guideline in flow chart form. As with any such pathway, there is no single correct method and no guaranteed correct answer. The construction of the pathway took into consideration the diagnostic efficacy of CT and MRI tests as determined through the literature review. One of the purposes of the algorithm and its supportive materials is to supply a protocol for patient selection that should increase the prevalence of the condition of interest, most often a herniated disc. In addition, it should decrease the use of testing that does little more than create diagnostic and therapeutic confusion and possibly cause the patient undue concern while contributing nothing to the management or outcome of patient care. Such testing may be inappropriate, only because a patient with neck or low back pain, possibly involving extremity pain, is slow to respond to conservative treatment. The questions suggested by Vosberg and colleagues[9] are worth reiterating:

Are the history and physical examination results adequately documented? Is the differential diagnosis supported? Consider the predictive value of the test for the diagnosis currently being favored. Try to limit problems of patient selection and prevalence. In the example given by Deyo et al,[10] the toss of a coin (50/50 chance) would perform better than MRI or CT scanning in uncovering the cause of nonspecific low back pain. If because of patient selection it is just as likely the patient has something else besides the condition under consideration, then the predictive value of the test and its value to patient management and outcome will be very low. Why perform the test?

Is the test able to discriminate amongst the conditions in the differential list? Is the possibly confirmatory information really required prior to initial or continued therapeutic intervention? CT or MRI scanning will not discriminate between extremity pain due to diabetic neuropathy or radiculopathy and pain of discal origin. Consider whether a different course of conservative management should be attempted or whether the patient may benefit from a course of pain management.

Will the doctor be able to explain to the patient the true significance of the test results? How will the test results be used to change the treatment and affect the outcome of care? As part of the move toward patient-centered management,[41] patients now expect to be told test results (and their significance) and to be active participants in decisions about treatment. As offered by Modic and Herzog, "... the imaging test should be ordered by the physician who will use it [the information] to change patient management."[1(p1765)] A patient's expectations are likely to be partly met if the physician seeks to increase certainty in reaching a definitive diagnosis and alters patient management to increase the chance of obtaining a favorable outcome.

This article has attempted to demonstrate that imaging tests intended to elucidate structural abnormalities do not necessarily correlate well with patients' clinical presentations. Additionally, they may provide potentially misleading information or information that has no impact on outcomes. To reduce their misuse, the authors reviewed the steps involved in deciding whether MRI and CT scans are appropriate for investigating the complaints of adults with back pain and developed a seed algorithm for review and potentially for local adaptation and implementation.

REFERENCES

1. Modic MT, Herzog RJ. Imaging corner: spinal imaging modalities, what's available and who should order them? *Spine.* 1994;19:1764–1765.
2. Cooper S, Chalmers TC, McCally M, Bernier J, Sacks HS. The poor quality of early evaluations of magnetic resonance imaging. *JAMA.* 1988;259:3277–3280.
3. Haldeman S, Chapman-Smith D, Petersen DM, eds. *Guidelines for Chiropractic Quality Assurance and Practice Parameters.* Gaithersburg, MD: Aspen Publishers; 1993.
4. Bigos SJ, Bowyer O, Braen G, et al. *Acute Low Back Problems in Adults.* Washington, DC: US Department of Health and Human Services, Agency for Health Care Policy and Research; 1994. Clinical Practice Guideline No. 14.
5. Christensen MG, ed. *Job Analysis of Chiropractic.* Greely, CO: National Board of Chiropractic Examiners; 1993.
6. Plamondon RL. A summary of 1991 ACA annual statistical survey. *J Am Chiro Assoc.* February 1992:59–65.
7. Shekelle PG, Brook RH. A community-based study of the use of chiropractic services. *Am J Public Health.* 1991;81:439–442.
8. Herzog RJ. The goal of spinal imaging. *Spine.* 1994;19: 2486–2488.
9. Vosburg CL, Koptor JA. Appropriate use of magnetic resonance imaging of the spine and extremities. *South Med J.* 1994;87:801–804.
10. Deyo RA, Haselkorn J, Hoffman R, et al. Designing studies of diagnostic tests for low back pain or radiculopathy. *Spine.* 1994;19:2057S–2065S.
11. Jensen MC, Brant-Zawadzki M, Obuchowski N, et al. Magnetic resonance imaging of the lumbar spine in people without back pain. *N Eng J Med.* 1994;331:69–73.
12. Wiesel SW, Tsourmas N, Feffer HL, et al. A study of computer assisted tomography: the incidence of positive CT scans in an asymptomatic group of patients. *Spine.* 1984;9:549–551.
13. Boden SD, Davis DO, Dina TS, et al. Abnormal MRI scans of the lumbar spine in asymptomatic subjects: a prospective investigation. *J Bone Joint Surg.* 1990;72:403–408.
14. Weinreb JC, Wolbarsht LB, Cohen JM, et al. Prevalence of lumbosacral disk abnormalities on MRI in pregnant and asymptomatic non-pregnant women. *Radiology.* 1989;170:125–128.
15. Powell MC, Wilson M, Szypryt P, et al. Prevalence of lumbar disc degeneration observed by MRI in symptomless women. *Lancet.* 1986;2:1366–1367.
16. Boden SD, Davis DO, Dina TS, et al. Abnormal magnetic resonance scans of the cervical spine in asymptomatic subjects. *J Bone Joint Surg.* 1990; 72:1178–1183.
17. Schellhas KP, Smith MD, Gundry CR, et al. Cervical discogenic pain. *Spine.* 1996;21:300–312.
18. Boos N, Rieder R, Schade V, et al. The diagnostic accuracy of magnetic resonance imaging, work perception, and psychosocial factors in identifying symptomatic disc herniations. *Spine.* 1995;20:710–714.
19. Fraser RD, Sandhu A, Gogan WJ. Magnetic resonance imaging findings 10 years after treatment for lumbar disc herniation. *Spine.* 1995;20:710–714.
20. Brightbill TC, Pile N, Eichelberger RP, et al. Normal magnetic resonance imaging and abnormal discography in lumbar disc disruption. *Spine.* 1994;19:1075–1077.
21. Schellhas KP, Smith MD, Gundry CR, et al. Cervical discogenic pain. *Spine.* 1996;21:300–311.
22. McCarron RF, Wimpee MW, Hudkins PG, et al. The inflammatory effect of nucleus pulposus: a possible element in the pathogenesis of low back pain. *Spine.* 1987;12:760–764.
23. Naftulin S, Fast A, Thomas M. Diabetic lumbar radiculopathy: sciatica without disc herniation. *Spine.* 1993;18:2419–2422.
24. Conley T, Schoenman K, Pudlik T. Cervical spondylitic myelopathy. *Top Clin Chiro.* 1995;2(3):48–53.
25. Coscia M, Leipzig T, Cooper D. Acute cauda equina syndrome: diagnostic advantages of MRI. *Spine.* 1994;19:475–478.
26. McGregor M, Mior S, Shannon H, et al. The clinical usefulness of flexion-extension radiographs in the cervical spine. *Top Clin Chiro.* 1995;2(3):19–28.
27. Deyo RA, Diehl AK. Cancer as a cause of back pain: frequency, clinical presentation, and diagnostic strategies. *J Gen Intern Med.* 1988;3(3): 320–328.
28. Deyo RA, Tsui-Wu YJ. Descriptive epidemiology of low back pain and its related medical care in the United States. *Spine.* 1987;12:264–268.

29. Sprangfort EV. The lumbar disc herniation. *Acta Orthop Scand.* 1972;142(suppl):1–95.
30. Hakelius A, Hindmarsh J. The comparative reliability of preoperative diagnostic methods in lumbar surgery. *Acta Orthop Scand.* 1972;43:234–238.
31. Kosteljanetz M, Esperen JO, Halburt H, et al. Predictive value of clinical and surgical findings in patients with lumbago-sciatica: a prospective study (part I). *Acta Neurochir (Wien).* 1984;73(1–2):67–76.
32. Supik LF, Broom MJ. Sciatic tension signs and lumbar disc herniations. *Spine.* 1994;19:1066–1069.
33. Jonsson B, Stromqvist B. The straight leg raising test and the severity of symptoms in lumbar disc herniation. *Spine.* 1995;20:27–30.
34. Van den Hoogen HM, Koes BW, Van Eijk J, et al. On the accuracy of history, physical examination and erythrocyte sedimentation rate in diagnosing low back pain in general practice: a criteria-based review of the literature. *Spine.* 1995;20:318–327.
35. Uchihara T, Furukawa T, Tsukagoshi H. Compression of brachial plexus as a diagnostic test of cervical cord lesion. *Spine.* 1994;19:2170–2173.
36. McCarthy KA. Improving the clinician's use of orthopedic testing: an application to low back pain. *Top Clin Chiro.* 1994;1(1):42–50.
37. Cox JM, Feller JA. Chiropractic treatment of low back pain: A multicenter descriptive analysis of presentation and outcome in 424 consecutive cases. *J Neuromusculoskeletal Syst.* 1994;2:178–190.
38. Yussen PS, Swatz JD. The acute lumbar disc herniation: imaging diagnosis. *Seminars in U/S, CT and MRI.* 1993;14(6).
39. Hansen DT, Mootz RD. Understanding, developing and utilizing clinical algorithms. *Top Clin Chiro.* 1994;1(4):44–57.
40. Simmons ED, Guyer RD, Graham-Smith A, Herzog R. Contemporary concepts in spine care: radiographic assessments for patients with low back pain. *Spine.* 1995;20:1839–1841.
41. Gatterman MI. A patient-centered paradigm: a model of chiropractic education and research. *J Alt Compl Med.* 1995;1:371–386.
42. Simmons ED, Guyer RD, Graham-Smith A, Herzog R. Contemporary concepts in spine care. Radiographic assessment for patients with low back pain. *Spine.* 1995;20:1839–1841.

Algorithm 1

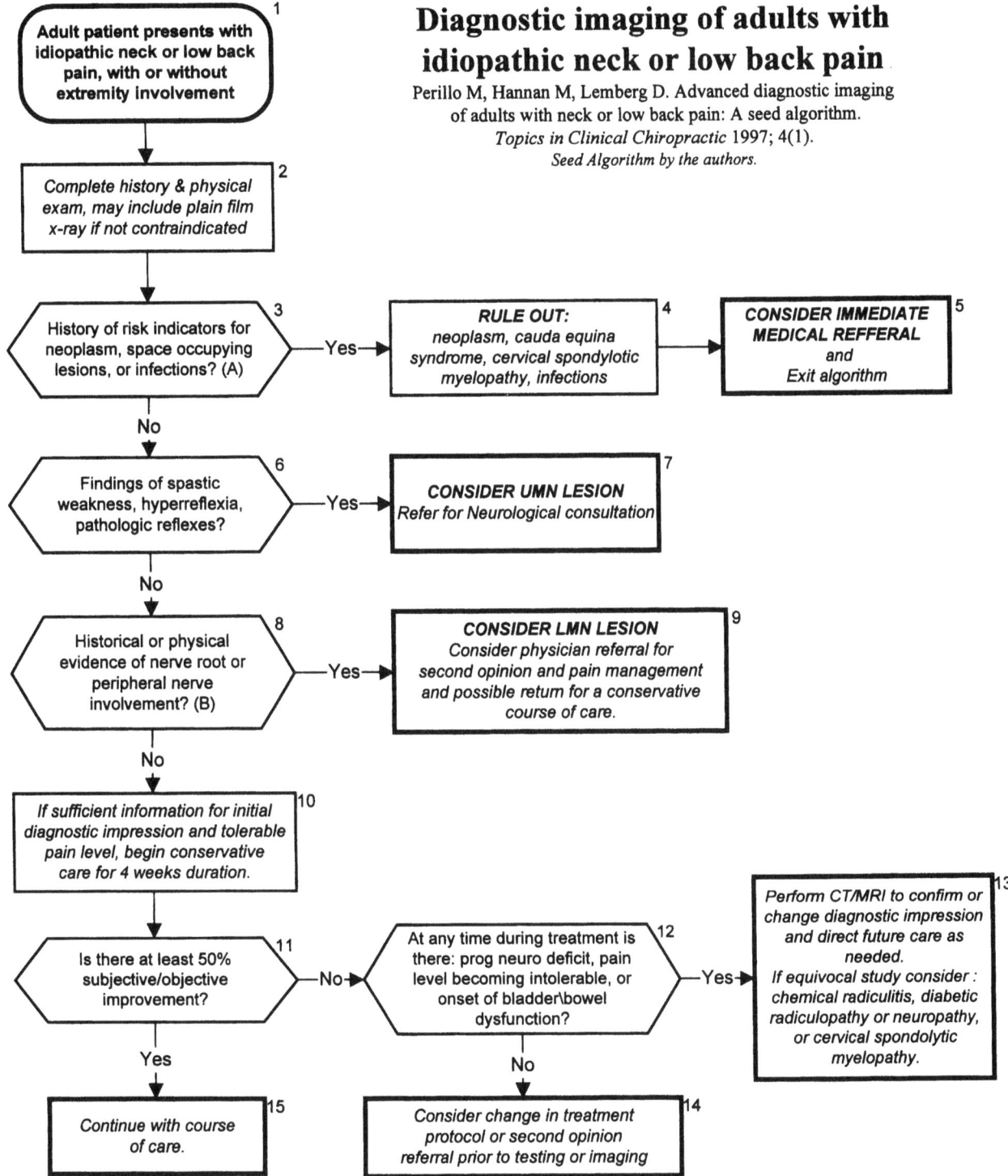

Diagnostic imaging of adults with idiopathic neck or low back pain
Perillo M, Hannan M, Lemberg D. Advanced diagnostic imaging of adults with neck or low back pain: A seed algorithm.
Topics in Clinical Chiropractic 1997; 4(1).
Seed Algorithm by the authors.

Annotations:
(A) e.g., pain>1mo, age >50 yrs old, pain not relieved by rest, unexplained weight loss, bilateral sciatica, saddle paresthesia, bowel/bladder involvement, urinary incontinence, retention, frequency, urgency.
(B) e.g., motor weakness, sensory deficit, diminished reflexes, and intolerable pain level, patient awakens with pain, cannot sit or stand due to pain, symptoms worsening 3-4 days.

11

Diagnostic Ultrasound of the Adult Spine: State of the Technology

Gary D. Schultz

Diagnostic ultrsound was first used in health care in the postwar 1940s. Its development followed the successful applications of sound technology in SONAR (SOund Navigation And Ranging).[1] Ultrasound technology is well suited for the evaluation of soft tissues, particularly deep soft tissues. While ultrasound has been applied successfully in a number of body regions, including the musculoskeletal system, certain applications, such as investigation of the adult spine, are quite controversial. Though it has been suggested that diagnostic ultrasound is a valuable and useful tool for evaluation of the spine in adults,[2] the American College of Radiology (ACR) and the American Chiropractic College of Radiology (ACCR) have discouraged widespread clinical application of this technology.[3,4] Controversy exists regarding the overt commercialization of the technology as well as the relative lack of methodologically sound supportive data for widespread application of ultrasound as an evaluative tool for examining the spine.[5]

DIAGNOSTIC ULTRASOUND OF THE MUSCULOSKELETAL SYSTEM

Ultrasound of the musculoskeletal system is a noninvasive, relatively efficient method for evaluating the bones, joints, and soft tissues of the musculoskeletal system.[6,7] Of particular interest is the use of ultrasound to visualize the rotator cuff as well as other extremity articulations that suffer from internal derangement.[8,9] While evaluation of the rotator cuff using diagnostic ultrasound is not completely without controversy,[10] there is evidence that diagnostic ultrasound compares favorably with other imaging modalities in the diagnosis of complete tears of the cuff and can thus obviate the need for more invasive and expensive additional studies.[11]

Applications of diagnostic ultrasound in the musculoskeletal system have expanded to include diagnosing nearly all soft tissue problems as well as some bone abnormalities. Infections have been successfully characterized in the soft tissues as well as osteomyelitis.[12–15] Ultrasound of the muscles and tendons of the extremities has received attention in the literature, and it appears that ultrasound might be useful as a noninvasive modality for the qualitative evaluation of these muscles and tendons.[16,17] Evaluation of the quantity of muscle may also be performed, although the unique diagnostic utility of this application has not yet been established.[18,19]

Ultrasound of muscle abnormalities has been criticized as being too operator dependent to be reliable, particularly for smaller anatomy, because of its small field of view and limited tissue contrast capability as compared with modalities such as computed tomography (CT) and magnetic resonance imaging (MRI).[20]

DIAGNOSTIC ULTRASOUND OF THE SPINE

Ultrasound of the spine has been limited to fetal, pediatric, and intraoperative applications in the past.[21,22] The first reported application of diagnostic ultrasound to the adult spine was by Porter and colleagues[23] in 1978. They applied diagnostic ultrasound using a posterior approach to measure the spinal canal. The oblique sagittal diameter of the spinal canal was reported for 73 symptomatic and 200 asymptomatic subjects. Unfortunately, the study did not evaluate diagnostic ultrasound for accuracy, but rather the differences between the symptomatic and asymptomatic group were analyzed.

More recent applications have sought to image tissues of the spine and paraspinal regions. The lumbar intervertebral discs have been evaluated in a small number of studies to

Reprinted from *Top Clin Chiro* 1997; 4(1):45–49
© 1997 Aspen Publishers, Inc.

determine the utility of diagnostic ultrasound for evaluating disc herniation. When diagnostic ultrasound has been compared with other imaging modalities for this clinical condition, its performance has generally been poorer than that of other modalities.

Kamei and coworkers[24] compared the performance of diagnostic ultrasound and myelography in the clinical diagnosis of 40 patients with surgically confirmed disc herniations. They used a posterior approach to perform the imaging and viewed the spinal canal through the "laminar window." They reported that ultrasound had a 78% sensitivity for disc herniation, as compared with 90% for myelography. There were approximately 5% false positives and 10% false negative results for ultrasound. Engel and coworkers[25] studied 67 low back pain sufferers and compared ultrasound (3.5 Mhz) and myelography using surgical confirmation as the gold standard in 19 patients. With a posterior approach, ultrasound was 89% sensitive and 100% specific for the diagnosis of disc herniation. Merx and coworkers[26] obtained sensitivities ranging from 63% to 78% using a transabdominal approach. Hagen[27] reported a range of 18% (L-2) to 70% (L-5) accuracy in diagnosing disc herniations with a transabdominal approach.

In summary, ultrasound has generally not performed as well as myelography or other advanced imaging modalities in the few studies performed to date. However, in and of itself, the performance of diagnostic ultrasound in this application appears worthy of additional study. The performance characteristics appear to be better using a posterior approach, and this might be an area of interest for future investigations. Too few patients have been studied overall to render strong conclusions about the ability of ultrasound to evaluate the disc. However, it appears clear that other modalities will probably outperform diagnostic ultrasound in the diagnosis of disc herniation. What remains to be seen is whether the additional cost and inconvenience of MRI and other types of studies are worth the added precision they provide.

Spinal canal size has been studied more extensively than disc herniation, and it appears that ultrasound has at least some validity evaluating spinal canal size. Legg and Gibbs[28] evaluated the interexaminer and interfacility reliability of measuring the spinal canal of 50 patients. There was 3.7% variability in interexaminer measurements and a 5.3% variability between facilities. The authors concluded that by using a standardized protocol for imaging they were able to achieve sufficient levels of reliability to perform future investigations. Porter and colleagues[29] used ultrasound to measure lumbar canal size and determined that the technique they advocated (15° angled from midsagittal between the spinous process and the facet structure) was reproducible because of the bony boundaries of the window. Kadziolka and colleagues[30] performed an in vitro study of 10 cadaveric spines and found ultrasound to vary slightly with the actual diameter. They were able to determine that the echoes found using ultrasound were the result of the dural tube margins. They concluded that myelography was a better method for evaluating canal size because it not only allowed for a more accurate evaluation of the size of the canal but also allowed the morphology of the canal to be visualized. Visualization could not be accomplished using ultrasound because of the narrow field of view provided by the "laminar window."

Engel and coworkers[25] found 95% sensitivity and 100% specificity in 19 cases of focal stenosis using a posterior approach. Studies have addressed the ability of diagnostic ultrasound to evaluate spinal canal diameter, at least in the 15° oblique diameter.[31-33]

Other authors, however, have questioned the reliability of this technique for accurately evaluating the spinal canal.[34,35] Howie and colleagues[36] reported that the sensitivity of diagnostic ultrasound was poor in their study of 17 patients with sciatica. They attempted to measure 50 sites in the spines and were unable to measure 15 of the 50. They only correctly located the stenotic area in 10 of the remaining 35 sites. All stenotic areas were confirmed surgically in their study population. They concluded that ultrasound was unreliable as a predictor of the location of stenosis. Porter's group[37] performed a prospective study in which they measured the spinal canal in 700 individuals over a 10-year period using ultrasound to evaluate the canal size. They compared spinal canal size with the development and severity of back pain. Unfortunately, their assessments did not include a follow-up regarding the accuracy of diagnostic ultrasound in evaluating the spine.

Ultrasound for the evaluation of skeletal muscle has been studied and reported in the peer-reviewed literature.[38-40] It appears that for volumetric and gross qualitative evaluation, ultrasound has potential value. Spinal applications of ultrasound for muscle evaluation are sparse and either relate to muscle cross-sectional size or the assessment of normal muscles.[41-44] There have been no tendon studies of the spine using diagnostic ultrasound.

The chiropractic literature has not provided any meaningful evaluation of diagnostic ultrasound to date. Stipkovich,[45] providing the only new information in the literature, describes a technique for examining the cervical spine and related soft tissues of the neck. This is the only information available addressing the use of diagnostic ultrasound in examination of the neck. Stipkovich's article focused on the cervical lymph nodes and did not comment on the paraspinal muscles, spinal canal, or discs specifically.

CONTROVERSIES AND PITFALLS

Diagnostic ultrasound is a dynamic modality and as such is extremely operator and technology dependent. Methodological difficulties in evaluating the performance potential of diagnostic ultrasound arise because of the hardware and the imaging technique employed in various studies. Some authors recommend the use of a 7.5- or 10-Mhz head, while others utilize 3.5- or 5-Mhz frequencies for spinal imaging. Still others have employed much lower frequencies (1.5 Mhz). Additionally, the skill of the equipment operator is rarely known. Given the operator dependency of diagnostic ultrasound, the generalizability of results becomes narrowly restricted. This has been particularly true for spinal applications of diagnostic ultrasound.[5]

Another difficulty is the issue of anisotropy. This is the phenomenon of lowered signal from a structure (such as a tendon) caused by the ultrasound beam striking the area of interest at an angle other than 90°. This false lowering of echogenicity may create the appearance of abnormality when indeed it is not present.[46,47]

CONSENSUS STATEMENTS

In response to the contemporary initiatives for guidelines and practice policies, authoritative groups have produced formal consensus statements regarding the use of diagnostic ultrasound in clinical practice. The Mercy Commission[48(p28)] conferred an "established" rating for ultrasound's limited applications in diagnosing musculoskeletal conditions outside the spine; for its promise as a noninvasive, inexpensive alternative to MRI and arthrography; and for its appropriateness as a modality for the evaluation of many intraabdominal and pelvic organs. Additionally the American College of Radiology[3] and the American Chiropractic College of Radiology[4] have produced practice policies regarding diagnostic ultrasound of the adult spine that have emerged from formal development processes. The policy statement of the American College of Radiology is as follows:

> The use of diagnostic spinal ultrasound in the evaluation of pain or radiculopathy syndrome (facet joints and capsules, nerve and fascial edema, and other subtle paraspinous abnormalities) currently has no proven clinical utility as a screening, diagnostic, or adjunctive imaging tool.

The policy statement of the American Chiropractic College of Radiology, which was submitted for review and ratification by the House of Delegates of the American Chiropractic Association, is as follows:

> Diagnostic ultrasound has been shown to be a useful modality for evaluating certain musculoskeletal complaints. Fetal, pediatric, and intra-operative applications have been published in the scientific literature.
>
> The quality of ultrasound images is extremely dependent on operator skill. The resolution abilities of the equipment may have an impact on diagnostic yield, and accuracy. Consequently, the importance of training to establish technologic as well as interpretive competency cannot be overstated. The application of diagnostic ultrasound in the adult spine in areas such as disc herniation, spinal stenosis, and nerve root pathology is inadequately studied and its routine application for these purposes cannot be supported by the evidence at this time.

CONCLUSION

Diagnostic ultrasound is a well-established modality for the evaluation of abdominal and retroperitoneal soft tissues. Musculoskeletal applications in the extremities have been reviewed extensively in the literature, and they appear to have the potential for a limited role in clinical practice. Spinal ultrasound has been found useful in pediatric, interventional, and intraoperative applications, although the range of applications is of limited scope. Adult spinal ultrasound has been the least studied of all musculoskeletal applications. With the exception of ultrasound for the evaluation of spinal canal size, there are too few studies to recommend frequent use of diagnostic ultrasound. The data provided to date are not altogether encouraging, but there is enough information to warrant further study of the ability of ultrasound to evaluate the lumbar spine. Preliminary studies of its ability to evaluate the cervical spine need to be performed before its potential in this area can be assessed (see Table 1).

Table 1. Technology assessment of diagnostic ultrasound

Application	Assessment
Soft tissues	Well established for evaluation of the abdominal and retroperitoneal soft tissues
Musculoskeletal, extremity	Limited role for articulations and muscles and tendons
Musculoskeletal, spine	Limited pediatric, interventional, and intraoperative applications
	MRI, CT, and myelography outperform DU for diagnosis of disc herniation
	May have limited usefulness in assessing spinal canal size in lumbar spine
	Insufficient evidence to assess usefulness of DU for spinal muscles or tendons

Key: MRI = magnetic resonance imaging, CT = computed tomography, DU = diagnostic ultrasound

The main clinical advantages of ultrasound are probably noninvasiveness and the ease with which the technology can be acquired.[49] However, these alone are not enough to warrant its clinical application, especially in light of how its performance compares with that of other imaging modalities.

The clinical disadvantages include extreme operator dependency and possible technical variability among different machines (the degree of variability is unknown). Given the lack of sufficient quantity and quality of supportive data in the literature and the clinical disadvantages that exist, it would appear that the position statements of the ACR and ACCR are currently appropriate. Further study of low back applications is needed, and there are no data supporting any cervical spine application to date. As new information emerges on the appropriateness of this technology in different clinical circumstances, it may be necessary to change existing policies and guidelines on the use of diagnostic ultrasound. The chiropractic physician will do well to stay abreast of advances in this technology, keeping in view where its application fits into the "best practice" for the patient.

REFERENCES

1. Curry T, Dowdey J, Murry R. *Christensen's Physics of Diagnostic Radiology*. 4th ed. Malvern, PA: Lea & Febiger; 1990.
2. Stipkovich N. The use of chiropractic diagnostic ultrasonography for case monitoring. Orthopedic notes. Arlington, VA: Council for Chiropractic Orthopedics; 1994. AANID001.
3. Neiman H. ACR Commission on Ultrasound. ACR Bulletin 2-96.
4. American Chiropractic College of Radiology. *Policy Statement on Diagnostic Ultrasound of the Adult Spine*. American Chiropractic Association House of Delegates, December 1995.
5. Barry M, Brandt J, Christensen K, et al. Facts and fallacies of diagnostic ultrasound of the adult spine. *Dynamic Chiro*. 1996;14(9):1.
6. Van Holsbeek M, Introcaso J. Musculoskeletal ultrasonography. *Radiol Clin N Am*. 1992;30:907-925.
7. Chhem R, Kaplan P, Dussault R. Ultrasonography of the musculoskeletal system. *Radiol Clin N Am*. 1994;32:275-289.
8. Crass J, Craig E, Feinberg S. Ultrasonography of rotator cuff tears: a review of 500 diagnostic studies. *J Clin Ultrasound*. 1988;16:313-327.
9. Moss G, Dishuk W. Ultrasound diagnosis of osteochondromatosis of the popliteal fossa. *J Clin Ultrasound*. 1984;12:232-233.
10. Burk DL, Karasick D, Kurtz AB, et al. Rotator cuff tears: prospective comparison of MR imaging with arthrography, sonography, and surgery. *AJR*. 1989;153:87-92.
11. Lund P, Nisbet J, Valencia F, et al. Current sonographic applications in orthopedics. *AJR*. 1996;166:889-895.
12. Aisen A, McCune W, McGuire A, et al. Sonographic evaluation of the cartilage of the knee. *Radiology*. 1984;153:781-784.
13. Abiri M, Dirpekar M, Ablow R. Osteomyelitis: detection with US. *Radiology*. 1988;169:795-797.
14. Young J, Kostrubiak I, Resnick C, et al. Sonographic evaluation of bone production at the distraction site in Ilizarov limb-lengthening procedures. *AJR*. 1990;154:125-128.
15. Lund P, Heikel A, Maricic M, et al. Ultrasound imaging of the hand and wrist in rheumatoid arthritis. *Skeletal Radiol*. 1995;24:591-596.
16. Gershuni D, Gosink B, Hargens A, et al. Ultrasound evaluation of the anterior musculofascial compartment of the leg following exercise. *Clin Orthop*. 1982;167:185-190.
17. Hicks J, Shawker T, Jones B, et al. Diagnostic ultrasound: its use in the evaluation of muscle. *Arch Phys Med Rehabil*. 1984;65:129-131.
18. Reimers K, Reimers C, Wagner S, et al. Skeletal muscle sonography: a correlative study of echogenicity and morphology. *J Ultrasound Med*. 1993;2:73-77.
19. Nishimura M, Nishimura S, Yamada S. Ultrasound imaging of the muscle in muscular dystrophy. *No To Hattatsu*. 1989;21:234-237.
20. El-Khoury G, Brandser E, Kathol M, et al. Imaging of muscle injuries. *Skeletal Radiol*. 1996;25:3-11.
21. Rubin J, DiPietro M, Chandler W, et al. Spinal ultrasonography: intraoperative and pediatric applications. *Radiol Clin N Am*. 1988;26:1-27.
22. Raghavendra N, Epstein F. Sonography of the spine and spinal cord. *Radiol Clin N Am*. 1985;23:91-105.
23. Porter R, Hibbert C, Wicks M. The spinal canal in symptomatic lumbar disc lesions. *J Bone Joint Surg*. 1978;60B:485-487.
24. Kamei K, Hanai K, Matsui N. Ultrasonic level diagnosis of lumbar disc herniation. *Spine*. 1990;15:1170-1174.
25. Engel J, Engel G, Gunn D. Ultrasound of the spine in focal stenosis and disc disease. *Spine*. 1985;10:928-931.
26. Merx J, Thijssen H, Meyer E, et al. Accuracy of evaluation of lumbar intervertebral discs by an anterior approach. *Neuroradiology*. 1989;31:386-390.
27. Hagen A. Transabdominal ultrasound tomography of the lumbar intervertebral discs and the lumbar canal. *Zentralbl Neurochir*. 1987;48:273-279.
28. Legg S, Gibbs V. Measurement of the lumbar spinal canal by echo ultrasound. *Spine*. 1984;9:79-82.
29. Porter R, Wicks M, Ottewell D. Measurement of the spinal canal by diagnostic ultrasound. *J Bone Joint Surg*. 1978;60B:481-484.
30. Kadziolka R, Asztely M, Hanai K, et al. Ultrasonic measurement of the lumbar spinal canal: the origin and precision of the recorded echoes. *J Bone Joint Surg*. 1981;63B:504-507.
31. Chovil A, Anderson D, Adcock D. Ultrasonic measurement of lumbar spinal canal diameter: a screening tool for low back disorders? *South Med J*. 1989;82:977-980.
32. Porter R, Bewley B. A 10-year prospective study of vertebral canal size as a predictor of back pain. *Spine*. 1994;19:173-175.
33. Battie M, Hansson T, Engel J, et al. The reliability of measurements of the lumbar spine using ultrasound B scan. *Spine*. 1986;11:144-148.
34. Stockdale H, Finlay D. Use of diagnostic ultrasound to measure the lumbar spinal canal. *Br J Radiol*. 1980;53:1101-1102.
35. Finlay D, Stockdale H, Lewin E. An appraisal of the use of diagnostic ultrasound to quantify the lumbar spinal canal. *Br J Radiol*. 1981;54:870-874.
36. Howie D, Chatterton B, Hone M. Failure of ultrasound in the investigation of sciatica. *J Bone Joint Surg*. 1983;65B:144-147.

37. Porter R, Hibbert C, Wellman P. Backache and the lumbar spinal canal. *Spine.* 1980;5:99–105.
38. Grubb N, Fleming A, Sutherland G, et al. Skeletal muscle contraction in healthy volunteers: assessment with Doppler tissue imaging. *Radiology.* 1995;194:837–842.
39. Van Holsbeeck M, Introcaso J. Sonography of muscle. In: Van Holsbeeck M, Introcaso J, eds. *Musculoskeletal Ultrasound.* St. Louis: Mosby; 1991.
40. Harcke T, Grissom L, Finkelstein M. Evaluation of the musculoskeletal system with sonography. *AJR.* 1988;153:1253–1261.
41. Hides J, Cooper D, Stokes M. Diagnostic ultrasound imaging for measurement of the lumbar multifidus muscle in normal young adults. *Physiother Theory Pract.* 1992;8:19–26.
42. Soltani A, Kallinen M, Malkia E, et al. Ultrasonography of the neck splenius capitis muscle: Investigation in a group of young healthy women. *Acta Radiologica.* 1996;37:647–650.
43. Hides J, Stokes M, Saide M, et al. Evidence of lumbar multifidus muscle wasting ipsilateral to symptoms in patients with acute/subacute low back pain. *Spine.* 1994;19:165–172.
44. Kennaly K, Stokes M. Pattern of asymmetry of paraspinal muscle size in adolescent idiopathic scoliosis examined by real-time ultrasound imaging. *Spine.* 1993;18:913–915.
45. Stipkovich N. Musculoskeletal ultrasonographic examination of the cervical spine and surrounding tissues including normal lymph nodes. *J Am Chiro Assoc.* December 1994:33–37.
46. Lund P, Nisbet J, Valencia F, et al. Current sonographic applications in orthopedics. *AJR.* 1996;166:889–895.
47. Fornage B. The hypoechoic normal tendon: a pitfall. *J Ultrasound Med.* 1987;6:19–22.
48. Haldeman S, Chapman-Smith D, Petersen D, eds. *Guidelines for Chiropractic Quality Assurance and Practice Parameters.* Gaithersburg, MD: Aspen Publishers; 1992.
49. Stewart H, Moore R. Development of health risk evaluation data for diagnostic ultrasound: a historical perspective. *J Clin Ultrasound.* 1984;12:493–500.

12

Optimizing Clinical Use of Radiography and Minimizing Radiation Exposure in Chiropractic Practice

Robert D. Mootz, Lisa E. Hoffman, and Daniel T. Hansen

Spinal radiographic imaging has long been associated with the chiropractic profession. In fact, radiographic imaging appears to have been incorporated into chiropractic as early as 1908, a mere 13 years after the discovery of X-rays.[1] Considerable instructional time in chiropractic education is devoted to radiographic procedures, diagnosis, and clinical use. As there are potential risks of ionizing radiation, considerable attention in the chiropractic literature has been given to minimizing exposure to radiation.[2-5] In order to best reduce radiation exposure, the clinical circumstances surrounding the decision to obtain radiographic images need to be carefully assessed.

Three distinct clinical judgment components should be considered:

1. The purpose for taking a radiograph in a particular clinical situation should be established.
2. The clinician must assess the potential value of the radiograph (eg, will the information provided have a worthwhile impact on patient management).
3. If radiography is warranted, appropriate technical procedures must be followed to prevent retakes, reduce primary radiation exposure, obtain a high-quality image, and protect the patient from primary radiation exposure outside the area of interest as well secondary radiation during the exposure.

The chiropractic profession as a whole plays an important role in setting standards for utilization of all clinical procedures. Not only do educational institutions set the tone for how students think about radiography, state and national societies as well as government regulatory agencies can establish standards and guidelines for clinical procedures. In recent years, accountable units on the delivery side, including hospitals, physician groups, and health services purchasers, have become involved in the promulgation of radiographic guidelines.

USEFULNESS OF RADIOGRAPHIC IMAGING

Chiropractors have many rationales for the clinical use of radiography.[6-8] It is generally considered a valuable diagnostic tool for determining the presence of pathology and contraindications for spinal manipulative therapy (SMT).[8-11] The challenges regarding the diagnostic significance of radiography for identifying pathology are not unique to chiropractors, and discussion of the value of radiography is common in the medical literature.[12,13] Identifying contraindications to the comparatively safe practices of spinal and extremity manipulation, however, is a purpose that belongs only to practitioners of manual therapies, especially DCs.

Chiropractors have frequently incorporated spinal imaging techniques in order to assess specific pathomechanical alterations amenable to the application of SMT.[14,15] This radiographic role appears to be uniquely chiropractic, at least in modern-day practice. Additionally, radiography has been used as a monitoring device to assess outcomes of management and therapeutic progress.[16] Unfortunately, the use of chiropractic radiography for biomechanical interpretations is not standardized and remains a source of controversy.[3]

The authors thank Carol Farber for assistance with manuscript preparation; William C. Meeker, DC, MPH, for earlier work reviewing validity and reliability of radiograph-marking systems; Alan H. Adams, MS, DC, and Gary Schultz, DC, for provision of literature; and Philip C. Sollecito, DC, for provision of IPA data.

VALUE OF RADIOLOGY AS A DIAGNOSTIC TOOL

Wyatt and Schultz[2] emphasized the need to determine in advance the likely "yield" that can be obtained from a radiograph. Specifically, a determination needs to be made regarding how a radiographic study will impact the diagnosis or course of care. Even though the results of diagnostic imaging may help rule in or rule out a diagnosis, unless the information somehow impacts patient management decisions, it probably is not clinically indicated. For example, an older female patient with clear current clinical indications of and previous chiropractic management of mechanical spinal dysfunction but no other pathological "red flags" has a reasonable probability of demonstrating some radiographic evidence of early bone demineralization and degenerative changes in the spine. Yet these findings may not significantly impact how such a patient would be managed with manipulation. It has been suggested that indicators such as trauma, advanced age, neuromotor deficit, and other historical findings constitute the main reasons for using radiography.[17,18] In the absence of such indicators, the diagnostic yield (clinical usefulness) of the radiograph is quite low and rarely affects therapy. Radiography is useful in the diagnosis of neoplasm, infection, trauma, and ankylosing spondylitis—all conditions that are likely to be suspected from history and physical examination.[19]

Halvorsen and Swanson[13] offer radiography guidelines for general practitioners based on general diagnostic yield considerations according to patient presentation. They emphasize that in addition to general attributes of appropriate patient selection, optimizing radiographic technique, and adequate interpretation, criteria for determining the need for radiography may be different for symptomatic versus asymptomatic individuals. Table 1 summarizes some of the key considerations that have been identified in determining appropriateness of radiology for diagnosis generally and for extremity and spine disorders specifically.[5,13,20,21]

VALUE OF RADIOLOGY FOR BIOMECHANICAL ASSESSMENT

A number of chiropractic techniques have incorporated routine biomechanical analysis of spinal radiographs for establishing manual care plans.[22] However, the usefulness of

---

Table 1. Criteria for using plain film radiography for diagnostic purposes

General issues
- Will radiography provide desired information regarding internal anatomy and physiology?
- Are results expected to be important in managing the patient (even when studies are normal)?
- Will results affect diagnostic level of certainty in a clinically meaningful way?
- Does the suspected pathology exhibit adequate incidence, severity, or contagiousness to warrant radiation exposure?
- Does the radiographic study under consideration have adequate reliability, sensitivity, and specificity to produce useful information in the given situation?
- Are the time and cost requirements for obtaining the study justifiable?
- What are the consequences to the patient if a given condition goes untreated?

Indications for extremity radiography in symptomatic patients having corresponding trauma
- Bone deformity, instability, crepitation, or point tenderness
- Severe upper extremity swelling
- Moderate to severe pain with weight bearing in a hip or thigh
- Knee pain
- Abnormal tendon or neurovascular function on examination
- Palpable mass
- History suggesting fracture risk (eg, cancer, Paget's disease)

Indications for extremity radiography in symptomatic patients without trauma
- Disturbances in skeletal maturation, osseous dysplasia
- History or findings of metabolic or endocrine disease affecting bone (eg, Cushing's disease, malnutrition)
- History of bone tumors, metastasis, infection, or cysts with growth potential
- History of joint disease (eg, arthritides, chondromatous tumors)
- Paget's disease

Indications for spine radiography in symptomatic patients
- History of trauma
- Cancer red flags (eg, unexplained weight loss, 1-month pain duration, conservative treatment failure, over age 50)
- Osteomyelitis red flags (eg, history of IV drug use, skin or urinary tract infection)
- Radicular pain distribution
- Clinical suspicion of spinal stenosis (eg, claudication, advanced age)
- Clinical suspicion of ankylosing spondylitis

Indications for spine radiography in asymptomatic patients
- Scoliosis evaluation and monitoring in those that are skeletally immature
- No other generally accepted criteria exist for spinal radiography in asymptomatic individuals

such approaches has long been the source of controversy within the chiropractic profession.[2,3,23] The nature of positional and distortional factors, along with biological asymmetry, complicates the task of radiographic evaluation of spinal biomechanics. Published radiographic protocols have proposed positioning precision[24,25] and minimizing error margins.[26,27] Several studies have varied position of radiographic phantom models in an attempt to examine the validity and reliability of some radiographic marking systems.[28-31]

Validity considerations

Studies of the validity of chiropractic radiographic marking systems have attempted to determine if radiographic markings can truly identify what is being measured. An earlier review in the chiropractic literature summarized some of these.[32] Rupert[28] examined bony symmetry by measuring dried specimens and concluded that asymmetry appeared to be the rule rather than the exception. Some landmarks appeared to vary relatively little when compared to their total size, but caution should temper any clinical decision based on listing systems. However, Zengle et al[29] attached rods to the vertebral end-plates of dry specimens radiographed, in known disrelationships and determined that off-centering and rotation produced no measurable effect on the position of constructed lines and therefore may be considered valid indicators of vertebral wedging.

Davis and Rozeboom[30] radiographed a model with controllable position factors and predetermined misalignments to compare known parameters with those identified radiographically using the Logan procedure. Pelvic anteriority and true sacral anteriority were subject to large error margins for rotational malpositioning of the model. Schram, Hosek, and Silverman[33] also altered dry specimen position to evaluate Gonstead marking systems. Rotation about the vertical axis produced greater error than rotation about a horizontal axis (tilt), because the latter errors are projected symmetrically. Tilt errors could, however, invalidate comparison for sequential studies.

Reinert and Davis[34] reported that shifts in the symmetry of weight bearing produced marked changes in pelvic listings on human subjects, suggesting that such listings may be a function of weight bearing instead of actual bony position. Triano and Marinelli[35] presented a study that assessed reliability and validity of radiographic assessment of facet orientation at the L-5/S-1 level on 22 cadavers that were subsequently dissected. A comparison of radiographic appearance, anatomical orientation, curve index, and curve eccentricity for each articulation revealed that radiographic appearance did not correlate well with actual anatomical measurements. Awareness of limitations regarding assumptions about the validity of static radiography is prompting promoters of radiation-intensive chiropractic techniques to reconsider strategies for using radiography.[36]

Reliability issues

The reliability of radiographic marking systems is a mixed bag. Rozeboom[37] evaluated inter- and intrarater reliability of the Logan marking system by taking two films of the same subject while allowing the subject to move and be repositioned between exposures. Both films were blindly analyzed by the same person with identical procedures. Analysis showed that several standard parameters of pelvic measurements varied from 40% to 90% upon measurement of the second film, casting doubt on the clinical usefulness of such measurements for clinical purposes. Over half of the time the average clinical measurement fell within the margin of error. Sigler and Howe[38] studied upper-cervical analysis of atlas rotation by comparing the measurements of three observers on a set of 20 films. The average measurement was 1.8°. The three observers agreed with the each other within 0.5° only 10% of the time. They only reached agreement 95% of the time if the range of variance was 3.5°. Given that 70% agreement is clinically sufficient, then a reliability variance of 1.5° must be accepted. However, this figure was 82% of the average clinical measurement.

Phillips[39] compared three chiropractic marking procedures for pelvic misalignment listings. The various methods indicated a wide range of findings, and he concluded that the lack of correlation between the systems suggested that the interpretation of spinal radiography for this purpose appears to be subjective. Bronfort and Jochumsen[40] evaluated measurement accuracy and sources of error in a single-plane functional evaluation of lumbar motion. By utilizing a digital analyzer, they were able to identify and measure instrument error, error in radiographic positioning by two different examiners, biological variation during a 1–5 day interval, and biological variation between sitting and standing radiographs. The smallest total error was 1.7° (at a 95% confidence level) of difference between two radiographic exams. The largest error was determined to be 2.9°, indicating that differences in mobility noted on pre- and posttests less than 1.7° are just as likely to be due to errors in measurement as to the treatment. They concluded that sitting, lateral bending, and standing flexion/extension examinations demonstrated the least variation. They also reported a high positive correlation between functional radiographic measurement and cineradiography.

Owens,[41] performing a qualitative literature review of studies on line drawing analysis of static cervical radiographs, concluded that reliability studies[42,43] have adequately demonstrated that lateral and rotational displacements of C-1 can accurately be measured within a 1° margin of error. Radiographic marking methods that use relative angular measurements of skeletal positioning seem to minimize the effects of radiographic distortion. However, it is still uncertain how this translates into three-dimensional movement or to what extent changes in pre- and postadjustment measurements might be due to changes in patient positioning in clinical applications.

Plaugher and his coworkers[44,45] have attempted to evaluate the reliability and significance of radiographic parameters commonly used in Gonstead technique protocols. Marking of femur head height was measured on 71 full spine radiographs twice by two different examiners. High concordance levels were reported, with intraexaminer agreement consistently better than interexaminer agreement.[43] Plaugher also demonstrated minimal variations for several radiographic pelvic markings in the repositioning of 37 relatively asymptomatic subjects at 1-hour and 18-day intervals using a feet-positioning grid.[44] Measurements included femur head height, right and left ileum height, pubis deviation, and sacral base heights (right and left side). However, another well-designed intra- and interrater reliability study of Gonstead marking procedures had promising results but relatively weak Kappa scores (it used the standard line marking procedures to determine specific levels of biomechanical lesions).[46] Although Plaugher's design included careful specification of which marking attributes were considered, Burk's work utilized practicing DCs who used the methodology to determine where to adjust, a theoretically important component of chiropractic care.

When radiography is used for biomechanical assessment, it should tell the clinician conclusively whether a mechanopathology is present or absent. Furthermore, the interpreter should be able to repeat the measurements with minimal variance, and different interpreters should be able to reproduce the same results. Many studies appear to suggest that radiographic interpretation may be a source of significant error in biomechanical assessment. However, when proper anatomical landmarks and well-trained interpreters are used, a number of markings do appear to have reasonable reliability.

VALUE OF RADIOLOGY FOR MONITORING THERAPEUTIC PROGRESS

Given the inherent limitations in reliability for many measurements, particularly if the interpreters are inexperienced, the usefulness of such markings may be questioned. However, since some measurements are reliable, the issue of whether or not they can be used as indicators of therapeutic progress must also be addressed. It is important to emphasize that reliability of a measurement does not imply any sort of construct validity. For example, just because segmental retrolisthesis can be reliably measured does not mean that any changes in retrolisthesis that occur are due to a therapeutic intervention or that such changes are clinically meaningful.

In a study by Plaugher and coworkers,[47] 49 full spine (AP and lateral) postural studies were evaluated for measurement of cervical and lumbar lordosis, segmental retrolysthesis, sacral base angle, and scapular angle before and after chiropractic adjustment. The reliability of the marking system was demonstrated for cervical lordosis and segmental retrolisthesis. A 34% reduction in retrolisthesis was demonstrated after treatment. No pre- and posttreatment changes were reported with cervical or lumbar lordosis angles, sacral base angles, scapular angles, or Cobb's angles.

Saggital spinal curvatures have been common targets of clinical assessment and follow-up by many investigators. As these are vertical measurements, the possibility exists that these evaluations may have some reliability. Jochumsen[48] devised a quantitative method of measuring lordosis and kyphosis and used it to evaluate 100 asymptomatic and 400 symptomatic individuals. Fifty-six percent of the symptomatic group displayed saggital curve straightening while 36% of the asymptomatic group displayed straightening, thus supporting the contention that cervical hypolordosis may be associated with neck symptoms. Jochumsen also concluded that trauma was not a main contributor toward a tendency for cervical straightening. He followed up with a descriptive trial of spinal manipulation and cervical pillow use. In the case of 20 patients treated with spinal manipulation alone, there was minimal change. Forty patients treated with both SMT and a cervical pillow had a reported 33% increase in lordosis. Unfortunately, the details of the statistical assessments were not reported.

Leach[49] reported a controlled study of the effect of spinal manipulation on hypolordosis of the cervical spine in 29 patients with complaints in the cervical area. He attempted to control for positional errors and anatomic anomalies (such as short pedicles, etc) and used a quantitative measurement system. The group of patients receiving SMT for hypolordosis (directed at the midcervical area) was compared to a hypolordotic control group receiving SMT in the upper cervical region. The mean change in the treatment group was statistically better than the mean change in the control group ($p = 0.01$). Leach also used a cervical pillow to treat six patients, but the results were less satisfactory than those of the SMT-alone group.

A RADIOLOGIC DIAGNOSIS AND BIOMECHANICAL ASSESSMENT REALITY CHECK

Even if radiograph diagnoses can be made accurately, even if certain biomechanical measurements prove reliable, and even if chiropractic intervention can be shown to reproducibly make alterations in reliable radiographic indicators, an underlying challenge remains to be met. Perhaps the most significant issue confronting clinicians, patients, and policy planners alike relates to the concept of *value per health care dollar spent*. Does having the information from a radiograph improve the overall outcome of treatment in a significant way that would not be possible without it? Developments in health care accountability and policy planning include a recent move away from clinical progress indicators toward such relevant outcomes questions.[50,51]

This is essentially the same question posed to DCs by Wyatt and Schultz[2] in 1987; how does the information provided by a radiograph affect patient management? If observer bias and errors in measurement can be determined and eliminated, then radiographic evidence of abnormal spinal alignment can be quantitatively linked to clinical processes. Unfortunately, no definitive data yet exist that would support the notion that reductions in misalignment factors are causally related to a reduction of symptoms or improvement in overall patient progress. This is not to say that chiropractic intervention has not been shown to be beneficial in the treatment of patients suffering from a variety of musculoskeletal conditions; in fact, both data and expert clinical opinion support manipulation in patients with neck and back pain.[52,53]

However, two significant questions remain that will require further research within the chiropractic community: (1) What tangible quality of care benefits accrue from having the clinical information gained from any given radiographic study (eg, does the patient get better faster? return to work sooner? avoid more costly or risky additional care? etc). (2) What other cheaper or less invasive alternatives to radiographic studies exist? Using plain film imaging, single studies result in relatively insignificant radiation dosages and expense. However, both dosages and expense can become significant with repeat studies and retakes.

Medical irradiation remains the source of greatest exposure to artificial radiation, accounting for 12% of radiation from all sources.[54] Although only 1–2% of all cancers have been attributed to medical radiology,[55] limitations in long-term follow-up may mean the radiation-cancer association and life-time cancer risks have been underestimated many times over.[56] Radiation poses small but significant health risks, and long-term effects remain inadequately studied. Quality of care concerns mandate that it be used sparingly and wisely.

Practitioners have reasonable resources at their disposal to assist in determining the appropriateness of radiography for diagnostic purposes. Diagnosis and therapeutic yields for biomechanical assessment remain less clear, and the comparative contribution of biomechanical radiographic analysis to meaningful patient outcomes has yet to be studied. Chiropractors whose techniques require little to no radiography to achieve patient outcomes equivalent to those of DCs using radiographic-intensive procedures may find themselves favored by policy planners and consumer advocates and hence at a competitive advantage in the years ahead.

TECHNICAL STRATEGIES FOR QUALITY ASSURANCE AND EXPOSURE REDUCTION

As part of the decision to use radiography, a number of strategies to assure quality and maintain technical excellence should be considered. Lowering patient exposure dose is critical.[4,53] Maintaining vigilance in the operation and maintenance of radiographic equipment and facilities is also essential.[57] In addition, quality assurance requirements regarding radiography are being implemented by government agencies and accreditation organizations.[58]

Retakes

Improper technique on the part of the operator is probably the single greatest culprit in necessitating retakes. Estimation of exposure factors may be a relatively common occurrence in many practices. Such an approach is unlikely to minimize exposure, since poor images will compel the taking of a second exposure. Therefore, devices such as the "Super-Tech" should be used in establishing technique charts for all new or relocated equipment. Technique charts developed for the exact equipment and routine use of accurate patient measurement are essential for minimizing retakes. Another practice to avoid is routinely increasing exposure time (MAS) instead of penetration (KVP) when darkroom chemicals weaken.

A common source of easily preventable error is improper patient or equipment positioning. Every DC has forgotten to close a bucky, load a film, or center the patient to the central ray at least once, which leads to making a second exposure. An investment of the extra time and energy required for careful thought and double-checking will minimize the need for retakes. Regular maintenance of the darkroom and developing materials is another technical activity that can increase film quality. Meticulous practices regarding these factors reduce costs and radiation exposure in the long run.

Patient protection

There are several ways the patient can be protected or shielded from the primary beam while avoiding a decline in the clinical usefulness of the resulting radiograph.[4] Obvious standard methods include minimal total tube filtration and beam limitation devices (collimation). Additional technical upgrades are available that not only reduce radiation but enhance film quality. High-speed rare earth screens, shielding devices, supplemental tube filtration, compensatory filtration, and high-frequency X-ray generators can all reduce the ionizing radiation that reaches a patient during exposure.

Shielding devices should be used routinely and placed properly. Regular use and proper placement of shields rest in the hand of the machine operator, and doctors need to ensure that they or their staff do not fail to use them. Shielding areas outside of the primary beam is essential, especially for the radiation sensitive tissues in the eyes, breasts, thyroid, and gonads. Although most jurisdictions require radiography rooms to be stocked with lead aprons and glasses, it is always the responsibility of the operator to insist on their regular use. Scuderi[4] recently reviewed X-ray filtration and shielding devices, delineating the relative advantages and disadvantages of several currently available products.

INFLUENCING CLINICAL BEHAVIORS

What strategies can and should be employed to optimize radiology practices in the field? Obviously, the medical and chiropractic literature contains important information for minimizing patient radiation exposure and appropriate utilization recommendations. However, it is a challenge for clinicians to stay abreast of new developments. Continuing education involving radiology is recommended, as is seeking out general reviews in the literature (many of these have been cited here). For the most part, chiropractic educational institutions have taken a responsible approach to teaching appropriate decision-making and clinical judgment processes.[3,4,59] However, many artificial incentives exist within chiropractic that significantly hinder responsible practice.

One incentive that impacts provider habits beginning in the educational setting consists of the numbers-based graduation requirements of the Council on Chiropractic Education. While it is clear that apprenticing is one of the best methods for learning clinical techniques, competency-based approaches need to supplement or supplant the arbitrary numbers game that currently exists. Clerkship rotation options, simulated patient assessment, laboratory radiographic reading opportunities, and individually tailored competency assessments are all legitimate approaches that could substitute for the dubious practice of having students take radiographs on real patients for nonclinical purposes, such as graduation requirements.

An example of an external incentive that fosters harmful patient practices is the Medicare reimbursement requirement that a patient's vertebral subluxation be demonstrated on a radiograph annually. This arbitrary requirement not only runs counter to standard medical and chiropractic practice, it violates the explicit policy recommendations of the American Public Health Association against the use of radiographs for insurance purposes only. Further, such a requirement may be clinically and scientifically bankrupt, since, as described previously, radiographs may be diagnostically unreliable.

A further absurdity of this harmful federal policy is seen in the ludicrous prohibition of Medicare reimbursement for radiography performed by chiropractors; not only do Medicare patients have to be irradiated needlessly in many instances, they have to pay for it themselves. However, before rushing to blame uncaring federal bureaucrats for the problem, remember that the original recommendations for this Medicare policy were made by the political leadership within chiropractic in the 1970s. A useful lesson here is that chiropractors need to be wary of letting their political leaders codify attributes of clinical practice driven by shortsighted reimbursement goals.

Responsible chiropractors should advocate at all levels (ranging from their individual practices to national organization's political agendas), for patient-centered decision making and policy planning. Given that individual initiative, training, peer pressure, and reimbursement incentives together influence much of the practice behavior surrounding imaging, much work is still needed in the health services and clinical research arenas.

Another more direct (but sometimes confrontational) route for influencing clinical behaviors is through guidelines and policies promulgated by professional trade associations. Legislative or regulatory edicts can influence clinical practices, as evidenced by the fact that some regional jurisdictions have restricted chiropractic utilization of radiography for the purpose of minimizing radiation exposure. Third-party payers often have an impact on clinical practices as well, through various peer review mechanisms and internal coverage guidelines. Sadly, they are sometimes motivated more by fiscal considerations than quality assurance concerns. It is far better for the profession and the practitioners to take the lead in ensuring responsible radiology practices than for outside government agencies to single out DCs for regulatory changes.

Professionwide contributions toward the rational utilization of radiography, however well intentioned, fail to address a major concern of practicing clinicians. Suggesting to an experienced clinician that a time-tested, widely used diagnostic procedure suddenly has severe clinical limitations poses the problem of finding potential alternatives. Emphasis must be placed on the development of other clinical resources, skills, and procedures for alternative types of diagnostic and biomechanical assessment. The reliability and validity of a great many orthopaedic, neurologic, and chiropractic evaluation procedures remain to be established as well. There is a certain amount of comfort provided by the nice black-and-white visual image afforded by a radiograph.[13] Clinicians of all stripes need resources for and guidance in synthesizing the vast amount of information they are expected to process.

EXAMPLES OF IMAGING GUIDELINES

Demands from the health reimbursement industry for more accountability and auditability in the purchase of expensive technologies and high-volume services have increased in recent years. Although they are partially driven by economic considerations, quality of care issues also come into play.[3,4,17] For example, given the high equivalent rates of disc herniation (on symptomatic and asymptomatic patients) evidenced on CT and MRI imaging,[60] nonspecific low back pain patients may be incorrectly diagnosed and put at risk for ineffective management, including further unnecessary high-risk diagnostics and questionable surgical interventions.

One approach to establishing guidelines for CT and MRI studies comes from a state workers' compensation regulatory agency.[61] Using a process of qualitative literature review and community-based physician input, criteria for MRI and repeat MRI of the lumbar spine were developed and implemented for injured worker care (Table 2). Although these guidelines focus on noninvasive MRI, they represent a regulatory agency's effort to ensure appropriate utilization of an expensive imaging technology. The process used also illustrates how a provider community can interact constructively with regulators to incorporate information from the literature as well as expert and community-based physician input into guidelines that impact provider practices.

The Agency for Health Care Policy and Research (within the US Department of Health and Human Services) issued recommendations for the use of imaging in the management of adult low back pain patients.[20] These guidelines recommend use of plain film radiographs only in the presence of clinical "red flags" for risk of cancer, spinal osteomyelitis, herniated disk, spinal stenosis, or ankylosing spondylitis. Advanced imaging was recommended when recovery from acute low back pain exceeded 1 month and only in the presence of clear indications of radiculopathy or systemic disease.

Table 2. Washington State Workers' Compensation criteria for MRI of the lumbar spine

Indications for MRI of the lumbar spine
- Any neurological deficit, evidence of radiculopathy, cauda equina compression (eg, sudden bowel/bladder disturbance) OR
- Suspected systemic disorder (eg, to r/o metastatic or infectious disease) OR
- Localized back pain with no radiculopathy (leg pain), clinical history of lumbar spine or strain, and failed 6-week course of conservative care

Indications for repeat MRI of the lumbar spine
- Significant change in clinical finding (eg, new or progressive neurological deficit)

Note: The primary physician is strongly encouraged to coordinate with a subspecialist (ie, a board-certified spine specialist, orthopedist, or radiologist) before ordering a repeat MRI of the lumbar spine.
Source: Reprinted with permission from Office of the Medical Director. *Medical Treatment Guidelines.* Olympia, WA: Washington State Department of Labor & Industries; 1996.

Minimization of radiation exposure is an important quality assurance goal.[4] The Radiologic Health Branch of the California Department of Health Services recently issued guidelines for establishing radiographic quality control and assurance programs for anyone involved in the operation and maintenance of radiographic equipment.[57] California requires operator certification separate from professional licensure for the operation of radiographic equipment. Technical topics ranging from certification of operators to specific requirements for repeat film and film-processing records to darkroom requirements are covered. Ensuring technical quality to minimize exposure has also been a focus of recommendations in the chiropractic literature.[56]

The Council on Diagnostic Imaging of the American Chiropractic Association recently published a general review of clinical decision-making processes involved in determining which patients should have diagnostic imaging.[62] The guidelines recommend a careful look at the potential diagnostic and therapeutic yield, followed by a consideration of accuracy, predictive value, performance, and benefits versus risks, before the selection of imaging. Although conceptually well founded, these guidelines suffer from minimal dissemination and an emphasis on attributes of diagnostic sensitivity and specificity, which may not be appreciated by the general chiropractic clinician.

While numerous attempts have been undertaken to implement clinical guidelines for the use of imaging technologies in government and medicine, for the most part national and regional chiropractic professional organizations have not filled the need to provide implementable guidelines that would predictably control for variations in the use of diagnostic imaging. However, examples of the implementation of such guidelines in chiropractic settings can be found. Parameters for the appropriate use of radiography have been attempted at a professionwide level but remain a source of some controversy, perhaps because the effort occurred before practitioners and the chiropractic leadership had much experience with such exercises.[63]

The Los Angeles College of Chiropractic has implemented a series of criteria necessary for both plain film and stress radiographs.[58] The criteria, some of which are patterned after Deyo and Diehl's recommendations,[17] appear in Table 3.

EFFECTIVENESS OF IMAGING GUIDELINES IN CHIROPRACTIC: A CASE STUDY

Responses to demands for quality and appropriateness in the use of imaging technologies are emerging from chiropractic managed care organizations. Implementable guidelines for utilization of diagnostic and treatment procedures are appearing in established regional and local chiropractic independent practice associations (IPAs). One such chiropractic

Table 3. Film ordering criteria of the Los Angeles College of Chiropractic

Criteria for plain film radiographs
- Age greater than 50 years
- Trauma sufficient to cause fracture
- Neuromuscular deficit
- Unexplained weight loss
- Suspicion of or confirmed inflammatory arthritis
- Drug or alcohol abuse
- History of cancer
- Use of steroids
- Fever of unknown origin greater than 100°
- Scoliosis
- History of regional surgery
- Failure to improve without prior radiographs
- Medicolegal or government regulations

Indications for stress radiographs
- Degenerative instability
- Traumatic instability (early or late)
- Inflammatory instability
- Failed surgical fusion
- Osseous fracture (congenital or acquired)
- High-risk ligamentous laxity population
- Scoliosis evaluation in growing skeleton

network identified the need for plain film radiograph and special imaging guidelines for application on new and established patients in an attempt to control quality and costs.[64] Chiropractic Network Services is a statewide IPA providing managed chiropractic care in Washington state. In 1994, a "seed" guideline for utilization of diagnostic imaging on IPA patients was prepared following review of existing evidence-based guidelines[20,62] and then refined through a Delphi consensus exercise involving representative end-users and experts. The final guideline was disseminated throughout the network and implemented through its utilization management system (Table 4).

By policy, the IPA acknowledges that

> diagnostic imaging procedures are vital to diagnosis and case management for doctors of chiropractic, just as they are for other healing arts specialists. The use of these procedures must be based on clinical judgment of the doctor, and guidelines/recommendations are difficult to establish. Only the person who takes the history, performs the examination, and is charged with the responsibility for diagnosis and case management has all of the facts leading to his/her decision on whatever diagnostic imaging procedure may be most beneficial.[65]

The IPA identified key protocols for inclusion in the guideline that address criteria for decision making, justification for initial study, and weighing benefits versus risks. And it underscores the need for auditability by requiring the necessity for imaging to be documented in the patient's chart notes.

Table 5, which presents basic statistics for a recent 4-year period, shows there was an increase in the volume of patients, an increase in the number of providers, and a decrease in the proportion of new patients. Considering the guideline was implemented late in 1994, effects of the guideline implementation may be realized in subsequent years. Data for the

Table 4. Imaging guidelines from a chiropractic IPA

All diagnostic imaging services for new patients are to be based on clinical necessity. When no recent radiographs of the area in question are available from another provider, it may be appropriate to expose new films if at least one of the following is present and documented in the record:
- Significant subjective pain/impairment findings specific to the area to be imaged
- Significant objective findings specific to the area to be imaged
- History indicating the possibility of infection, neoplasm, inflammatory process, or other potential contraindication for manipulative therapy
- Recent significant trauma (any age), recent mild trauma (patient over 50), history of long-term steroid use, osteoporosis, patient over age 70

All diagnostic imaging services for established patients are to be based on clinical necessity. When no recent radiographs of the area in question are available from another provider, it may be appropriate to expose new films if at least one of the following is present and documented in the record:
- Significant worsening in subjective pain/impairment findings specific to the area to be imaged
- Significant worsening in objective findings specific to the area to be imaged
- Significant new injury/aggravation in a previously imaged area
- Significant pain/impairment findings in an area not previously imaged
- History indicating the possibility of infection, neoplasm, inflammatory process, or other potential contraindication for manipulative therapy
- Lack of response to treatment of problems not previously imaged
- Previous imaging showed possible fracture or pathology

Billings for radiology services must be accompanied by chart documentation of necessity. Radiology services lacking documentation of necessity will not be paid.

Note: Guideline developed explicitly and finalized through consensus exercise (Delphi) of representative end-users.

Source: Reprinted from PC Sollecito, *Chiropractic Network Services Provider Manual*, p. G3–4, © 1995, Chiropractic Network Services with permission from Triad Healthcare Network, Plainville, Connecticut.

Table 5. Four-year characteristics of a regional chiropractic independent practice association

	1992	1993	1994	1995
Total IPA doctors	127	161	150	205
Total patients	2,057	2,907	3,642	6,155
Total new patients	913	1,289	1,472	2,049
Percentage of new patients	44.4	44.3	40.4	34.0
Percentage of new patients radiographed	61.2	58.3	55.6	44.9
Percentage of established patients radiographed	8.0	8.5	7.8	6.1

Source: Reprinted from PC Sollecito, *Chiropractic Network Services Provider Manual*, p. G3–4, © 1995, Chiropractic Network Services with permission from Triad Healthcare Network, Plainville, Connecticut.

1996 benefit year were not available for this report. It should be emphasized that all patient care in the IPA in these 4 years was for general medical benefits through PPOs and HMOs (some gatekeeper activity) and does not include any activity related to industrial or auto injury cases. In this network, diagnostic imaging did not require preauthorization, but necessity had to be documented in a retrievable patient record.

The utilization of radiographic services in the years prior to and after implementation of the imaging guideline in the IPA is summarized in Table 6. The data are sorted according to the proportion between new patients and established patients and the number of radiographic codes billed per patient per year. The data demonstrate an overall decrease in the use of imaging in patient management.

The data show a general tendency toward conservatism in billing for imaging services, but since the implementation of the guideline, the degree of conservatism appears to be even greater. Although the use of one radiographic code did not change significantly, a trend toward marked reduction in the combined utilization of three or more codes occurred following the implementation of the guideline. There also may be a trend toward decreasing rates of utilization of imaging for established patients.

This information is only observational in nature, and no conclusive comments can be made regarding the effectiveness of the guideline compared to sentinel effects from other sources, such as continuing education or reimbursement incentives outside the IPA. However, this case study provides a look at trends when a guideline is implemented within a network of chiropractic practitioners, and it shows that changes may be occurring in the clinical behavior of chiropractic practitioners. Evaluation of the network providers' and patients' demographic characteristics, the patients' records (for case mix considerations), and the providers' practice attitudes and behaviors is needed before any conclusions can be generalized. Further investigations could provide insight into practice behaviors inside and outside of managed care organizations.

CONCLUSION

There are many ways that doctors of chiropractic may attempt to reduce the radiation exposure experienced by their patients. The primary method is by utilizing a radiographic procedure only when the results of the procedure will significantly impact patient management. More biomechanical, clinical, and health services research is needed to determine the value of

---

Table 6. Utilization of radiographic services in a regional chiropractic independent practice association

	1992 (2,057 patients)		1993 (2,907 patients)		1994 (3,624 patients)		1995 (6,023 patients)	
	% NP	% EP	% NP	% EP	% NP	% EP	% NP	% EP
Total patients	44.4	55.6	44.3	55.7	40.6	59.4	34.8	65.2
Patients with 0 X-ray codes	38.1	91.9	41.7	91.4	44.4	92.0	55.1	93.9
Patients with 1 X-ray code	33.0	4.9	33.4	4.9	31.9	5.8	31.4	4.2
Patients with 2 X-ray codes	19.3	1.6	16.3	2.3	19.0	1.4	11.6	1.9
Patients with 3 X-ray codes	8.5	1.4	7.1	1.3	3.7	0.6	1.6	0.1
Patients with 4+ X-ray codes	0.4	0.2	1.6	0.1	1.0	0.1	0.3	0.0
All patients with any X-ray codes	61.2	8.0	58.3	8.5	55.6	7.9	44.9	6.1

Key: NP = new patients, EP = established patients
Source: Reprinted from PC Sollecito, *Chiropractic Network Services Provider Manual*, p. G3–4, © 1995, Chiropractic Network Services with permission from Triad Healthcare Network, Plainville, Connecticut.

many radiographic procedures in common use. Many evidence- and expert-based criteria and guidelines are available as resources to assist clinicians making decisions about imaging. Their use is likely to increase, particularly if research demonstrates that it results in reductions in the use of unnecessary films, has no detrimental effect on desired outcomes of care, and leads to cost savings. Technical strategies such as filtration, beam limitation, shielding, use of optimal radiographic techniques, and adherence to quality assurance standards also help to ensure minimal radiation exposure when films are needed. Medicolegal concerns are real. Implementation and adherence to protocols or guidelines may reduce liability. The bottom line is this: if radiography is to be performed, optimum diagnostic quality should be the goal so that maximum benefit is obtained at minimum risk.

Chiropractors continue to receive high patient satisfaction marks,[66] and they have a reputation for being among the most caring providers in the health care system. The natural tendency of chiropractic toward patient-centered practice and its clinical strategies aimed at optimizing recovery from disease and dysfunction should place the profession at the forefront when it comes to providing the safest and most conservative health care options available, including radiation-minimizing technologies and practices.

REFERENCES

1. Canterbury R, Krakos G. Thirteen years after Roentgen: the origins of chiropractic radiology. *Chiro Hist.* 1986;6:25–29.
2. Wyatt LH, Schultz GD. The diagnostic efficacy of lumbar spine radiography: a review of the literature. In: Hodgson M, ed. *Current Topics in Chiropractic.* Sunnyvale, CA: Palmer College of Chiropractic-West; 1987.
3. Mootz RD, Meeker WC. Minimizing radiation exposure to patients in chiropractic practice. *J Chiro.* 1989;26(4):65–74.
4. Scuderi DJ. Minimizing patient radiation exposure during radiographic examination. *Top Clin Chiro.* 1994;1(3):33–38.
5. Taylor JAM, Resnik D. Imaging decisions in management of low back pain. In: Lawrence DJ, Cassidy JD, McGregor M, et al, eds. *Advances in Chiropractic.* Vol 1. St Louis: Mosby; 1994.
6. Howe J. Facts and fallacies, myths and misconceptions in spinography. *J Clin Chiro* (Archives ed 2). 1972;2:34–45.
7. Hildebrandt R. Chiropractic spinography and postural roentgenology, II: clinical basis. *J Manipulative Physiol Ther.* 1981;4:191.
8. Howard BA, Rowe L. Spinal X-rays. In: Haldeman S, ed. *Principles and Practice of Chiropractic.* 2nd ed. Norwalk, CT: Appleton & Lange; 1992.
9. Peterson C. Standards for diagnostic imaging. In: Vear H, ed. *Chiropractic Standards of Practice and Quality of Care.* Gaithersburg, MD: Aspen Publishers; 1992.
10. Maurer E. *Clinical Roentgenology.* Baltimore: Williams & Wilkins; 1983.
11. Yochum TR, Rowe LJ. *Essentials of Skeletal Radiology.* 2nd ed. Baltimore: Williams & Wilkins; 1996.
12. Deyo RA, Diehl AK. Cancer as a cause of back pain: frequency, clinical presentation, and diagnostic strategies. *J Gen Intern Med.* 1988;3:230–238.
13. Halvorsen JG, Swanson D. Indications for office radiographs. *J Fam Pract.* 1990;31:521–529.
14. Gregory R. Mechanical and manual adjusting: a comparison. *The Upper Cervical Monograph.* 1983;3(6):1–3.
15. Plaugher G. *Textbook of Chiropractic: A Specific Biomechanical Approach.* Baltimore: Williams & Wilkins; 1993.
16. Stillwagon G. The posterior inferior cervical and the lorphoshis. In Suh CH, Coyle BA (eds). *Proceedings, 13th Annual Biomechanics Conference on the Spine.* Sunnyvale, CA: Palmer College of Chiropractic-West, 1982.
17. Deyo R, Dial A. Lumbar spine films in primary care. *J Gen Intern Med.* 1986;1:20–25.
18. Kelen G. Guidelines for the use of lumbar spine radiography. *Ann Emerg Med.* 1986;15:245.
19. Hall F. Routine oblique projections of the lumbar spine in evaluation of chronic low back pain. *Radiology.* 1980;137:209–210.
20. Bigos S, Bowyer O, Braen G, et al. *Acute Low Back Problems in Adults.* Washington, DC: US Department of Health and Human Services, Agency for Health Care Policy and Research; 1994. Clinical Practice Guideline No. 14.
21. Brand DA, Frazier WH, Kohlhepp WC, et al. A protocol for selecting patients with injured extremities who need X-rays. *N Engl J Med.* 1982;306:333–339.
22. Plaugher G. The role of radiography in chiropractic clinical practice. *Chiro J Aust.* 1992;22:153–161.
23. Hildebrandt R. The chiropractic spinography issue. *J Manipulative Physiol Ther.* 1981;4:171–172.
24. Coehlo L. Spinal radiation technique, quality assurance and radiation safety. In: Haldeman S, ed. *Modern Developments in the Principles and Practice of Chiropractic.* New York: Appleton-Century-Crofts; 1980.
25. Gregory R, Seeman R. An analysis of some hypotheses about the atlas subluxation complex. *Dig Chiro Econ.* January–February 1976:21–23.
26. Suh C. Analysis of three-dimensional multi-rigid-body of dynamic model for spinal systems. In: Suh CH (ed). *Proceedings, 10th Annual Biomechanics Conference on the Spine.* Davenport, IA: Palmer College of Chiropractic; 1979.
27. Schram S. Analysis of errors in X-ray measurement of cervical vertebrae. In: Suh CH (ed). *Proceedings, 10th Annual Biomechanics Conference on the Spine.* Boulder, CO: University of Colorado; 1980.
28. Rupert R. Anatomical measures of standard chiropractic skeletal references (a preliminary report). In: Suh CH (ed). *Proceedings, 10th Annual Biomechanics Conference on the Spine.* Boulder, CO: University of Colorado; 1980.
29. Zengle F, Davis B, Rozeboom D. Lack of effect of projectional distortion on Gonstead vertebral endplate lines. In: *Proceedings of Advances in Conservative Health Sciences Conference.* St. Louis: Logan College of Chiropractic Academic Press; 1982.
30. Davis B, Rozeboom D. A model to test the radiographically determined pelvis subluxation. In: *Proceedings of Advances in Conservative Health Sciences Conference.* Lombard, IL: National College of Chiropractic Academic Press; 1983.

31. Jepsen L, Oestreich, Bolton JE. The effect of phantom rotation on apparent difference in femur head height on a standard AP-lumbopelvic radiograph. *Eur J Chiro.* 1990;38(3):109–113.
32. Meeker W, Mootz R. Evaluating the validity, reliability, and clinical role of spinal radiography. In: Coyle B, ed. *Current Topics in Chiropractic.* Sunnyvale, CA: Palmer College of Chiropractic-West; 1985.
33. Schram S, Hosek R, Silverman H. Spinographic positioning errors in Gonstead pelvic X-ray analysis. *J Manipulative Physiol Ther.* 1981;4:179.
34. Reinert O, Davis B. Radiographic analysis of pelvic/spinal biochemical response to weight-bearing. In: *Proceedings of Advances in Conservative Health Sciences Conference.* Lombard, IL: National College of Chiropractic Press; 1983.
35. Triano J, Marinelli C. Radiographic reliability of facet orientation. In Coyle BA, Chase D, Furda MA, et al (eds). *Fourth Annual Conservative Health Science Research Conference.* Sunnyvale, CA: Palmer College of Chiropractic-West, 1985.
36. Harrison DD, Harrison DE, Troyanovich SJ, et al. The anterior-posterior full spine view: the worst radiographic view for determination of mechanics of the spine. *Chiro Technique.* 1996;8:163–170.
37. Rozeboom D. Reliability of full spine X-ray analysis. In: *Proceedings of Advances in Conservative Health Sciences Conference.* Lombard, IL: National College of Chiropractic; 1983.
38. Sigler D, Howe J. Intra- and inter-examiner reliability of the upper cervical X-ray marking system. *J Manipulative Physiol Ther.* 1985;9:75–80.
39. Phillips R. An evaluation of the graphic analysis of the pelvis on the A-P full spine radiograph. *J Am Chiro Assoc.* 1975;12:139–148.
40. Bronfort G, Jochumsen O. The functional radiographic examination of patients with low back pain: a study of different forms of variations. *J Manipulative Physiol Ther.* 1984;7:89–97.
41. Owens EF. Line drawing analysis of static cervical X-ray used in chiropractic. *J Manipulative Physiol Ther.* 1992;15:442–449.
42. Jackson BL, Barker W, Bentz J, et al. Inter- and intra-examiner reliability of the upper cervical marking system: a second look. *J Manipulative Physiol Ther.* 1987;10:157–163.
43. Grostic J, DeBoer K. Roentgenographic measurement of atlas laterality and rotation: a retrospective pre- and post-manipulation study. *J Manipulative Physiol Ther.* 1982;5:63–71.
44. Plaugher G, Hendricks AH. The inter- and intraexaminer reliability of the Gonstead pelvic marking system. *J Manipulative Physiol Ther.* 1991;14:503–508.
45. Plaugher G, Hendricks AH, Doble RW, et al. The reliability of patient positioning for evaluating static radiologic parameters of the human pelvis. *J Manipulative Physiol Ther.* 1993;16:517–522.
46. Burk JM, Rhudy TR, Ratliff CR. Inter- and intra-examiner agreement using Gonstead line marking methods. *Am J Chiro Med.* 1990;3:114–117.
47. Plaugher G, Cremata EE, Phillips RB. A retrospective case analysis of pretreatment and comparative radiologic parameters following chiropractic adjustment. *J Manipulative Physiol Ther.* 1990;13:498–506.
48. Jochumsen O. The curve of the cervical spine. *J Am Chiro Assoc.* 1970;8:49–55.
49. Leach R. An evaluation of the effect of chiropractic manipulative therapy on hypolordosis of the cervical spine. *J Manipulative Physiol Ther.* 1983;6:17–23.
50. Mootz RD, Shekelle DT, Hansen DT. The politics of policy and research. *Top Clin Chiro.* 1995;2(2):56–70.
51. Hansen DT, Mootz DT. Formal processes in technology assessment: a primer for the chiropractic profession. *Top Clin Chiro.* 1995;2(4):71–83.
52. Bronfort G. Effectiveness of spinal manipulation and adjustments. In: Haldeman S, ed. *Principles and Practice of Chiropractic.* 2nd ed. Norwalk, CT: Appleton & Lange, 1992.
53. Vernon H. Spinal manipulation and headaches: an update. *Top Clin Chiro.* 1995;2(3):34–47.
54. Fung K. Lowering patient dose on single phase X-ray units. *Radiol Technol.* 1995;66:159–164.
55. Kohn H, Fry RJ. Radiation carcinogenesis. *N Engl J Med.* 1984;310:504–511.
56. Krain LS. Some thoughts about the importance of X-ray exposure history. *Med Hypotheses.* 1992;37:225–231.
57. Taylor JAM, Lawson DM. Quality assurance in chiropractic radiology. *Top Clin Chiro.* 1994;1(4):58–66.
58. Radiologic Health Branch. *Guidelines for Establishing Radiographic Quality Assurance and Quality Control Programs.* Sacramento, CA: Department of Health Services; 1994.
59. Schultz G, Phillips RB, Cooley J, et al. Diagnostic imaging of the spine in chiropractic practice: recommendations for utilization. *Chiro J Aust.* 1992;22:141–152.
60. Jensen MC, Brandt-Zawadski MN, Obuchowski N, et al. Magnetic resonance imaging of the lumbar spine in people without back pain. *N Engl J Med.* 1994;331:69–73.
61. Office of the Medical Director. *Medical Treatment Guidelines.* Olympia, WA: Washington State Department of Labor & Industries; 1996.
62. Marquart DJ. A review of the cognitive process used to decide which patients require diagnostic imaging. *Roentgen Briefs* (Council of Diagnostic Imaging American Chiropractic Association). 1992;7(3):1–6.
63. Haldeman S, Chapman-Smith D, Petersen D, eds. *Guidelines for Chiropractic Quality Assurance and Practice Parameters.* Gaithersburg, MD: Aspen Publishers; 1992.
64. McElheran LJ, Sollecito PC. Delivering quality care in a managed care setting. *Top Clin Chiro.* 1994;1(4):30–39.
65. Sollecito PC, ed. *Chiropractic Network Services Provider Manual.* Lynnwood, WA: Chiropractic Network Services; 1995.
66. Coulter ID, Hays RD, Danielson CD. The chiropractic satisfaction questionnaire. *Top Clin Chiro.* 1994;1(4):40–43.

13

Quality Assurance in Chiropractic Radiology

John A.M. Taylor and Douglas M. Lawson

The objective of a quality assurance program in chiropractic radiology is to obtain the highest quality image while minimizing patient exposure to ionizing radiation. Recommendations for the safe and effective use of diagnostic radiology have been established by the National Council on Radiation Protection (NCRP).[1-4] The laws and regulations governing the use of diagnostic radiology, however, are established by individual state and provincial radiation protection authorities. All chiropractic radiographic facilities are expected to implement the NCRP recommendations and are required to abide by the state laws and regulations in their respective jurisdictions.

In addition to established laws and regulations, each health profession is charged with the responsibility of establishing practice guidelines and standards of practice. In chiropractic, the "Mercy document"[5] in the United States and the "Glenerin document"[6] in Canada briefly outline standards of practice for radiographic quality assurance. Chiropractic regulatory boards in certain jurisdictions such as Alberta[7] and Ontario[8] have established detailed quality assurance programs for chiropractic radiology. The following presentation incorporates the Mercy and Glenerin recommendations and provides a brief discussion of each quality assurance procedure.[9]

A comprehensive quality assurance program should include

1. documentation;
2. analysis of processing and darkroom procedures;
3. inspection, analysis, and maintenance of image receptors;
4. analysis and calibration of generator and control equipment; and
5. analysis and modification of radiographic techniques.

Reprinted from *Top Clin Chiro* 1994; 1(4): 67–71
© 1994 Aspen Publishers, Inc.

The radiography quality assurance program for chiropractic installations outlined in this article is not all-inclusive, but serves as a guideline for some of the more commonly employed procedures.

DOCUMENTATION

Every radiographic facility should maintain radiographic log books. Recommended log books include radiographic exposure log, quality assurance and maintenance log, and processing log.

The *radiographic exposure log* should document every exposure taken.[7] Log entries should include the date, patient name, radiograph or patient number, projections obtained, thickness (in centimeters), peak kilovolt (kVp), milliampere (mA), exposure time, and the quality of each radiograph. The *quality assurance and maintenance log* should include the dates of every quality assurance inspection, repair, maintenance, and calibration procedure performed. The *processing log* is used to document the findings of sensitometer/densitometer tests and other quality assurance tests used to assess processing and darkroom procedures. It is also a record of processor maintenance. This processing log can be one component of the quality assurance and maintenance log or it can be a separate document.

These records are used by office staff, radiation protection authorities, and service personnel to ensure radiographic quality and the safety of patients and office staff.[7]

PROCESSOR AND DARKROOM: ANALYSIS AND MAINTENANCE

It is estimated that 90% of radiographic errors occur in the darkroom.[10] Many of these common errors can be avoided by paying careful attention to detail in all radiographic processing and darkroom procedures. This attention to detail will result in higher quality radiographs with minimal patient exposure. Every radiographic installation must have a detailed schedule of maintenance and film analysis to ensure optimum processing quality.[7,10]

The processor rollers and crossover racks should be cleaned daily using a clean, damp sponge. Processor chemical levels should also be checked (and replenished if necessary) daily. Once the processor is warmed up, sensitometry strips should be obtained and the densitometric readings compared with a master film.[7,9,10]

Processor temperature and replenishments levels should be checked weekly. At the same time, the processor should be examined for evidence of fluid leaks, unusual noises, and broken parts such as gears and belts. Also during the weekly inspection, the darkroom should be examined for light leaks. This procedure requires remaining in the darkroom for at least 5 minutes in order to allow the eyes adequate time to adapt to the dark.[7,9,10]

In addition to daily and weekly procedures, the processor should be thoroughly cleaned monthly. Many chiropractors rely on service technicians for all maintenance, however, many of these simple procedures can be performed by the doctor or the office staff. A thorough processor cleaning includes draining of all chemistry including water, fixer, and developer; cleaning thoroughly all tanks, rollers, and racks with special solutions available from radiographic supply centers; and refilling the tanks with fresh water, developer, and fixer. Water filters, if present, are replaced, and processor replenishment rates are checked and adjusted accordingly. A detailed examination and lubrication of processor components are also performed monthly. A sensitometer strip is then obtained, and the densitometric readings are documented. This sensitometer strip serves as the master for comparison for the following month.

It is also appropriate to perform a repeat film analysis on a monthly basis. This process involves reviewing all radiographs that required "re-takes" due to technical errors. The reasons for poor quality radiographs should be identified and corrected.[7]

Every 6 months, each processor should undergo a major inspection, cleaning, and lubrication. Commercial cleaning solutions are available from radiographic equipment dealers. Extensive sensitometric evaluation of film speed and contrast should be performed every 6 months. This evaluation involves comparing densitometric readings of present film speed and contrast with earlier densitometric readings. These diagnostic tests can indicate a processing problem as well as a diminishing efficiency (speed) of intensifying screens.[7,10]

IMAGING RECEPTORS

Modern intensifying screens with rare earth phosphors offer excellent resolution and dramatic reduction in radiation exposure.[11] Intensifying screens should be examined monthly for evidence of dust, dirt, artifacts, and damage. Cleaning with commercially available screen cleaning solutions should be performed as necessary. Abrasive or lint-producing materials should be avoided when cleaning screens. Also, adequate time should be allowed for each intensifying screen to dry thoroughly before closing cassettes.[10]

Because the efficiency (speed) of intensifying screens gradually diminishes with time, the film/screen combination speed should be checked every 6 months. This procedure uses standardized exposures of a phantom taken at 6-month intervals. The densitometric readings are then compared with previous readings. Damaged or inefficient screens should be replaced.[7,10]

Loss of film/screen contact occurs as a result of damaged or overused cassettes. The film/screen contact should be tested every 6 months. A simple method is to distribute a box of paper clips evenly on the outside front surface of each cassette loaded with film and then take an exposure. (It is essential to use brand new paper clips that are not bent or twisted.) All images of the paper clips should be sharp. Evidence of blurred images indicates inadequate film/screen contact. Cassettes with poor film/screen contact must be replaced.[7,9,10]

GENERATOR AND CONTROL APPARATUS: ANALYSIS AND CALIBRATION

The major cost of a radiographic installation is the radiographic generator and control hardware. Once the equipment has been initially installed and calibrated, it only requires inspection and re-calibration every 6 to 12 months or whenever an obvious breakdown occurs. Most chiropractors (even those who choose to maintain their own processors) rely on radiographic service technicians or even radiation physicists to analyze and calibrate the generator and control apparatus. Furthermore, it is unsafe for the inexperienced to tamper with the electronic components of the radiographic equipment. Some tests are simple to perform and require little or no specialized equipment; other tests are more complicated and require sophisticated electronic equipment.[9]

Every radiographic installation requires an accurate exposure factor technique chart. Unfortunately, no two radiographic installations produce the same quantity of radiation photons. Even identical radiographic units from the same manufacturer have different radiation outputs and require their own personalized exposure techniques. Radiation output is measured in terms of milliroentgen per milliampere-seconds (mR/mAs). The mR/mAs value varies according to the tube potential (kVp), size and capacity of the tube, and the amount of inherent and added filtration. The mR/mAs output is measured using a dosimeter, a procedure usually performed by the radiation engineer or physicist. The radiation output should be measured at installation, whenever major equipment repair or calibration is performed, and on a routine basis every 6 to 12 months.

The exposure factor technique chart is only as accurate as the control settings on the radiographic equipment. One of the most important diagnostic tests is mA/mAs linearity. The linearity test determines the output of the tube for various mA and time station combinations. For example, an exposure taken at 100 mA for 1 second should produce the same output (optical density) as an exposure taken at 50 mA for 2 seconds, all other factors being equal. The linearity test compares different mA-time (mAs) combinations by assessing the optical density produced by various exposures or by directly measuring the mR/mAs output. The service engineer then calibrates either the mA station or the timer to correct variations in linearity.[9]

The kVp accuracy can be measured in two ways. The modified Adran and Crookes cassette (Wisconsin radiographic test cassette)[9,12] is a specially designed standardized cassette that requires a series of test exposures. Optical densities of these exposures are measured with a densitometer, and the actual kVp is calculated from the readings. A quicker and less cumbersome method is the electronic kVp meter. This device is placed directly in the radiographic field where it measures the energy of the radiographic beam and provides a digital display of the actual kVp. Both methods measure tube potential to an accuracy of 1 or 2 kVp. Usually, the radiographic engineer will adjust the autotransformer in the radiographic control panel to calibrate kVp accuracy.[9,12]

Timer accuracy is just as essential as kVp accuracy and mA/mAs linearity in producing consistently good quality radiographs. Most modern timers are electronic and can produce exposures at millisecond increments. Testing timer accuracy of single-phase radiographic units can be performed using a simple metal spin-top equipped with a tiny pin hole in its periphery.[9,13,14] The spin-top device is available from any radiographic supply dealer. Exposures at various timer settings are obtained of the spinning top. Because X-ray photons are emitted in "pulses," the resultant image appears as a series of radiopaque dots distributed in a circular pattern representing the X-rays passing through the pin hole. A single-phase, fully-rectified radiographic unit should emit 120 pulses per second. A 0.1 second exposure should produce 12 pulses per second. A simple count of the number of pulses on the test film reveals the accuracy of the timer. For three-phase and medium- or high-frequency radiographic generators, a more sophisticated electronic timer must be employed.[9] Most modern electronic timers rarely require calibration, but are usually tested routinely whenever kVp and mA stations are tested (ie, once every 6 to 12 months or when a specific problem arises).[9,13,14]

Half-value layer (HVL) is an indirect measure of the amount of filtration in the X-ray beam. It is defined as the amount of aluminum, measured in millimeters, necessary to reduce an exposure to one half of its original value, assuming kVp and mAs remain fixed.[9,13,14] The higher the HVL (and hence the more filtration present), the less the entrance exposure to the patient. Although the minimum HVL for radiographic units is 2.5 mm at 90 kVp, at least 4 mm is more appropriate to minimize radiation exposure. The HVL is obtained by taking successive mR dosimeter readings following the addition of known thicknesses (1 mm, 2 mm, 3 mm, and so forth) of aluminum. Once the original X-ray beam has

Table 1. Radiographic quality assurance and maintenance schedule

Daily
  Clean processor rollers and crossover racks
  Check and replenish processor chemical levels
  Compare sensitometer strips with master
Weekly
  Check developer temperature
  Compare exposure step-wedge with master
  Inspect processor for leaks, noises, broken parts
  Check processor replenisher levels
Monthly
  Check processor replenishment rates
  Replace fresh water filter (if present)
  Replace fixer and developer in processor
  Clean processor thoroughly
  Examine processor components in detail
  Examine intensifying screens
  Lubricate processor
  Check darkroom for light leaks
  Repeat film analysis and radiographic technique modification
Every 6 to 12 months
  Processing
    Perform major cleaning and lubrication
    Perform major sensitometry comparison: film speed and contrast
  Image receptors
    Check film/screen combination speeds
    Clean all screens (replace if necessary)
    Check film/screen contact
  Generator and control components
    mR/mAs output
    mA/mAs linearity
    kVp accuracy
    timer accuracy
    collimator alignment
    half-value layer
    focal spot resolution
    calibration of generator and control components
    grid alignment and servicing
    radiographs of radiation protection garments to detect leaks

kVp, peak kilovolt; mR/mAs, milliroentgen per milliampere-seconds; mA/mAs, milliampere per milliampere-seconds.

been attenuated by one half, the total thickness of added aluminum represents the HVL. The HVL should be measured at initial installation, routinely every 6 to 12 months, whenever the collimator or radiographic tube is replaced or serviced, or whenever filtration is added or removed.[9]

Collimator alignment should also be checked at initial installation, routinely every 6 to 12 months, when the collimator or tube is replaced or serviced, and whenever collimator lights are replaced. The purpose of the collimator alignment test is to ensure that the actual radiographic field (the collimated area of exposure) coincides with the light field emitted from the collimator (the area illuminated by the collimator light). This test is performed simply by taping coins to the front of a loaded cassette along the periphery of the illuminated collimator light field. Without moving the cassette, a small exposure is taken and the film developed. The coins should be aligned with the perimeter of the exposed area. Discrepancies in the light field and radiographic field can be corrected by adjusting the leaves of the collimator or the collimator bulb. Because the adjustment of the collimator can be meticulous work and can lead to serious electric shocks, it is usually left to the experienced technician or service personnel.[9,10]

In addition to the specific tests outlined above, focal spot resolution and grid alignment and servicing should be performed annually or whenever a specific problem arises. Furthermore, all radiation protection garments such as gloves, shields, and aprons should be radiographed annually to detect radiation leaks.[7,9]

Calibration of generator and control components is usually performed by service personnel at the time of quality assurance testing. An efficient radiographic engineer will quickly identify any problems and adjust or calibrate the equipment during the same service call.

RADIOGRAPHIC TECHNIQUES: ANALYSIS AND MODIFICATION

When all processor, generator, and control components are functioning according to specifications and a reliable radiographic exposure technique chart is developed and functioning, a mechanism must then be developed to maintain top quality radiographs. One method used in quality control of radiographic quality is the detailed repeat analysis.[7,9,15] This analysis involves recording the details of all radiographs that are not of excellent quality and that require retakes. The patient's name and number and exposure factors should be included as well as the radiographic problem such as over- or underexposure, over- or underdevelopment, positioning, artifacts, and so forth. At the end of each month, the films and recorded notations should be reviewed and analyzed. Any recurring or repeated errors should be corrected, and the exposure factor technique chart should be modified or updated if necessary. Radiographic vendors and service representatives often are helpful in diagnosing and troubleshooting errors in quality assurance.

SUMMARY

The comprehensive chiropractic radiographic quality assurance program includes several components. Table 1 summarizes a schedule of some diagnostic and maintenance tests recommended for radiographic quality assurance. Before attempting to establish an exposure factor technique chart for radiographic installations, it is essential to test and correct any problems in darkroom and processing procedures, imaging receptors, and generator and control equipment.

REFERENCES

1. National Council on Radiation Protection and Measurements. *Basic Radiation Protection Criteria: NCRP Report #39*. Washington, DC: NCRP; 1974.
2. National Council on Radiation Protection. *Medical X-ray and Gamma-Ray Protection for Energies up to 10 MeV: Equipment Design and Use, NCRP Report #33*. Washington, DC: NCRP; 1975.
3. National Council on Radiation Protection. *Recommendations on Limits for Ionizing Radiation Exposure. NCRP Report #91*. Washington, DC: NCRP; 1987.
4. Sinclair WK. Trends in radiation protection—a view from the NCRP. *Health Physics*. 1988;55:149–157.
5. Haldeman S, Chapman-Smith DA, Petersen D, eds. *Guidelines for Chiropractic Quality Assurance and Practice Parameters*. Gaithersburg, Md: Aspen Publishers, Inc; 1992.
6. Henderson D, Chapman-Smith D, Mior S, Vernon H, eds. Clinical guidelines for chiropractic practice in Canada. *J Can Chiro Assoc*. 1994;38(1)suppl:22–42.
7. College of Chiropractors of Alberta, Practice Review Board. *X-ray Quality Assurance Manual*. Edmonton, Alberta: College of Chiropractors; 1994.
8. *Healing Arts Radiation Protection Act, Revised Statutes of Ontario*. Ottawa, Ontario: Government Printer; 1980.
9. Gray JE, Winkler NT, Stears J, et al. *Quality Control in Diagnostic Imaging*. Rockville, Md: Aspen Publishers, Inc; 1983.
10. Sherman R, Bauer F. *X-ray X-pertise—From A–X*. Fort Worth, Tex: PCRF; 1982.
11. Skukas J, Gorski J. Application of modern intensifying screens in diagnostic radiology. *Med Radiogr Photogr*. 1980;56:25–36.

12. Jacobson AF, Cameron JR, Siedband MP, et al. Test cassette for measuring peak tube potential of diagnostic x-ray machines. *Med Phys.* 1976;3:19–25.
13. Buschong SC. *Radiographic Science for Technologists: Physics, Biology, and Protection.* 3rd ed. St. Louis, Mo: Mosby; 1984.
14. Curry TS, Dowdey JE, Murry RC. *Christensen's Physics of Diagnostic Radiology.* 4th ed. Philadelphia, Pa: Lea & Febiger; 1990.
15. Goldman LW. *Analysis of Retakes: Understanding, Managing, and Using an Analysis of Retakes Program for Quality Assurance.* Washington, DC: US Dept of Health, Education, and Welfare; 1979. DHEW publication FDA 79-8097.

Part III

Therapeutic Technologies

14

The Use of Expert Panel Results: The RAND Panel for Appropriateness of Manipulation and Mobilization of the Cervical Spine

Ian D. Coulter, Paul G. Shekelle, Robert D. Mootz, and Daniel T. Hansen

A key question in contemporary health care research is how to determine that a given service or course of treatment is appropriate or necessary. Questions of appropriateness, however, involve judgment calls, particularly in those areas where research evidence does not allow for a definitive resolution. However, where evidence does exist it must itself be evaluated and interpreted. Therefore, a key issue in developing appropriateness criteria is the method by which the criteria are developed. One approach that has been used to address this issue is the RAND appropriateness method.[1]

THE RAND APPROPRIATENESS METHOD

The RAND method has been described extensively elsewhere.[2-5] One of the essential features of the RAND approach is an emphasis on clinical experts over scientific authorities.[6] This is in contrast to approaches used by the National Institutes of Health where principally scientific and research experts make recommendations based on the literature.[7] The RAND appropriateness method has also been previously described in the chiropractic literature;[8] therefore, only a brief overview is presented here.

A RAND panel typically consists of a group of nine clinical experts. Experience in small group dynamics has shown that meaningful discussion among participants is difficult with more than nine members. Panelists are normally chosen to reflect a geographic distribution as well as a spectrum of clinicians and academics so that any given specialty does not dominate the panel. The objective is to have an array of individuals who encounter the given disease or procedure at different points in the treatment cycle with no more than five out of the nine panelists being individuals who perform the procedure under review.

The overall process used involves a modified Delphi consensus method where panelists are provided with a literature review of the procedure(s) in question along with a list of clinical scenarios (or indications). Participants are asked to rate the appropriateness of the procedure for a given scenario on their own. These ratings are scored and returned to the panelists for their review. Next, a second round utilizes a nominal small-group process where the panel is convened in person to discuss areas of disagreement amongst themselves and re-rate appropriateness a second time. Thus, panelists receive feedback from the first round of ratings about how the group rated the indications prior to re-rating them in the second round.

Literature review and indications list development

An extensive literature synthesis is the first step. Published reports on the procedure are identified and gathered, then systematically evaluated. This initial review is used by the project staff to develop an initial clinical indications list. The indications categorize patients in terms of their symptoms, past medical history, and the results of previous diagnostic tests, resulting in a brief, yet comprehensive clinical scenario. The objective is to create lists that include adequate detail so that the patients characterized in a given category

---

A number of key individuals on the research team played important roles in making this study possible, including Eric Hurwitz, DC, Peter Aker, DC, William C. Meeker, DC, MPH, Alan H. Adams, DC, and Barbara Genovese.

This project was funded by the Consortium for Chiropractic Research.

are relatively homogeneous. This is to ensure that the procedure would be equally appropriate for all patients who would meet the criteria identified in the scenario. To be comprehensive they must include all the indications for doing the procedure that occur in practice. However, they must be short enough that the panelists can complete them within a reasonable time.

First round "modified-Delphi" methodology

The literature synthesis and completed indications list are circulated to the panelists, who are asked individually to rate the appropriateness of a given procedure for a patient characterized by each indication or scenario. Appropriateness is rated on a scale from 1 to 9, with 1 representing extremely inappropriate and 9 extremely appropriate. "Appropriate" is defined to mean that the expected health benefits to the patient (relief of symptoms, improved functional capacity, and reduction of anxiety) exceed expected health risks (pain and discomfort) by a sufficiently wide margin that the procedure is worth doing. The panelists are instructed to evaluate the risks and benefits based on commonly accepted, best clinical practice for the year in which the panel is conducted. Considering an average group of patients with each listed indication, presenting to an average practitioner in the United States, the ratings should reflect the panelist's own best clinical judgment. Panelists return their ratings to the project staff, where an individual report is prepared for each panelist showing both the rating he or she gave for each indication along with the average score for the entire group.

Second round "nominal group" methodology

Next, the panelists are brought together and the results of the ratings from the first round are distributed. Each panelist is shown his or her rating for each indication and the distribution of the ratings of the panel for each indication. Only the panelist knows his or her individual rating, but all know the group's ratings. Following group discussions and revising of the indications, the panels re-rate the indications. From the second rating it is possible to determine the degree of agreement in the panel and to calculate the average median ratings and the average dispersion measures (differences between scores of panelists) for the procedures. In most instances the dispersion decreases during the second rating as the panelists come closer to a consensus. Using this method, criteria for measuring the appropriateness or inappropriateness of a procedure are established. Ideally, these criteria can then be used to measure the proportion of "appropriate" or "inappropriate" care being given in practice by assessing care actually received by patients and comparing it against the criteria.

MEASURING CONSENSUS

RAND has utilized two approaches to characterize the dimensions of consensus on appropriateness. In the first, the raters agree if all their responses fall within one of the three, three-point regions of the scale (ie, 1–3; 4–6; 7–9). This is operationalized to mean that the raters agreed that the procedure should not be done (inappropriate); they agreed that it was questionable (uncertain); or they agreed that it was worth doing (appropriate). The second method characterizing consensus defines agreement when all the panelists' ratings for a given indication fall within any three-point range. Furthermore, agreement can be determined using both methods but first rejecting one extreme high or low rating.

Similarly, disagreement can be calculated using two methods. If at least one rater chose a 1 and one chose a 9; or if at least one rater fell in the lowest three-point region and at least one in the highest, a conclusion regarding disagreement can be reached. As with the methodology for agreement, the extreme ratings can be discarded. Thus, a procedure is considered inappropriate for a given indication if its median rating is in the range 1 to 3 and without disagreement. The procedure is considered uncertain if the median rating is in the range 4 to 6 or if the panelists disagreed on the proper rating. Finally, a procedure for a given indication is considered clearly appropriate if it is 7 to 9 without disagreement.

RESEARCH ON THE APPROPRIATENESS METHOD

Of the approaches used for the problem of appropriateness and the establishment of consensus, none has been more extensively researched than the RAND method. Numerous studies have investigated the reliability of the ratings[9–14]; face and content validity[15–20]; and construct validity.[21–24] Research has also examined the relationship between the literature and the ratings.[25] These studies have demonstrated that the appropriateness method results have a reasonable level of test-retest reliability, as well as content and construct validity. However, as Brook notes,[26] although the published work is extensive, there is still much more research needed to expand knowledge about the process.

APPROPRIATENESS OF SPINAL MANIPULATION AND MOBILIZATION OF THE CERVICAL SPINE

Methods

The expert panel held for mobilization and manipulation of the cervical spine followed the RAND procedures as outlined previously. A review of the medical and chiropractic literature was conducted to summarize knowledge about efficacy, complications, and indications for manipulation and mobilization for the cervical spine. From this literature and clinical experience, a set of patient clinical scenarios (indications) was created for manipulation and mobilization for neck pain, headache, and other clinical syndromes.

A panel was convened of neck pain experts from the disciplines of orthopaedics, chiropractic, neurosurgery, internal medicine, family medicine, and neurology to rate for appropriateness the indications for spinal manipulation and mobilization. The panel included four chiropractic physicians, three medical physicians, one osteopathic physician, and one individual holding both an MD and DC credential. The panel was co-chaired by a medical and chiropractic physician. The set of indications derived from the literature and informed sources was circulated to the panel to be rated individually by each panelist for appropriateness for manipulation and mobilization (first modified-Delphi rating round). The panel of experts was convened to rate the same indications for the cervical spine following reporting and discussion of the previous ratings (second nominal group rating round).

Results

Table 1 describes the average median, the mean absolute deviation from the median, and the percentage of agreement for the initial and final appropriateness ratings for spinal manipulation or mobilization for neck pain and headache. The table shows that the ratings changed from an initial median of 4.60 to a final median of 4.02. The table also shows a decrease in dispersion between the initial and final ratings.

The preferred definition of "agreement" is that after discarding one extreme high and one extreme low rating, the remaining seven fall within any three-point range. According to this definition, at the conclusion of the process, panelists agreed on the ratings in 40% of the indications. The preferred definition of "disagreement" is that, after discarding one extreme high and one extreme low rating, at least two of the remaining seven fall in the lowest three-point region (1 to 3) and at least two fall in the highest. Table 1 shows that the panelists disagreed on the ratings in only 2% of the indications. For comparison, using the same definition for disagreement, a similar multidisciplinary panel of experts had disagreement on 3% of 1550 indications for manipulation of the lumbar spine. However, the level of panel disagreement for cervical manipulation and cervical mobilization were distinctly different.

Indications were also classified into one of three categories of appropriateness: inappropriate, uncertain, or appropriate. An indication was classified as "uncertain" for either of two reasons: The benefits and risk of doing the procedure were considered roughly the same (a median rating of 4 to 6), or the panelists disagreed on the proper rating. An indication was called "appropriate" if the panelists assigned a median rating in the 7 to 9 range without disagreement, and it was "inappropriate" if they assigned a 1 to 3 rating without disagreement. Table 2 categorizes the final indications by their appropriateness ratings. Of the indications, 43% were rated inappropriate. Appropriate and uncertain indications each accounted for 16% and 41% of the total, respectively.

The previous analysis represents aggregate values for both mobilization and manipulation. As seen in Table 3 there were differences in the ratings of these two forms of therapy. More indications were rated as inappropriate for manipulation than for mobilization, and the category of uncertain was larger for mobilization.

With respect to the level of disagreement, this also differed when manipulation and mobilization were considered independently. For mobilization, the panel disagreed on 0.9% of indications while for manipulation, there was disagreement on 3.3% of indications. When compared with the level of disagreement observed for the multidisciplinary panel that rated the appropriateness of lumbar spinal manipulation, the level of disagreement for cervical spinal manipulation is slightly more, which could be expected given the larger amount of evidence in the literature regarding manipulation and low back pain. Interestingly, given the option to utilize the similar but gentler mechanical therapy of mobilization, there was a clear trend of the panel toward a higher appropriateness rating for some indications.

Table 1. Median ratings and extent of agreement and disagreement on appropriateness ratings for spinal manipulation or mobilization

Item	Initial rating	Final ratings
Number of indications	1171	1436
Average median	4.60	4.02
Mean absolute deviation from median	1.51	1.14
Percentage of agreement	19.98%	39.97%
Percentage of disagreement	10.08%	2.09%

Table 2. Categories of appropriateness of 1436 indications for cervical manipulation and mobilization

Category	Number of indications	Percentage of indications
Inappropriate	623	43%
Uncertain	586	41%
Appropriate	122	16%

Table 3. Categories of appropriateness of indications for cervical manipulation and mobilization

	Cervical manipulation		Cervical mobilization	
Category	Number of indications	Percent of indications	Number of indications	Percent of indications
Inappropriate	424	57.6%	199	28.4%
Uncertain	230	31.3%	356	50.9%
Appropriate	82	11.1%	145	20.7%
Total	736	100%	700	100%

DISCUSSION

What do these results mean and how should they be used?

These results indicate that a multidisciplinary group of neck pain experts can agree on both appropriate and inappropriate uses of cervical spine manipulation and mobilization. The low average median and large number of indications rated inappropriate found in this study do not necessarily suggest inappropriate care is being rendered. It may be the case that in practice, manipulation or mobilization is used for highly appropriate indications. It will require the collection of clinically detailed patient level data on persons presenting with symptoms referable to the cervical spine to understand the frequency of appropriate use of cervical spine mobilization and manipulation.

In general, patients who present with clinical situations that are similar to indications rated as appropriate are good candidates for cervical spine manipulation or mobilization, while patients who present with clinical situations that are similar to indications rated as inappropriate are not. In actual practice, any individual patient may have additional clinical circumstances that warrant a departure from such expert recommendations. In other words, the use of cervical spine manipulation or mobilization may be appropriate in a patient with a certain clinical indication when this indication was rated as inappropriate and vice versa. However, this should not be seen in the majority of patients with a given presentation.

These results do not address the relative effectiveness of one practitioner type compared to another or the cost-effectiveness of cervical spine manipulation or mobilization or the practitioners who provide these treatments. In addition, these results do not support or refute any particular hypothesis of illness or disease. There simply is not enough data to draw conclusions about these issues.

Utility of such appropriateness ratings by chiropractors

The impact of the RAND low back appropriateness studies[18,19] has been seen in the development of single-discipline practice policies[27] and common domain clinical guidelines,[28] especially with regard to spinal manipulative management of uncomplicated mechanical back pain and non-progressive lumbar radiculopathy. It is reasonable to expect that these policies and guidelines might be implemented broadly in the health delivery arena, but thus far there is no evidence that such new information has changed either chiropractic or medical practitioner's clinical behavior. Further synthesis of the low back evidence and consensus results is showing up as practice policies that can be implemented directly into portal of entry management of low back conditions in the managed care environment.[29]

The RAND panel results for cervical spine and headache will likely experience a similar sequence of dissemination and implementation. The degree of application of these findings into practice will depend on efforts of individual professionals, professional organizations, and other interest groups such as managed care organizations. Public expectations for proper implementation includes effective dissemination and training of individuals in the proper and reliable use of the guidelines.[30]

Dissemination and implementation of findings

It has been documented that physicians require substantial help in meeting current science information needs.[31] Increase in such resources as "validated reviews" or "expert networks" might help meet these needs.[31,32] The RAND appropriateness study, by its design and format, partially serves the needs as a validated review. The end product of the study is not very user friendly for practical application by the portal of entry practitioner and will likely need further synthesis into applications that more efficiently assist in clinical decision making. Although there may be a tendency for generalization from the collection of evidence and consensus of this study, care must be taken to include descriptions of inclusion/exclusion modifications for different patient conditions, complications, or preferences.

For the practitioner, the results of this cervical spine study may lead to modifications in current practice. It should provide confidence in the areas of cervical spine management where there is some science and high levels of consensus. It may also cause a change in diagnostic or therapeutic protocols considering the level of scientific study quality and high consensus. On the other hand, there has to be recognition for those elements of clinical management for which there is a lack of scientific evidence and high levels of disagreement. This effort can result in an inventory of what is known, what is agreed on, and what is disagreed on for the use of manipulation for cervical spine problems and headache.

Acknowledgment of "process"

Since this study is now the second major RAND product of evidence-based and formal consensus methodology that contributes to increasing social acceptance for the chiropractic profession, the results should provide confidence that evidence-based methodology can help characterize clinical issues. Such explicit, evidence-based and consensus processes can be used to lay out a reasonable description of whether a procedure or method is a "good thing" or "bad thing" for common application by practitioners and practitioner groups.[32] Defining appropriateness of a clinical procedure is consistent with "playing by the rules," which means that now professionals using manipulation for the management of cervical spine conditions and headaches will likely be guided in some manner by the results of the RAND study. However, there continues to be a relative lack of sensitization of chiropractic practitioners to evidence-based guidelines, especially compared to the efforts of their medical counterparts.[33]

Clinical decision making

When considering the results of this study, it is important to recognize that the panel established specific definitions to characterize terminology used in the indications list (see glossary of selected terms in Table 4). The panel of experts carefully differentiated appropriateness of manipulation as compared to mobilization for over 700 patient indications. It is important to emphasize that there were significant differences in the ratings of these two forms of therapy (Table 3). A deeper analysis of the full report[34] suggests indications of manipulation show greater appropriateness scores and higher levels of agreement for subacute and chronic cervical pain presentations, especially in patients who have had previous success with spinal manipulation and in whom serious cervical spine pathology has been excluded.

Mobilization was rated to be more appropriate for acute cervical pain. However, there was more uncertainty among the panelists for its application. Thus, factoring for patient selection issues, complications and available patient clinical data will influence the physician decision whether to utilize manipulation, mobilization, both, or neither since some of the more common patient presentations occur when there is agreement from the appropriateness panel. Those factors that produce a lack of panel agreement should not be considered strongly in clinical decision making.

Value of appropriateness studies to the chiropractic profession

Appropriateness ratings are directed at individual clinical conditions and ideally should give clinicians insight into what the science says and what the experts believe regarding whether a particular procedure may be of value in a given clinical circumstance. Although recommendations like those in the cervical spine study need some clinical synthesis to be put in a more useful format for a physician, they also offer some valuable insight for the chiropractic profession detailing what the landscape looks like regarding what is known and believed about certain procedures at the time the study was conducted. Table 5 summarizes key issues involved in the utilization of appropriateness ratings by key constituents.

Table 4. Selected glossary of terms used in the cervical spine appropriateness study

Acute neck pain—pain or condition present less than 3 weeks (to include acute episodes of an intermittent condition).

Cervical manipulation—a controlled, judiciously applied dynamic thrust (adjustment), that may include combined extension and rotation of the upper cervical spinal segments, of high or low velocity and low amplitude force directed to spinal joint segment within patient tolerance. These procedures often take joints into the "paraphysiological" space resulting in joint cavitation.

Cervical mobilization—a controlled, judiciously applied force of low velocity and variable amplitude directed to spinal joint segment(s). These procedures usually do not take joints beyond the passive range of motion and do not result in joint cavitation.

Cervical SMT—spinal manipulative therapy (SMT), a generic label for a family of procedures that includes manipulation and mobilization.

Chronic neck pain—pain or condition present for more than 13 weeks.

Favorable response to prior SMT—patient has received SMT to the neck for a similar complaint and experienced positive clinical benefit.

Neck pain—pain in the region of the cervical spine including the occipital-cervico and cervico-thoraco junctions.

No or unfavorable response to prior SMT—patient has received SMT to the neck for a similar complaint and experienced equivocal or no clinical benefit.

No prior spinal manipulative therapy—the patient has never received SMT to the neck for a similar complaint.

Subacute neck pain—pain or condition present for more than 3 but less than 13 weeks.

Table 5. Utilization of cervical spine appropriateness ratings by key constituents

For chiropractic providers
- serves as information synthesis resource
- provides insight for procedure appropriateness in clinical situations
- reports appropriateness for rated indications (where rating and reports agreement are high)
- provides insight into situations where procedure may be inappropriate
- helps providers develop reasonable clinical guidelines
- ratings do not address relative effectiveness of practitioner type, cost effectiveness, or support or refuse any theories of disease

For the chiropractic profession
- serves to inventory what is known and believed about certain clinical procedures at the time of study
- helps prioritize research agenda and resource allocation
- when used realistically, helps promote credibility and willingness to engage in self-scrutiny
- promotes comfort with evidence processes to assess current practices
- provides input into guideline development
- ratings do not serve as a springboard for over extrapolation or exaggeration for public relations purposes

Non-physician constituencies
- assists policy makers and health planners regarding utility of cervical manipulation and mobilization in clinical situations
- develops patient-centered guidelines to provide consumer information for informed patient choice

---

This should be of strategic significance to the profession's researchers, foundations, and academic institutions. For instance, these guidelines showed strong trends toward favoring mobilization over manipulation for some of the more acute or complex cervical spine conditions.[34] In contrast, it has been suggested that manipulation might be of greater therapeutic benefit than mobilization in some low back conditions.[35,36] Additionally, cervical spine manipulation has been linked to rare but significant complications.[37] Given the fact that cervical manipulation is in such widespread use by chiropractors, sorting out these inconsistencies through prospective research in a systematic fashion would be of significant value. The profession could use this report to serve as a springboard to earmark resources to perform clinical trials comparing manipulation to mobilization in a population of patients experiencing acute neck problems and with nonprogressive radicular symptoms.

Just as has happened with information gleaned from the RAND low back panel, elements of this inventory may likely find their way into practice policies such as future iterations of practice parameters, federal guidelines on neck pain and headache, or into care pathways for interdisciplinary management strategies in the public domain and in managed care settings. Ideally, such an inventory can be used to establish an agenda for further critical study into the appropriateness of these conservative care approaches (e.g., randomized clinical trials). Thus, laying out the landscape of intra- and interprofessional agreement and disagreement about manipulation in the cervical spine is important internally to the chiropractic community in setting policy and determining future research and funding priorities. The results of this study should affect planning by chiropractic college researchers, chiropractic research foundations, and political organizations.

Further, these kinds of efforts demonstrate a willingness to engage in evidence-based critical appraisal of chiropractic methods. When done with the support and involvement of the chiropractic community, both academic and political credibility is enhanced. (This project was funded by the Consortium for Chiropractic Research, and DCs served on the panel, co-chaired it, and were on the research team.) It wasn't all that long ago that many people expected experts in medicine and chiropractic to be in substantial disagreement about the appropriateness of spinal manipulation. The use of a structured evidence-based consensus process for the RAND low back study[18,19] showed that practitioners from both of these very different clinical approaches were in agreement more than they were not.

These kinds of appropriateness studies should provide chiropractors with confidence that evidence-based processes are not only valuable to researchers, but they contribute to profession-wide political and social needs as well. Through identification of what is known from science, what is believed through consensus, and what has yet to be determined, the profession can responsibly move forward to improve and enhance its clinical contributions to patient care.[38]

Utility of such appropriateness ratings by non-physicians

Non-physician end users will also be likely to find value in the information contained in the review of literature and ratings for appropriateness. Health care administrators, insurance adjusters, medical directors for insurers and managed care organizations, as well as various types of providers, will find value in the summarized information from this study. Key issues of technology utilization, complications, and therapeutic benefit can be used in administrative and clinical oversight, especially as conservative manual methodologies are incorporated into more insurance programs. As has been urged previously, proper implementation of these study results requires appropriate education and dissemination.[30,33] Ultimately, development of patient-centered guidelines will provide accessible information to assist patients in making informed decisions on the application of manual methods.

How are patient preferences incorporated into decision making using these results?

RAND appropriateness criteria are constructed on a net health benefit scale, and formal patient preferences have not been incorporated into the process. However, some assumptions are made by the panelists when rating appropriateness, for example, that death is less preferable than major morbidity, which is less preferable than minor morbidity, which is less preferable than good health. Clearly, patients value some outcomes over others and clinicians should seek to maximize those health outcomes important to their patients.

The issue of particular treatment preferences on the part of a patient can also affect a clinician's decision making. Therefore, patient preference might influence the appropriateness ratings of the panel. It is conceivable that patient preferences could render some appropriate care inappropriate and considerable uncertain care as either appropriate or inappropriate, but it is not likely that patient preferences could render much inappropriate care as appropriate. Patient preferences are another of the additional clinical factors that are considered by clinicians, along with the available scientific literature and expert panel appropriateness ratings when deciding upon a course of care to recommend. Given an increasing political focus being placed on the need for a decision-making partnership between patients, physicians, purchasers, and policy makers,[33,38,39] in the future it may also be worthwhile to study the impact on expert panelist's ratings of incorporating patient preference information into clinical indications lists.

Placing it all in perspective

The vast amount of scientific and clinical information that confronts providers, policy makers, and physicians cannot be reasonably synthesized and managed by a single individual. The issues of variation in research study quality along with variation in clinical opinion and practice confound matters further. Given that health care costs continue to increase during a time of shrinking resources to pay for them, it is important for providers to have tools for efficient synthesis and integration of quality clinical information in order to serve the needs of the community. Appropriateness methodologies such as those used by RAND provide one such tool. Perhaps McGuire summed it up best[40(p707)]:

> Our medical procedural intensity has been sometimes referred to as a "technologic imperative," with multiple forces giving it astonishing momentum. The words "imperative" and "emperor" have a common root. Our problem is not that the emperor has no clothes, but because the emperor is increasingly supported at public expense, we must give him guidelines that make his clothes fit our needs as well as his. To do so, many of us will need to gain a rough qualitative sense of the magnitudes and probabilities of clinical gains relative to their costs and refrain from regarding small differences in the outcomes of different strategies as occasions for heated debate. We must also learn to see ourselves not solely as health care consumers, providers, or managers, but as members of a society prepared to accept some personal constraints for community gains.

REFERENCES

1. Coulter ID, Shekelle P, Hurwitz E, Adams A. Impact of varying panel membership on ratings of appropriateness in consensus panels. A comparison of a multi- and single disciplinary panel. Accepted for publication HSR; 1995.
2. Park RE, Fink A, Brook RH, Chassin MR, Kahn KL, Merrick N, Kosekoff J, Solomon DH. Physician ratings of appropriate indications for six medical and surgical procedures. *Am J Public Health.* 1986;76:766–772.
3. Fink A, Kosekoff J, Chassin M, Brook R. Consensus methods: Characteristics and guidelines for use. *Am J Public Health.* 1984;74:979–983.
4. Brook RH. Appropriateness: The next frontier. *British Med J.* 1994;308:218–219.
5. Brook RH. The RAND/UCLA Appropriateness method. In McCormack KA, Moore SR, Siegel RA, eds. *Clinical Practice Guideline Development.* Methodology Perspectives. US Department of Health and Human Services. AHCPR; 1994:59–65.
6. Brook RH, Chassin MR, Fink A, Solomon DH, Kosekoff J, Park RE. A method for the detailed assessment of the appropriateness of medical technologies. *Int J Technology Assessment in Health Care.* 1986;2:53–63.
7. Fink A, Kosekoff J, Chassin M, Brook R. Consensus methods: characteristics and guidelines for use. *Am J Public Health.* 1984;74:79–81.
8. Coulter ID, Adams AH. Consensus methods, clinical guidelines, and the RAND study of chiropractic. *J Chiropractic.* 1992;Dec:52–61.
9. Park RE, Fink A, Brook RH, et al. Physician ratings of appropriate indications for six medical and surgical procedures. Santa Monica, CA: RAND. RAND R-3280-CWF/HF/PMT/RWJ; July 1986.
10. Merrick NJ, Fink A, Park RE. Derivation of clinical indications for carotid endarterectomy by an expert panel. *Am J Public Health.* 1987;77(2):187–190.
11. Brook RH, Park RE, Winslow CM, et al. Diagnosis and treatment of coronary disease: comparison of doctors' attitudes in the USA and the UK. *Lancet.* 1988;1:750–753.
12. Chassin M. How do we decide whether an investigation or procedure is appropriate? In Hopkins A, ed. *Appropriate investigation and treat-*

ment in clinical practice. Royal College of Physicians, London, England; 1989.

13. Leape LL, Park RE, Kahan JP, et al. Group judgments of appropriateness: the effect of panel composition. *Quality Assurance in Health Care.* 1992;4(2):151–159.

14. Kahn KL, Park RE, Vennes J, et al. Assigning appropriateness ratings for diagnostic upper gastrointestinal endoscopy using two different approaches. *Medical Care.* 1992;3:1,016–1,028.

15. Chassin MR, Fink A, Brook RH, et al. *Indications for selected medical and surgical procedures—a literature review and ratings of appropriateness: Coronary artery bypass graft surgery.* Santa Monica, CA: RAND Corporation, R-3204/2-CWF/HF/HCFA/PMT/RWJ; 1986b.

16. Kahn KL, Park RE, Brook RH, et al. The effect of comorbidity on appropriateness ratings for two gastrointestinal procedures. *Clinical Epidemiology.* 1988;41(2):115–122.

17. Hilborne LH, Leape LL, Kahan JP, et al. *Percutaneous transluminal coronary angioplasty: A literature review and ratings of appropriateness and necessity.* Santa Monica, CA: RAND Corporation, JRA-01-CWF/HF; 1991.

18. Shekelle PG, Adams AH, Chassin MR, et al. *The appropriateness of spinal manipulation of low-back pain: indications and ratings by a multidisciplinary expert panel.* Santa Monica, CA: RAND Corporation, R-4025/2-CCR/FCER; 1991.

19. Shekelle PG, Adams AH, Chassin MR, et al. *The appropriateness of spinal manipulation of low-back pain: indications and ratings by an all chiropractic expert panel.* Santa Monica, CA: RAND Corporation, R-4025/3-CCR/FCER; 1992.

20. Bernstein SJ, McGlynn EA, Kamberg CJ, et al. *Hysterectomy: a literature review and ratings of appropriateness.* Santa Monica, CA: RAND Corporation, JR-04; 1992.

21. Merrick NJ, Fink A, Brook RH, et al. *Indications for selected medical and surgical procedures—a literature review and ratings of appropriateness: carotid endarterectomy.* Santa Monica, CA: RAND Corporation, R-3204/6-CWF/HF/HCFA/PMT/RWJ; 1986.

22. Chassin MR, Kosecoff J, Park RE, et al. *The appropriateness of use of selected medical and surgical procedures and its relationship to geographic variations in their use.* Ann Arbor, MI: Health Administration Press; 1989.

23. Brook RH, Park RE, Chassin MR, et al. Predicting the appropriate use of carotid endarterectomy, upper gastrointestinal endoscopy, and coronary angiography. *New England J Med.* 1990;323:1,173–1,177.

24. McClellan M, Brook RH. Appropriateness of care: a comparison of global and outcome methods to set standards. *Medical Care.* 1992;30(7):565–586.

25. Fink A, Brook RH, Kosecoff J, et al. Sufficiency of the clinical literature for learning about the appropriate uses of six medical and surgical procedures. *West J Med.* 1987;147(5):609–615.

26. Brook RH. The RAND/UCLA "Appropriateness Method." In: *Clinical practice guideline development: methodologic perspectives.* AHCPR, Rockville, MD: Public Health Service; 1993.

27. Haldeman S, Chapman-Smith D, Petersen D, eds. *Guidelines for chiropractic quality assurance and practice parameters.* Gaithersburg, MD: Aspen Publishers; 1993.

28. Bigos S, Bowyer O, Braen G, et al. *Acute low back problems in adults.* Clinical Practice Guideline No. 14. Washington, DC: US Department of Health and Human Services, Agency for Health Care Policy and Research; December, 1994.

29. Zografos PT, Thompson J, Gienapp T, Hansen DT. Algorithm: portal of entry management of the adult patient with back pain. In Mootz RD, Haldeman S. The evolving role of chiropractic within mainstream health care. *Top Clin Chirop.* 1995;2(2):72.

30. Audet AM, Greenfield S, Field M. Medical practice guidelines: current actions and future directions. *Ann Int Med.* 1990;113:709–714.

31. Williamson JW, German PS, Weiss R, Skinner EA, Bowes F. Health science information management and continuing education for physicians: a survey of US primary care practitioners and their opinion leaders. *Ann Int Med.* 1989;110:151–160.

32. Mootz RD. The impact of health policy on chiropractic. Proceedings, 1995 Chiropractic Centennial, Washington, DC. July 4–9, 1995 Toronto, World Federation of Chiropractic, 1995.

33. Hansen DT. Prospects for the future of chiropractic guidelines. In Lawrence DL, ed: *Advances in chiropractic,* Volume 1. Chicago, IL: Mosby–Year Book; 1994.

34. Coulter ID, Hurwitz E, Adams, et al. *The appropriateness of spinal manipulation and mobilization of the cervical spine: indications and ratings of a multidisciplinary expert panel.* Santa Monica, CA: RAND; 1995.

35. Anderson R, Meeker WC, Wirick B, Mootz RD, Kirk D. A meta-analysis of clinical trials of spinal manipulation. *J Manip Physiol Therap.* 1992;15(3):181–194.

36. Meade TW, Dyer S, Browne W, Townsend J, Fran AO. Low back pain of mechanical origin: randomized comparison of chiropractic and hospital outpatient treatment. *Br Med J.* 1990;300:1,431–1,437.

37. McGregor M, Haldeman S, Kohlbeck FJ. Vertebrobasilar compromise associated with cervical manipulation. *Top Clin Chirop.* 1995;2(3):63–73.

38. Mootz RD, Shekelle PG, Hansen DT. The politics of policy and research. *Top Clin Chirop.* 1995;2(2):58–70.

39. Harkin T. The importance of alternatives to health care reform. *J Alternative Compl Med.* 1995;1(1):5–8.

40. McGuire LB. A long run for a short jump: Understanding clinical guidelines. *Ann Int Med.* 1989;113:705–708.

15

Assessment of Chiropractic Techniques and Procedures

Robert Cooperstein and Michael S. Schneider

The cumulative impact of recently published studies on the effectiveness and appropriateness of spinal manipulation[1-4] and, most recently, the recommendations found in federal guidelines on management of adults with acute low back pain,[5] have added strength to the debate on whether chiropractic will occupy a significant share of the health care market in the future. It certainly can. The extent, however, to which chiropractic becomes integrated into the mainstream of health care will depend on the degree to which its technology assumes acceptable levels of standardization and predictability and meets the needs of the consumer community. For the chiropractic profession, this technology takes the form of procedures, devices, and protocols of care generally found in chiropractic practice.

TECHNOLOGY ASSESSMENT AND ACCOUNTABILITY

Technology assessment is a form of policy research that evaluates procedures, devices, and protocols for providing decision makers with information on different policy options.[6] It is clearly important to determine whose interests it serves, who should perform it, and who the target audience is. "Technology" consists not only of the physical hardware and office procedures, but also the analytic engine the doctor uses to formulate a diagnosis, design a treatment plan, select appropriate outcome measures, and choose the means to manage the case.

In the medical profession, new treatment methods and technologies routinely arise from the teaching hospitals and research departments of medical schools that are affiliated with major universities. A common exception is the development of new drugs, which typically arises from within the pharmaceutical industry. All new drugs and many clinical procedures are subjected to intense research scrutiny, including clinical trials and complex analytic synthesis of experimental data, before they are approved for use on patients. Further study is required before drugs find their way to general distribution for over-the-counter purchase by consumers. Technology assessment in the medical disciplines also involves procedures that are expensive, invasive, controversial, or that may affect special populations (eg, pediatric or geriatric).

By comparison, new chiropractic procedures typically arise from field doctors and technique entrepreneurs who rarely subject them to any serious level of scientific investigation before marketing them to other providers and patients. Generally, the colleges do what they can to investigate a selected subset of these procedures, but must constantly struggle to prevent the more outlandish of them from taking hold among the students through exploitation of their inexperience.[7]

So long as the doctor was the sole arbiter of the doctor-patient relationship, it did not matter that the technology was mostly unstudied and that the science was largely theoretical. The lack of substantive underpinning virtually rationalized the unbridled belief in chiropractic that played such a pivotal role in the profession's survival strategy, insulating it from potentially contradictory evidence. True believers need research to "prove chiropractic" about as much as a minister needs the space program to prove the existence of God.

The situation changes when another level of decision making—employers, third-party payers, managed care organizations, and governmental agencies—begin to require culpability in the determination of appropriateness, safety, clinical efficacy, and cost-effectiveness of health care procedures, including those found in chiropractic care. This transition marks the end of laissez-faire chiropractic technique attitudes and is consistent with the transition from physician-centered to patient-centered case management.[8] In recent years, the answer sought then becomes which individuals or entities could, would, or should assume the primary responsibility, not if chiropractic technology is to be assessed. This article addresses some of these issues in relation to three of the primary entities that currently appear to be the most active in this area: the chiropractic colleges, entrepreneurial technique developers, and some managed care organizations. Although state licensing authorities and the national chiropractic organizations are clearly interested in technique assessment, the diverse nature of their constituencies, and lack of scientific expertise and resources, often results in their seeking rather than offering guidance.

PREVIOUS ATTEMPTS AT CHIROPRACTIC TECHNOLOGY ASSESSMENT

There have been several attempts to begin the process of evaluating technique systems and procedures in the chiropractic profession. Drs Herb Magee and Ted Shrader were instrumental in bringing into existence the Panel of Advisors to the American Chiropractic Association (ACA) Council on Technique. Its first meeting took place during October 1983.[9] The panel has been actively involved over the years clarifying issues directly related to chiropractic technique in the areas of terminology, practice, education, research, and evaluation. Another pioneering effort was the publication in 1987 of what has become known as the Kaminski model for the evaluation of chiropractic techniques.[10] The 1990 Seattle Consensus Conference on the Validation of Chiropractic Methods[11,12] and the subsequent follow-up Conferences on Research and Education (CORE) symposia at Monterey in 1991, Palm Springs in 1992, and Monterey in 1993, were instrumental in establishing an ongoing process for the evaluation of chiropractic technique. These conferences brought in representatives from various named technique systems, chiropractic and nonacademicians, and leaders in chiropractic organizations and educational institutions for a series of panel presentations and subsequent discussions. Although an attempt was made to foster debate and discussion—and even consensus—about various treatment and diagnostic procedures, the conferences did not get much beyond agreeing to follow the scientific processes and use consensus methods.

Later, the CORE symposia convened both formal consensus panels and less formal procedure panels on a wide array of topics covering many chiropractic diagnostic and therapeutic procedures. In each instance, experts prepared critical reviews of the literature as a backdrop for the invited presentations. Testimony from academic and clinical experts was also presented, followed by attempts at finding agreement on whether the technologies satisfy the various attributes of social and scientific acceptability.

This process, of course, was far from trivial. The various technique developers, by participating at all, implicitly acknowledged the need for consensus processes and conforming to the methods of explicit science and experimental research, rather than continued reliance on anecdotal, individual case experience, and in some instances, reckless hyperbole. Although it is not yet obvious, the passage of time will confirm that these conferences marked the passing of control of chiropractic technique from the proprietary advocates of named technique systems to the colleges and independent research organizations. This change is a welcome one that will become especially critical for those chiropractors who will decide to seek integration into the mainstream of health care delivery.

The entire August 1990 issue of *Chiropractic Technique* was devoted to coverage of the Seattle consensus conference. The proceedings[13-15] of the 1990 to 1993 CORE symposia sponsored by the Consortium for Chiropractic Research contain many detailed reviews of the literature pertaining to chiropractic technology, such as stress radiographs, full-spine radiographs, short/long lever nonspecific contact adjustments, leg length insufficiency, specific contact adjusting, surface electromyography (EMG), videofluoroscopy, motion palpation, static radiograph line marking, and thermography. Table 1 lists these reviews. All of these literature reviews have been published in the *Journal of Manipulative and Physiological Therapeutics* and are retrievable; the summaries of the majority of

Table 1. Technology assessments sponsored by the Consortium for Chiropractic Research

Chiropractic procedure	Reviewer	Year
Leg length insufficiency measurement	Mannello	1991
Static cervical radiograph analysis	Owens	1991
Lumbar motion palpation	Panzer	1991
Skin temperature assessment	Plaugher	1991
Short lever specific contact procedures	Bergmann	1991
Short lever manual force mechanically assisted procedures	Bergmann	1991
Short and long lever manual force mechanically assisted procedures	Bergmann	1991
Short lever mechanical force manually assisted procedures	Osterbauer	1991
Bending/stress radiograph analysis	Mick	1992
Full spine radiograph analysis	Taylor	1992
Short/long lever nonspecific contact adjusting	Bergmann	1992
Surface electrode electromyography/lumbar spine	Meyer	1993
Videofluoroscopy of the cervical spine	Schultz	1993
Chiropractic terminology project	Gatterman & Hansen	1993

the CORE procedure panels have been published in *Chiropractic Technique*.

In 1989, the Congress of Chiropractic State Organizations set in motion a process that eventually led to the Mercy Center Consensus Conference of 1992. The proceedings document that emerged, generally known as the Mercy Guidelines,[16] featured sections that described and rated both chiropractic diagnostic methods and treatment methods in common use. Rather than citing specific named technique systems, the Mercy Guidelines recognized generic descriptions of procedures slightly modified from those proposed by Bartol.[17] The Mercy Guidelines should be understood as being an inventory of chiropractic procedures in common use, and not a set of condition-specific clinical guidelines. The fact that the literature cited by the conferees most often involves low back patient presentations is not surprising given that there is a greater amount of such literature compared to other spinal and body regions. Unfortunately, this reliance has sometimes given the false impression that the Mercy Guidelines would confine chiropractic to the treatment of acute low back pain. Nothing could be further from the truth.

Two other Mercy-like parameters of care documents have also been produced. The Canadian chiropractic profession, under the aegis of the Canadian Chiropractic Association, used similar evidence scales and consensus methods for their Glenerin Document[18] of 1993. In that same year, the World Chiropractic Alliance convened a conference in Arizona, out of which emerged the Wyndham Document.[19] Bell,[20,21] in comparing the Mercy Guidelines and Wyndham Document praised the former for its reliance on substantive research, but condemned the latter for having postulated the "inviolability" and "final authority" of the individual practitioner's clinical judgment—that is, the explicit rejection of the very idea of practice guidelines.

Support provided by the Consortium for Chiropractic Research (CCR) and the Foundation for Chiropractic Education and Research resulted in the production of two appropriateness studies regarding spinal manipulation and low back pain by RAND, a California-based health policy think tank.[1,2] Although these reports addressed only one aspect of chiropractic technology (manipulation) and only one specific condition (low back pain), they did much to legitimize chiropractic, given that manipulation and chiropractic are so strongly associated in the public mind. Another appropriateness study on the manipulative treatment of the cervical spine funded through CCR and published by RAND has recently been completed.[22]

Between 1993 and 1995 the ACA Council on Technique cosponsored three national symposia on the comparison of chiropractic treatment procedures.[23-25] Invited guests, representing a number of named chiropractic technique systems, were asked to discuss and debate their respective clinical approaches to specific clinical conditions. The moderator at these symposia used the Bartol classification of chiropractic techniques[26] for the characterization of chiropractic adjustive procedures in order to extract the baseline (generic) commonalities among the technique systems. The primary goal was to raise the level of critical thinking among the participants as well as the audience. More recently, members of the Panel of Advisors to the ACA Council on Technique have published overviews (not to be construed as full technology assessments) of chiropractic technique systems in *Chiropractic Technique*.[27-31] Table 2 lists the technique overviews published to date.

TECHNOLOGY ASSESSMENT AND THE CHIROPRACTIC COLLEGES

Although it would seem obvious that the chiropractic colleges, just like the medical schools, would play a leading role in technology development and assessment, they have usually responded more reactively than proactively to chiropractic methods including those developed by the named technique proprietors. The primary reason for this response is financial; unlike a medical school, the chiropractic college is by and large tuition dependent for revenues and receives little or no direct public support. Indirectly, tuition dollars come in large measure by way of government-secured student loan programs. Still, students more than the health care consuming public, tend to be viewed as the "customer" by chiropractic colleges. Apart from the obvious budgetary way in which tuition dependence limits the quantity of research the colleges can undertake, it imposes more subtle constraints on the colleges' capabilities and desires in the area of technology assessment. They vary considerably in terms of their chiropractic orientations, technique programs, financial status, and human resources. Some colleges or college technique departments may not be well suited or strongly motivated to play an important role in technology assessment.

Equipment manufacturers often donate, sell, or loan (on liberal terms) devices to the chiropractic colleges. In return the manufacturers may expect endorsements or free research and development, particularly publications that may aid in

Table 2. List of chiropractic technique overviews published by the Panel of Advisors to the ACA Council on Technique

Technique	Author	Year
Receptor-tonus (Nimmo)	Schneider[30]	1994
Logan Basic	Filson & Johnson[31]	1994
Applied Kinesiology (AK)	Perle[29]	1995
Thompson Technique	Cooperstein[28]	1995
Chiropractic Biophysics (CBP)	Cooperstein[27]	1995

their merchandising efforts. Some colleges tend to accept such equipment, often with strings attached; others decline. There are historical examples of colleges having been involved in direct marketing of equipment to students and field doctors, which creates an obvious conflict of interest and taints the interpretation of research findings on the utility of such devices. Keating[32] describes BJ Palmer's heavy-handed efforts to market the neurocalometer beginning in 1924, an archetypal example of this type of bias.

Another factor that may drain the motivation of the chiropractic college to evaluate technique unbiasedly is the chilling effect of negative studies. Although the chiropractic colleges have evaluated many of the examination procedures and outcome measures in their core curricula through small-scale intra- and interexaminer reliability studies, results have often been quite disappointing. Those standard examination procedures and outcome measures that have shown poor reproducibility include static and dynamic palpation, leg checks, radiograph line marking, thermography, galvanic skin response, manual muscle testing, and so forth. A few representative examples are provided as references.[33–43] Functional outcome measures and "soft" survey instruments are currently viewed as more useful than many of the more structural "hard" measures (eg, range of motion, joint alignment) that chiropractors have traditionally stressed.[44] These results are not encouraging ones to bring back to the students and alumni, who wonder aloud why the colleges would undermine confidence in their own core curricula. The resulting cynicism on the campuses has no doubt led some administrators and faculty to ask themselves the same question. In an ideal world, the proverbial "search for the truth" would be paramount, but in the world such as it is, the satisfaction of the immediate consumers of chiropractic education—the students—cannot be ignored, not when college revenues are so highly tuition dependent.

Although many of the colleges and individual faculty have shown great integrity and perseverance in assessing chiropractic technology, the overall collegiate ambiance for this line of inquiry seems distinctly less supportive than it was, even in the recent past. There is an oft-repeated proviso that, confronted with the reality of negative studies, the colleges can at least teach the students how they might "practice with uncertainty." Although offered sincerely enough, this approach lacks the zeal and dedication of the more traditional mission to "prove chiropractic"[45] with all of its flourish and testimony. To compound the matter, there is no going back to a simpler time when many of the colleges more or less agreed with field doctors that anecdotal evidence, clinical experience, and patient satisfaction could adequately establish that "chiropractic works." Having accepted the importance of research in chiropractic, and having taken many initial steps down that path, the chiropractic colleges cannot now find the mission unimportant. In short, colleges today are confronting the challenges of charting a path between the Scylla of an initially disappointing run at technology assessment and the Charybdis of an anachronistic faith in chiropractic procedures. Thus, chiropractic colleges may not be as ideally suited to become extensively involved in technology assessment as one might suppose.

There are also technical obstacles to conducting clinical research in the colleges. There is no question that the proverbial "asymptomatic chiropractic students" have been very generous, even magnanimous, in offering up their bodies to serve as subjects in a great variety of research studies. Unfortunately, using subjects such as these creates the possibility that examiners in a reliability study may have poor concordance not primarily due to inherent problems in the measuring apparatus, but rather the low signal intensity of the phenomenon they are trying to detect among asymptomatic experimental subjects. For this reason, investigators who report negative findings generally recommend repeating the study using symptomatic, non-student subjects.

On the other hand, it is fairly difficult to move such studies from the research laboratories to the college's outpatient clinic, where a greater number of symptomatic patients might be found. All the usual difficulties in recruiting subjects and acquiring data are compounded by additional difficulties that are inherent within the pedagogic environment itself. A number of common issues arise: the student doctors may not be trained adequately enough to perform the diagnostic test under investigation or have barely more than a naive competency in a given technique and they may fear losing academic credits and/or even the experimental subject as a patient when faculty members or more senior students are brought in to conduct the study. Moreover, the high rate of intern turnover and the variability of their clinic schedules further complicate the task of maintaining the short-term continuity and long-term follow-up that the study may require. Finally, clinic administrative and other support staff may find that the study unduly complicates their already hectic and complicated job duties.

INTERCOLLEGIATE TECHNOLOGY ASSESSMENT

Although an individual college may have its hands full attempting to perform technology assessment, an intercollegiate organization composed largely of individuals involved in chiropractic technique instruction or research might be in a better position to avoid some of the problems that have been discussed above. Enhanced capability for technology assessment may result from pooling of financial resources, facilities, equipment, and skilled personnel. Furthermore, attainment of a "critical mass" of dedicated investigators, risk sharing as to the impact of negative findings on college morale, cross-fertilization with new ideas, and sharing of relevant experiences can be had. Both the *Consortium for Chiropractic Research* and the Panel of Advisors to the *ACA Council on Technique* have been functioning in this manner for approximately a decade, and they have met with a significant amount of success as outlined previously. Nevertheless, there are some possible limitations in the intercollegiate assessment of chiropractic technology. The representatives of the colleges and the other participating organizations, because they often have divergent political agendas, institutional goals, and research priorities, may find it challenging to agree on matters pertaining to technology assessment.[46] In addition, the geographic dispersal of the collaborators and their lack of day-to-day contact constitute other impediments. Although intercollegiate collaboration has increased coordination, efficiency, and productivity, financial and personnel resources are limited in availability.

TECHNOLOGY ASSESSMENT AND TECHNIQUE ENTREPRENEURS

Proprietors of technique systems (named techniques) increasingly have the responsibility (but not necessarily the motivation) to assure the quality of the technology that they market through seminars, instructional materials, equipment, and certification programs. Some of these individuals and organizations are handling this responsibility with considerable professionalism, conducting well-designed and well-executed research, presenting results at recognized research symposia, and publishing their results in high-quality peer-reviewed journals. A few representative examples are provided.[47-52] Other vendors have been less successful in this regard, persisting in the type of behavior that has fully earned the epithet "technique peddling," replete with unsupported claims, lurid advertising, and published works in trade journals or popular press tabloids.

The technique system entrepreneurs, although no longer immune from the research imperative (at least since the time of the 1990 Seattle consensus conference and the follow-up CORE conferences), have an unfair advantage over the colleges in the area of technology assessment: they can get away with making virtually any unsubstantiated claim they want without fear of being damaged much by professional censure. A college is, after all, directly accountable to accrediting agencies and indirectly accountable to a variety of other constituencies: public health agencies, the scientific community, student loan granting agencies, alumni, students, and finally its own faculty. Technique vendors, by comparison, need only stay out of court and avoid being seen as fringe enough to have their practitioners barred from practicing the given technique by the state board or reimbursement agencies such as state workers' compensation systems.

Through it all, the field of discussion has very quietly gone beyond the "Gonstead vs SOT vs Logan" type of discourse and entered a more sophisticated arena in which the question is one of deciding whether a side-posture adjustment, a blocking procedure, or a light-force sacral contact would be more appropriate for facet syndrome, for example. In other words, there is a tendency, already partially evident in the way grand rounds were conducted during the recent Washington centennial meeting,[30] to stop pitting stand-alone technique systems against one another, in favor of comparing and contrasting the indications for generic technique procedures. Ironically, several of the most prominent of the proprietary technique organizations have played an important role in ushering in this change, by accepting the challenge to subject individual components of their diagnostic and treatment methods to clinical investigation. This acceptance implicitly suggests the feasibility of combining methods, of devising an evidence-based and generic chiropractic armamentarium. It would be both appropriate and timely, as the health care delivery system accelerates its rate of reform, demanding more attention to reducing practice variations, attaining uniformity of terminology, and achieving widespread agreement on what methods belong in the basic chiropractic toolkit.

Under the best of circumstances, technology assessment in the hands of technique entrepreneurs cannot be taken at face value, any more than can the scientific claims of drug companies that fund clinical research on their own drugs. The credibility of technique evaluation is clearly enhanced if the investigating party has no proprietary stake in the outcome. Although the entrepreneurs will continue to play an important role in technology assessment, the inevitable appearance of impropriety dictates that the primary responsibility will probably lie elsewhere.

TECHNOLOGY ASSESSMENT AND MANAGED CARE ORGANIZATIONS

Society's need for an affordable basket of health care services must be met by a rational allocation of its limited health care resources. The economic imperative is clearly identified as a question of optimization. Although the ongoing transformation in health care has been described in various ways, it is perhaps most illustrative to consider it a process of conglomeration, in which increasingly larger purchaser and provider units strive toward improving economies of scale, benefits of interchangeable parts, and efficiency of resources. In the past decade, the center of this transformation has been managed care organizations (MCOs), which seek to achieve cost containment through changes in access to physicians, discounted fees, and improved utilization management. Chief among the better MCOs' concerns is the ability to guarantee a certain level of consistency and quality in their health care products, including chiropractic. A given diagnostic entity is likely to be described using industry-standard terminology, treated using methods that are drawn from a widely shared clinical armamentarium, and the case managed in a predictable manner. MCOs, therefore, have an obvious and immediate interest in chiropractic technology assessment.

The managed care administrators earn their income by attempting simultaneously to lower the cost and raise the quality of health care. Although the pioneering environment of transforming the health care system has seen the establishment of many MCOs more focused on the bottom line than on quality patient care, clinical utility and cost containment are actually symbiotic needs. If businesses cannot obtain coverage that they can afford, at a benefit level their workers will accept, then they will take their business elsewhere. Much of the antagonism expressed by physicians to managed care, be they medical or chiropractic, stems from the mistaken belief that lowering the cost of health care inevitably leads to reducing the quality and even the quantity of care. In fact, managed care is most likely to funnel patients from inefficient to efficient providers. There is potential for this process to lead to a drastic increase in the total number of patients having access to chiropractic care.

Technology assessment is at the center of this process. Mootz and associates write:

> No one (especially an insurance company) wants to pay for clinical procedures that are ineffective, overpriced, or unnecessary, but how can these characteristics be determined? Surgeons believe surgery is necessary, and chiropractors believe spinal adjustments are necessary—but under what circumstances, and how much? . . . The advent of better technologies to synthesize research, establish professional consensus, and determine appropriateness has offered a reasonable alternative to the arbitrary and proprietary methods of the past.[6(p59–60)]

MCOs are not inclined to wait around for the chiropractic colleges, the technique entrepreneurs, or the licensing authorities to accomplish technology assessment and work out detailed practice guidelines. Market forces have brought them to the juncture that they are required to make immediate decisions as to the appropriateness of the various diagnostic and treatment methods for given patient presentations. They need to know which methods are mainstream and which are fringe, which seem plausible and which do not. To that end, the MCOs are already convening their own versions of community-based expert "consensus panels," privately inviting chiropractic consultants to participate in an ongoing series of meetings. Although there is no inherent reason why such panels could not come up with reasonable guidelines, the means by which they would be held publicly accountable for their guidelines are not as tangible as publication in peer-reviewed publications and exposure in a symposium setting. Like the technique entrepreneurs, MCOs must contend with the perception, widely shared among patients and doctors, that their contribution to technique assessment is potentially biased by their commercial positions. Still, the market forces and clinical necessity questions place immediate pressure on MCOs to perform technology assessment as part of an ongoing cost of doing business. The near future seems certain to see an increasing and broadening role for MCOs directly engaging in technology assessments and outcomes research on chiropractic procedures. The potential for interdisciplinary collaborations, comparative trials, and assessment of resource costs in providing chiropractic is extremely high.

CONCLUSIONS

The chiropractic profession is enjoying some good publicity for a change, mostly because federal-level guidelines endorse the clinical value of manipulation. However, the profession will soon discover itself once more on the defensive, as the chiropractic community is challenged to explain the wide fluctuations in chiropractic utilization that occur geographically, the large variation in the number of office visits and total expense of treating any common patient presentation, and the diverse number of methods in common use.[53,54] With greater public acceptance of chiropractic practice comes a proportionally greater degree of responsibility and accountability. It is not acceptable to offer the blanket assertion that "chiropractic works." Instead the explicit, evidence-based assessment processes are being mandated by government, third-party payers, and the consumer public.

Some of the issues confronting individual chiropractic colleges, technique developers, and MCOs in the area of technology assessment have been described. It is emphasized that economic and clinical imperatives demand that this critical work continue to move forward. The colleges may find their greatest opportunity in intercollegiate collaboration. It has become traditional for physicians to adopt a very pessimistic, fatalistic attitude toward the development of practice guidelines, as evidenced in the following representative remark: "what is clear is that if chiropractors do not develop [guidelines] for themselves, outside parties (such as third-party payers) will do it for them."[55(p53)] On the other hand, it is entirely possible that the external development of such guidelines, with significant physician input, represents a feasible and even welcome opportunity to get the job done with great dispatch.

In the present socioeconomic climate, no doctor has the medico-legal or ethical luxury of declining to participate in the struggle that inexorably ushers in the era of practice guidelines. "Not all practice styles can be right, and the profession has an obligation to find out which ones are."[56(p645)] Just as technology assessment must precede the formulation of guidelines, so must implementation of guidelines precede evaluation of validity. The ultimate test of chiropractic technology is always its predictive validity, the extent to which its adoption in clinical practice actually leads to better patient outcomes.[57]

REFERENCES

1. Shekelle P, Adams AH, Chassin MR, et al. *The Appropriateness of Spinal Manipulation for Low Back Pain: Indications and Ratings by an All-Chiropractic Expert Panel.* Santa Monica, Calif: RAND; 1992.

2. Shekelle P, Adams AH, Chassin MR, et al. *The Appropriateness of Spinal Manipulation for Low Back Pain: Indications and Ratings by a Multidisciplinary Expert Panel.* Santa Monica, Calif: RAND; 1991.

3. Manga P. *The Effectiveness and Cost-Effectiveness of Chiropractic Management of Low-Back Pain.* Richmond Hill, Ontario, Canada: Kenilworth Publishing; 1993.

4. Meade TW, Dyer S, Browne W, Townsend J, Fran AO. Low back pain of mechanical origin: randomized comparison of chiropractic and hospital outpatient treatment. *Br Med J.* 1990;300:1431–1437.

5. Bigos S, Boyer O, Braen G, Brown K, eds. *Acute Low Back Problems in Adults. Clinical Practice Guideline No. 14.* Rockville, Md: Agency for Health Care Policy and Research, Public Health Service, US Department of Health and Human Services; 1994.

6. Mootz RD, Shekelle PG, Hansen DT. The politics of policy and research. *Top Clin Chiro.* 1995;2(2):56–70.

7. Lawrence DJ. The challenges of teaching technique. *Chiro Tech.* 1989;1(1):6–8.

8. Hansen DT. Prospects for the future of chiropractic guidelines. In: Lawrence D, ed. *Advances in Chiropractic Volume 1.* Chicago, Ill: Mosby-Year Book; 1994.

9. Shrader TL. Technic council sponsors conference on fundamentals. *ACA J Chiro.* 1983;20:52–54.

10. Kaminski M, Boal R, Gillette RG, Peterson DH, Villnave T. A model for the evaluation of chiropractic methods. *J Manipulative Physiol Ther.* 1987;10(2):61–64.

11. Phillips RB. Summary of roundtable I: analytic/diagnostic methods. *Chiro Tech.* 1990;2(3):154.

12. Sawyer CE. Summary of roundtable II: treatment/therapeutic methods. *Chiro Tech.* 1990;2(3):155.

13. Hansen D, ed. Focus on health policy and technology assessment in chiropractic. In: *Proceedings of the Seventh Annual Conference on Research and Education.* Palm Springs, CA: Consortium for Chiropractic Research; 1992.

14. Hansen D, ed. Chiropractic science in health policy and research. In: *Proceedings of the Eighth Annual Conference on Research and Education.* Monterey, Calif: Consortium for Chiropractic Research; 1993.

15. Hansen D, ed. Emphasis on consensus. In: *Proceedings of the Sixth Annual Conference on Research and Education.* Monterey, Calif: Consortium for Chiropractic Research; 1991.

16. Haldeman S, Chapman-Smith D, Petersen DM, eds. *Guidelines for Chiropractic Quality Assurance and Practice Parameters.* Gaithersburg, Md: Aspen Publishers; 1993.

17. Bartol KM. A model for the categorization of chiropractic treatment procedures. *Chiro Tech.* 1991;3(2):78–80.

18. Henderson DJ. Towards the development of guidelines on chiropractic care and practice: an opportunity to enhance professional credibility. *J Can Chiro Assoc.* 1991;35:203–205.

19. Rondberg T, ed. *Practice Guidelines for Straight Chiropractic: Proceedings of the International Straight Chiropractic Consensus Conference.* Chandler, Ariz: World Chiropractic Alliance; 1993.

20. Bell DM. Guidelines for chiropractic quality assurance and practice parameters. *Abstr Clin Care Guidelines.* 1993;5(3): 7–10.

21. Bell DM. Practice guidelines for straight chiropractic. *Abstr Clin Care Guidelines.* 1993;5(3):10–14.

22. Coulter ID, Shekelle PG, Mootz RD, Hansen DT. The use of expert panel results: the RAND panel for appropriateness of manipulation and mobilization of the cervical spine. *Top Clin Chiro.* 1995;2(3): 54–62.

23. Bartol K, Schneider MS, eds. *Proceedings of the Third National Symposium on the Comparison of Chiropractic Treatment Procedures: The Cervical Subluxation Complex.* Seattle, Wash: ACA Council on Technique; 1995.

24. Bartol K, Schneider MS, eds. *Proceedings of the First National Symposium on the Comparison of Chiropractic Treatment Procedures: Emphasis on Sacroiliac Subluxations.* Milwaukee, Wisc: ACA Council on Technique; 1993.

25. Bartol K, Schneider MS, eds. *Proceedings of the Second National Symposium on the Comparison of Chiropractic Treatment Procedures: The Cervical Subluxation Complex.* Valley Forge, Pa: ACA Council on Technique; 1994.

26. Bartol KM. Algorithm for the categorization of chiropractic technique procedures. *Chiro Tech.* 1992;4(1):8–14.

27. Cooperstein R. Technique system overview: chiropractic biophysics technique (CBP). *Chiro Tech.* 1995;7(4):141–146.

28. Cooperstein R. Technique system overview: Thompson technique. *Chiro Tech.* 1995;7(2):60–63.

29. Perle SM. Technique system overview: applied kinesiology (AK). *Chiro Tech.* 1995;7(3):103–107.

30. Schneider M. Receptor-tonus technique assessment. *Chiro Tech.* 1994;6(4):156–159.

31. Filson RM, Johnson G. Technique system overview: Logan system of body mechanics assessment. *Chiro Tech.* 1994;6(3):98–103.

32. Keating JC. Introducing the neurocalometer: a view from the fountainhead. *J Can Chiro Assoc.* 1991;35(3):165–178.

33. Nansel DD, Jansen RD. Concordance between galvanic skin response and spinal palpation findings in pain-free males. *J Manipulative Physiol Ther.* 1988;11(4):267–272.

34. Plaugher G, Haas M, Doble RW Jr, Lopes MA, Cremata EE, Lantz C. The interexaminer reliability of a galvanic skin response instrument. *J Manipulative Physiol Ther.* 1993;16(7): 453–459.

35. Plaugher G, Lopes MA, Melch PE, Cremata EE. The inter- and intraexaminer reliability of a paraspinal skin temperature differential instrument. *J Manipulative Physiol Ther.* 1991;14(6):361–367.

36. Haas M, Peterson D, Hoyer D, Ross G. The reliability of muscle testing response to a provocative challenge. *Chiro Tech.* 1993;5(3): 95–100.

37. Haas M, Peterson D, Rothman EH, et al. Responsiveness of leg alignment changes associated with articular pressure testing to spinal manipulation: the use of a randomized clinical trial design to evaluate a diagnostic test with a dichotomous outcome. *J Manipulative Physiol Ther.* 1993;16(5):306–311.

38. Haas M, Peterson D, Panzer D, et al. Reactivity of leg alignment to articular pressure testing: evaluation of a diagnostic test using a randomized crossover clinical trial approach. *J Manipulative Physiol Ther.* 1993;16(4):220–227.

39. Haas M, Peterson D, Hoyer D, Ross G. Muscle testing response to provocative vertebral challenge and spinal manipulation: a randomized controlled trial of construct validity. *J Manipulative Physiol Ther.* 1994;17:141–148.

40. Falltrick DR, Pierson DS. Precise measurement of functional leg length inequality and changes due to cervical spine rotation in pain-free subjects. *J Manipulative Physiol Ther.* 1989;12(5):369–373.
41. Leboeuf C. The reliability of specific sacro-occipital technique diagnostic tests. *J Manipulative Physiol Ther.* 1991;14(9):512–517.
42. Rhudy T, Sandefur RM, Burk JM. Interexaminer/intertechnique reliability in spinal subluxation assessment: a multifactorial approach. *Am J Chiro Med.* 1988;1(3):111–114.
43. Rhudy TR, Burk JM. Inter-examiner reliability of functional leg-length assessment. *Am J Chiro Med.* 1990;3(2):63–66.
44. Cherkin DC. Patient satisfaction as an outcome measure. *Chiro Tech.* 1990;2(3):138–141.
45. Cooperstein R. Brand name techniques and the confidence gap. *J Chiro Educ.* 1990;4(3):89–93.
46. Cooperstein R. On hybrid vigor and creative disaccord: the panel of advisors to the ACA panel on technique. *Dynamic Chiro.* 1995;13(13):14, 20.
47. Osterbauer P, Derickson KL, Peles JD, DeBoer KF, Fuhr A, Winters J. Three-dimensional head kinematics and clinical outcome of patients with neck injury treated with spinal manipulative therapy: a pilot study. *J Manipulative Physiol Ther.* 1992;15(8):501–511.
48. Osterbauer PJ, Fuhr AW. The current status of activator methods chiropractic technique, theory, and training. *Chiro Tech.* 1990;2(4):168–175.
49. Jackson BL, Harrison DD, Robertson GA, Barker WF. Chiropractic biophysics lateral cervical film analysis reliability. *J Manipulative Physiol Ther.* 1993;16(6):384–391.
50. Schneider MJ. Soft tissue effects of sacroiliac lumbosacral joint manipulation. *Chiro Tech.* 1992;4(4):136–142.
51. Schneider MJ. Tender points/fibromyalgia vs trigger points/myofascial pain syndrome: a need for clarity in terminology and differential diagnosis. *J Manipulative Physiol Ther.* 1995;18(6):398–406.
52. Plaugher G, Hendricks AH, Doble RW Jr, Bachman TR, Araghi HJ, Hoffart VM. The reliability of patient positioning for evaluating static radiologic parameters of the human pelvis. *J Manipulative Physiol Ther.* 1993;16(8):517–522.
53. Cooperstein R. Contemporary approach to understanding chiropractic technique. In: Lawrence D, ed. *Advances in Chiropractic Volume 2.* Chicago Ill: Mosby-Year Book; 1995.
54. Bergmann TF. Various forms of chiropractic technique. *Chiro Tech.* 1993;5(2):53–55.
55. Coulter I, Adams A. Consensus methods, clinical guidelines, and the RAND study of chiropractic. *ACA J Chiro.* December 1992;29:50–61.
56. Fletcher RH, Fletcher SW. Clinical practice guidelines. *Ann Intern Med.* 1990;113(9):645–647.
57. Chassin MR. Standards of care in medicine. *Inquiry.* 1988;25:437–453.

16

Quantitative Functional Capacity Evaluation: The Missing Link To Outcomes Assessment

Steven G. Yeomans and Craig Liebenson

Outcomes assessment (OA) is a health care buzzword for the 1990s. Quality assurance in health services delivery requires that certain guidelines be followed and that measurable outcomes be used to document the appropriateness of care. Most methods of OA have been "high-tech," requiring substantial expenses of time and money. Due to the cost and the failure to demonstrate validity, a shift in emphasis to "low-tech" approaches has occurred. Modern methods of OA must be time efficient, economical, reliable, and valid.

Modern reporting on spinal pain patients requires a consensus-based classification approach, relevant historical data gathering, and reliable and valid OA of both subjective and functional parameters. Such an approach has great potential for future data collection and analysis and may even allow multiple high-quality care facilities to provide invaluable information for research purposes.

Physicians, insurance companies, medico-legal reviewers, and managed care organizations are becoming increasingly interested in OA and functional testing, because of the demand to objectify patient status and document patient progress during the course of treatment.[1] OA represents a method used to measure a change in a patient's health status as a result of some type of treatment approach.[2] OA instruments are also used as a tool for measuring treatment effectiveness regardless of methods used.[3] Moreover, OA plays an important role in steering quality care and cost containment. Algorithm 1 graphically indicates an outcomes assessment approach.

THE STATE OF THE ART IN OUTCOMES ASSESSMENT

OAs are primarily concerned with showing patient progress over time and objectifying patient status. There are a number of different types of OA instruments that can be performed at critical junctures of patient care. For example, in the acute stage (initial patient evaluation) baseline data can be collected by the subjective OA questionnaires concerning pain level, disability, general health, depression, work dissatisfaction, and others. In the subacute stage, functional outcomes become necessary. A quantifiable functional capacity evaluation using reliable and valid tests that can be compared to a normative database is essential before the patient has completed 4 to 6 weeks of care. This evaluation enables the patient, doctor, and third-party payer to have baseline levels of the patient's impairment or dysfunction and allows for comparison over time. A final type of OA, the work capacity evaluation (WCE), aims to establish return to work (RTW) goals. This evaluation is especially important in medico-legal situations and in instances where disability is involved.

The information gained about the acute patient through the use of subjective OA is critical for documenting, in a quantitative manner, the subjective information concerning how the injury or condition is affecting the patient. Most important, these instruments can be repeated at a future reexamination date and, by comparing the baseline or initial information gathered to that at follow-up, confident clinical decision making can occur that can lead to one of the following:

- continued care (if improvement is noted without reaching maximum therapeutic benefit);
- change in treatment approach, strategy, or goals (if no clinical improvement or change is noted and case resolution has not occurred);

- initiation of rehabilitation and reduction of passive treatment frequency (improvement without resolve and deconditioning is complicating further improvement); or
- referral to another health care provider if therapeutic benefit can be obtained or, simply, a discharge with or without permanent residual sequelae, disability, or impairment.

The ability of the treating health care provider to make the "next" case management decision in the unresolved case has been at the core of the problem regarding overutilization of passive care, doctor dependency, chronic pain behavior, and insurance company "nightmares."

Table 1 lists some of the more common and studied OA instruments[4-40] the health care provider can choose from to help gain the leverage needed to make intelligent clinical decisions. It is necessary to use the same OA instrument at follow-up in order to compare results at follow-up reexaminations. Note that there are many different OA instruments from which to choose and the list in Table 1 is not all-inclusive.

The method by which the subjective OA information is documented and reported is important so that the information derived from the OA can be reviewed easily. Ease of review serves the needs of the health care provider (to render appropriate care), the patient (for orientation and referencing his or her response to treatment in a report of findings), and the insurance company (to justify payment of a claim) as well as the attorney (in a medico-legal arena such as a malpractice suit). The form in Fig. 2 summarizes the various tools one may use. By summarizing the results of the various OA tools on one page, the information can be reviewed quickly, and clinical decisions can be driven in a prompt and efficient manner.

The common thread that ties the historical and subjective data to the objective quantitative functional capacity evaluation (QFCE) is the various OA instruments. Once the patient is subacute, it is essential to establish objective functional baselines. Safety in applying the functional tests must be determined before proceeding with functional testing. It should be noted that functional capacity testing is contraindicated in the acute stage of an injury when pain is more of a "chemical" nature than a "mechanical." Mooney and Matheson recommend that a physical capacity evaluation (PCE) be considered at 2 weeks' postinjury in order to determine the "weak functional link"[41] and at 4 weeks to perform their California Functional Capacity Protocol (Cal-FCP).[42] Triano (personal communication, May 1994) has reported that 4 weeks' postinjury is an appropriate time to initiate testing. Hart and associates[43] report indications for functional testing include the following:

Table 1. Assessment options*

Assessment goals	Instruments
1. General health	COOP charts,[4,5] HSQ,[††] SF-36,[6] SIP[7,8]
2. Pain perception	NPS,[9] VAS,[11-13] McGill[14-16]
3. Condition specific	
• Low back pain[20]	• Oswestry,[17,18] Roland-Morris,[19] Dallas,[21] lower back TyPEs[22]
• Neck	• NDI,[23] headache questionnaire[24]
• TyPE (from Health Outcomes Institute)[††]	• Asthma, CTS, COPD, depression, low back pain, hypertension/lipid disorders, osteoarthritis of the knee, rheumatoid arthritis, allergic rhinitis, smoking cessation, and others[††]
4. Psychometrics	HSQ (questions 37-39)[†,††] SF-36,[†,6] Waddell's signs,[‡25] SARS,[‡26] modified Zung,[27] modified somatic perception questionnaire,[28] SCL-90R,[29] Beck's depression scale,[30] DRAM,[31] FABQ[32]
5. Patient satisfaction	Chiropractic satisfaction questionnaire,[33] visit-specific questionnaire[34-37]
6. Job dissatisfaction	APGAR[38]
7. Disability	Vermont questionnaire,[39] FASQ[40]

COOP = Dartmouth COOP Health Charts; HSQ = Health Status Questionnaire; SIP = sickness index profile; NPS = numerical pain scale; VAS = visual analogue scale; NDI = neck disability index; CTS = carpal tunnel syndrome; COPD = chronic obstructive pulmonary disease; SARS = somatic amplification rating scale; DRAM = distress and risk assessment method; FABQ = fear-avoidance beliefs questionnaire; FASQ = functional assessment screening questionnaire; TyPE = technology of patient experience.

*Once an OA instrument is chosen, do not change to a different OA instrument at follow-up. Otherwise the baseline information cannot be compared to follow-up information.

†Only parts of the questionnaire relate to the categories.

‡These are physical examinations, not questionnaire tests.

§Cannot be scored (not quantitative, only qualitative).

††Available: Health Outcomes Institute, 2001 Killebrew Drive, Ste 122, Bloomington, MN 55425.

- plateau in treatment progress,
- discrepancy between subjective and objective findings,
- difficulty in returning the patient to gainful employment, and
- vocational planning or medico-legal case settlement.

As soon as the patient leaves the acute guarded stage, the QFCE not only provides ideal outcomes assessment information, but also identifies key functional pathologies that can be addressed with various treatment approaches such as manipulation, exercise, and patient education. Mooney reports that the functional capacity evaluation should be mandatory for any patient still suffering pain after 6 to 7 weeks.[41]

Functional testing serves as an objective OA method, thus complementing the subjective outcomes assessment instruments or questionnaires completed by the patient at various intervals of time during care. The objective functional tests measure factors such as flexibility, strength, coordination, endurance, aerobic capacity, posture, and balance. Functional tests, whether provocative or functional in nature, must follow certain criteria in order to be useful and reliable. Five issues that must be addressed in the selection and use of any functional test in a patient population have been described.[42] These issues, presented in hierarchical order, are

1. *Safety*: Given the known characteristics of the patient, the procedure should not be expected to lead to injury.
2. *Reliability*: The test score should be dependable across the evaluators, patients, and the date or time of administration.
3. *Validity*: The interpretation of the test score should be able to predict or reflect the patient's performance in a target work setting.
4. *Practicality*: The cost of the test procedure should be reasonable. Cost is measured in terms of the direct expense of the test procedure plus the amount of time required of the patient, plus the delay in providing the information derived from the procedure to the referral source.
5. *Utility*: The usefulness of the procedure is the degree to which it meets the needs of the patient, referrer, and payer.

High-tech instrumentation and dynametric assessment of the low back have been considered the "gold standard" of lumbar spine functional assessment. This view is largely due to their reliability and reproducibility. However, the validity of some of the high-tech testing approaches has recently become an issue of controversy. Grabiner and colleagues[44] have demonstrated, for example, that normal strength measurements from a high-tech approach do not necessarily correlate with normal human function. In this study, electromyography (EMG) was used during isometric trunk extension. The results revealed decoupling, or asymmetric lumbar paraspinal muscle activity, was present in low back pain subjects who were considered normal on high-tech dynametric testing. This decoupling phenomenon also differentiated between pain and non-pain subjects. This study suggests that musculoskeletal function involves not only strength, but also coordination during the performance of a specified task. Because spinal movement and coordination use complex neuromuscular functions, simple strength assessment by high-tech dynamometer does not necessarily correlate with assessment of spinal function. The EMG results illustrate the limitations of high-tech dynametric testing of muscle strength and endurance, and they also suggest that the often harsh criticism of low-tech evaluation approaches regarding strength and coordination may be inappropriate and unjustified.

Newton and Waddell[45] reported that no convincing evidence supports that isokinetic or any other type of iso-measure has greater utility in assessing the patient with low back pain than a clinical evaluation of physical impairment, isometric strength, a simple isoinertial lift, or psychophysical testing. Because of the inability to demonstrate high quality of spinal function assessment by high-tech methodologies, there has been insufficient evidence to suggest abandonment of lower tech quantifiable tests. Many low-tech approaches to identify functional pathology have been reported.[46-73] Valid and reliable information, often with a normative database, has been reported; hence, serves as excellent low-tech functional OA tools. Careful observation of the quality of movement during the test can give valuable insight to treatment prescription addressing functional pathologies such as muscle imbalance, joint stiffness, poor movement and coordination, and postural dysfunction.

Reliability has been reported in several low-tech tests that do not provide numerical quantification results. For example, the *National Institute for Occupational Safety and Health* (NIOSH) *Low Back Atlas* identifies 19 tests with significant reliability (<0.74 Cohen's Kappa and >0.79 coefficient for interclass correlation coefficient [ICC]).[63,69] Moffroid[70] studied the ability of the 53 NIOSH tests to discriminate between low back pain and non-pain subjects. It was found that 23 of the 53 tests could not discriminate adequately between the two groups and that when the 7 strongest tests were grouped together, a sensitivity of 87% and a specificity of 93% were obtained. Interestingly, the most important measurements were those that assessed passive mobility, dynamic mobility, strength, and symmetry. Reports[71] have recently been published that also suggest that **non-dynamometric tests correlate better with pain and disability** than those that deal with isokinetic testing. The authors were careful to point out that non-dynamometric tests are still useful in the clinical setting in spite of the development of more sophisticated and accurate methods of testing muscle strength.[69] Harding and Williams[72] reported a group of low-tech tests were determined safe, reliable, and valid for assessment of physical dysfunction in chronic pain subjects. A normative database segregated by age, gender, and vocation (blue collar vs white collar) were studied and found reliable when tests on over 500 individuals were carried out.[73] Hence, because validity and reliability have been established, as well as a normative database regarding several low-tech functional tests, it would appear natural to adopt these particular tests as representatives in a low-tech functional capacity evaluation setting.

THE QFCE

Achieving a low-cost, time-efficient, valid, and reliable method of evaluating functional capacity of a patient was the design goal in developing the QFCE instrument. This test is intended to allow the doctor to identify functional baselines for active rehabilitation in order to improve deconditioning and restore function. The QFCE introduces an OA instrument that can be used both as an objective barometer for measuring change in function over time ("descriptive"), as well as an aid in driving specific rehabilitation protocols ("prescriptive"). When coupled with the subjective OA instrument(s), the QFCE enables the provider to document changes in symptoms and function over time. It also provides a method for the health care provider to use in making a clinical decision (change treatment approach, refer, discharge with or without permanent residuals, and so forth), depending in part on the QFCE results. The QFCE is not designed to replace, but rather complement, other qualitative, less "objective" tests such as trigger point and end-feel palpation, postural and gait analysis, and observation of altered movement patterns.

The second goal is to incorporate the QFCE into a computerized format in preparation for establishing a large database for clinical as well as research objectives. Regardless of whether it is used in a computerized or noncomputerized format, the data derived from the QFCE can be used to generate reports for documentation reasons that can enhance communication with the patient when reporting findings, with insurance companies when supporting the need for rehabilitative care, and with the treating physician/therapist when facilitating the process of establishing maximum therapeutic benefit or maximum medical improvement (MMI) and thus support case closure or referral.

Each test of the QFCE is fully explained and referenced. When the original reference was unclear, the principal author who described the specific test was contacted and the clarifying information was incorporated into the text. Because low-tech functional testing is gaining interest in the research community, it is probable that the QFCE will be updated from time to time in order to stay current as well as to incorporate new valid and reliable approaches that measure function.

When performing the QFCE, it is important to perform each test as precisely as possible in the manner described. Such adherence is important for improving reliability. Ekstrand and coworkers[47] observed an improvement in the coefficient of variation (CV) from 7.5 ± 2.9 to 1.9 ± 0.7 after using the tests for 2 months and refining their technique. In particular they paid attention to the details regarding:

- standardizing inclinometer placement and allowing the pendulum of the gravity type to swing freely,
- stiffening up the examination table (plywood with straps),
- identifying bony anatomic landmarks (mark on skin), and
- standardizing examination bench height for each visit.

The following text describes each of the 21 tests that comprise the QFCE (in the order they are performed).

Initial and final test

1. Visual analogue scale

The visual analogue scale (VAS)[10–14] evaluates the patient's perception of his or her pain level on a 0 to 10 pain scale. It is completed at the beginning and conclusion of the QFCE. Pain is most commonly measured by intensity, frequency, and duration. The VAS is a 10-cm line with two pain descriptors at each end ("No pain" or "0" and "Unbearable pain" or "10"). For the purpose of the QFCE, the pain being rated is pain that is being perceived at the time the QFCE is administered. Scoring is completed by laying a transparent 10-cm ruler over the line and reading the centimeter and millimeter markings. More specifically, a 0 to 10 scale is used where 1 cm = 1/10 pain; 5.5 cm = 5.5/10 pain; and so forth.

Standing tests

2. Repetitive squat

The repetitive squat[71,73] evaluates the strength and endurance of those muscles required to perform a squat. The patient stands with his or her feet 15 cm apart and squats until the thighs are horizontal; the patient then returns to the upright position (Fig 1). Each repetition lasts 2 to 3 seconds in duration, and each test is repeated until a maximum number of repetitions is achieved or 50 repetitions are done, whichever occurs first. Observation of the quality of movement as well as the number of repetitions is important because information derived about the quality of movement gives rise to treatment and exercise prescriptions. Therefore, the quantitative information assesses outcomes while the qualitative data drive treatment goals. The normative data are age, gender, and occupational specific, as depicted in Table 2.[73]

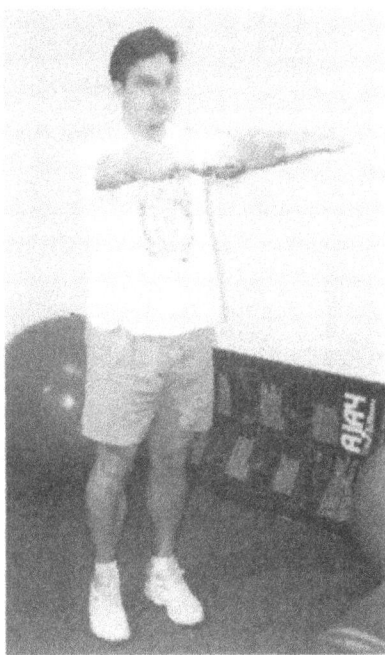
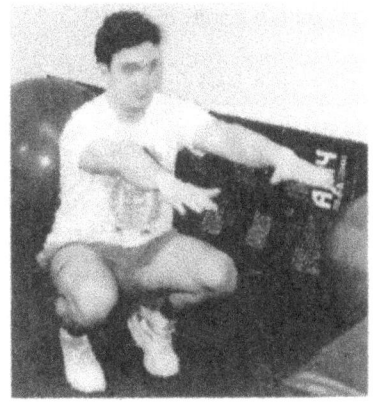

Fig 1. Repetitive squat test.

3. Range of motion: Lumbar

The range of motion (ROM): lumbar test evaluates the mobility of the lumbar spine.[57,74-80] An inclinometer is placed at T-12 and S-2. Sagittal plane movements (flexion/extension) are assessed by placing the inclinometer vertically perpendicular to the spine on the midline. Frontal plane motion (lateral flexion) is assessed by placing the base of the inclinometer horizontal so that the needle hangs freely. The end points of movement are recorded at both the T-12 and S-2, and the difference is calculated using the equation: T-12 – S-2. If the average of three consecutive readings falls within 5° or 10% of the average, the highest of the three readings is recorded. This procedure may be repeated a maximum of six times in an attempt to achieve this result.[57] Table 3 presents the normative data for the lumbar spine.[80]

4. Pain/tenderness (Waddell nonorganic low back pain test 1)

The Waddell nonorganic low back pain (LBP) signs evaluate for abnormal psychosocial issues.[25] More specifically, this test is performed by applying a light touch in a manner that should normally not provoke pain. A nonorganic pain response is reported when the patient describes or portrays pain. There are five categories (see Table 4) of the Waddell nonorganic LBP test (QFCE tests 4, 5, 8, 9, 10, 13), which are nonprovocative tests (ie, do not try to provoke a pain response such as when performing standard orthopaedic provocative tests). If a pain response occurs, this finding constitutes a positive (+) response. The practitioner should determine if there is a physiologic explanation and repeat the tests as many times as needed in order to assure evaluator objectivity. These tests are reported as positive or negative in terms of presence of nonorganic LBP rather than in terms of a number. The final score is documented as the total number of positive signs out of the five (eg, two out of five). When three or more of the five signs are positive, nonorganic LBP must be considered, and the psychosocial issues must be therapeutically addressed.

Test 1 is performed by standing or sitting behind the patient and a light touch or pinch is applied to the skin over the lumbar area. A deep type of palpation over a nonanatomic, wide area of pain not localized to one structure is also performed. Observation focuses on looking for a disproportionate or exaggerated response ("jump sign," verbal response, and so on).

5. Simulation (Waddell nonorganic low back pain test 2)

Axial compression

This test[25] is performed by standing behind the patient and placing a light pressure downward on the occiput, similar to a cervical compression test. However, it is performed in a manner that should not normally provoke pain. Nonorganic LBP is suggested if a pain response is obtained. Neck pain may occur with axial loading; hence, this approach may be contraindicated. If it occurs, downward pressure on the shoulders will simulate a similar test.

Table 2. Normative data for repetitive squatting test*

| | Males (n = 242) | | | | | | Females (n = 233) | | | | | |
| | Blue collar | | White collar | | All | | Blue collar | | White collar | | All | |
Age	x̄	SD	x̄	SD	x̄	SD	x̄	SD	x̄	SD	x̄	SD
35–39	39	13	46	8	42	12	24	11	27	12	26	12
40–44	34	14	45	9	38	13	22	13	18	8	20	12
45–49	30	12	40	11	33	13	19	12	26	13	22	13
50–54	28	14	41	11	33	14	13	10	18	14	14	11
35–54	33	14	43	10	37	13	20	12	23	12	21	12

x̄ = mean; SD = standard deviation.
*A maximum of 50 repetitions is allowed.
Source: Alaranta H, Hurri H, Heliovaara M, et al. Non-dynamometric trunk performance tests: reliability and normative data. Scand J Rehab Med. 1994;26:211–215.

Trunk rotation

This test[25] is performed by standing behind the weight-bearing patient. The pelvis is manually rotated at the hips in a manner that should not normally provoke a pain response. The patient is instructed not to rotate the shoulders beyond the movement being actively assisted by the evaluator at the pelvis. Nonorganic LBP is suggested if a pain response is obtained. (*Note:* If lumbar root pain is present, a false-positive response may be obtained. Therefore, it should be correlated with a straight leg raise and neurologic examination findings.)

The following two functional tests are included in this evaluation due to the importance of the ankle joint in maintaining balance and coordination and its important relationship to the "kinetic chain." In addition, the stability of the subtalar joint is highly dependent on the flexibility of the ankle and must be intact for proper proprioceptive function. Determination of the ROM at the ankle can also yield valuable information when correlated to the Dictionary of Occupational Titles (DOT) when assessment of work capacities is requested.[81]

6. Gastrocnemius/ankle dorsiflexion test (knee straight)

In this test,[46,47] the patient stands upright, feet parallel and knees straight. The inclinometer is positioned above the lateral malleolus and "zeroed" in the upright standing position. The patient leans forward, placing the hands on a wall to a point of maximum ankle dorsiflexion (DF), while keeping the heel down; the angle is then measured. The normative data reveal 22.5° ± 0.7°, intra-assay CV is 2.2%, and inter-assay CV is 2.5%.[47]

7. Soleus/ankle dorsiflexion test (knee flexed)

The patient position in this test[46,47] is standing with one leg on floor while the foot being tested is placed on a bench. The knee is flexed and the ankle is dorsiflexed to a maximum angle maintaining heel-to-bench contact. The normative data reveal 24.9° ± 0.8°, intra-assay CV is 2.2%, and inter-assay CV 2.6%.[47]

Sitting tests

8. Sitting vs supine straight leg raise/distraction (Waddell nonorganic low back pain test 3)

This test[25] evaluates for abnormal psychosocial issues. The patient is seated, and the doctor performs a sitting straight leg raise (SLR) test while distracting the patient by

Table 3. Normal ranges of lumbar motion in railroad workers

Motion	Mean ± SD*	Normal range	Percent of normal
True flexion	58 ± 9.6	65°	89.2
True extension	22 ± 9.7	30°	72.7
Pelvic flexion	60 ± 13.8	55°	109.1
Straight leg raise			
Right	77 ± 12.5	75°	102.9
Left	77 ± 12.0	75°	102.9
Right lateral flexion	24 ± 7.4	25°	96.9
Left lateral flexion	25 ± 8.2	25°	100.6

*Sample includes 160 male railroad workers; average age = 35 years ± 8 years; height = 70 in ± 3 in; weight = 187 ± 29 lbs.[8]
Sources: Mayer T, Tencer A, Kristoferson S, Mooney V. Use of noninvasive techniques for quantification of spinal range-of-motion in normal subjects and chronic low-back dysfunction patients. Spine. 1984;9:588–595. Mayer T, Gatchel RJ, Keeley J, Mayer H, Richling D. A male incumbent worker industrial database. Spine. 1994;19:762–764.

Table 4. Waddell nonorganic low back pain signs

Test	Assessment method	Reporting
Pain (superficial) Simulation	Light pressure to skin	+ or −
Axial compression	Light downward pressure on calvarium	+ or −
Trunk rotation	Minimal twisting of the pelvis without excess shoulder rotation	+ or −
Distraction	Sitting (distracted) SLR is nonpainful versus the nondistracted supine SLR	+ or −
Regional neurology	Nonanatomic findings during routine neurologic examination	+ or −
Exaggeration	Noted at any time during the physical examination	+ or −

SLR = straight leg raise.
Source: Waddell G, McCulloch JA, Kummel E, Venner RM. Nonorganic physical signs in low-back pain. *Spine.* 1980;5:117–125. © 1980, Lippincott Williams & Wilkins.

---

the performance of a plantar superficial reflex while rapidly extending the knee. A positive test occurs when there is little or no pain noted in the distracted sitting SLR position and a disproportionately high level of pain observed during the nondistracted supine SLR test (positive "flip" sign). Note that if a sciatic nerve tension sign exists, this test may be invalid. Also, the evaluator should be cautious regarding the speed at which the sitting SLR is performed if nerve tension is suspected. As with the other Waddell nonorganic LBP signs, this test is reported as positive or negative as it relates to nonorganic LBP rather than a number (Table 4).

9. Regional neurology (Waddell nonorganic low back pain test 4)

This test[25] evaluates for abnormal psychosocial issues. The health care provider performs a standard neurologic physical examination (deep tendon reflexes, muscle strength, sensory perception). A positive test is present when the neurologic examination reveals findings that do not follow an expected anatomic pattern or are highly inconsistent (or both). These findings may include altered motor functions where many muscle groups are weak. If the quality of weakness is of a "breakaway" variety, where the patient suddenly discontinues the strength test, one must differentiate between pain-induced weakness (physiologic) and a poor voluntary effort (nonorganic). Sensory changes may be of a nondermatomal variety, often with hyperpathia mixed with dysesthesia. Another differential diagnosis to consider is sclerotomal pain, which may arise from the posterior disc or joint structure usually described in the history as a deep, nonspecific, rather global distribution that does not follow any obvious anatomic pathway. In general, the evaluator should look for multiple signs of nonorganic LBP before feeling secure about this assessment. This test is reported as positive or negative as it relates to nonorganic LBP rather than as a number (Table 4).

10. Exaggeration/overreaction (Waddell nonorganic low back pain test 5)

This test[25] evaluates for abnormal psychosocial issues. It is not a specific test but rather inconsistent examination findings with overreaction noted at any time during the consultation or examination. Observation focuses on looking for disproportionate responses, such as tremor, crying out, and collapse. This test is reported as positive or negative as it relates to nonorganic LBP rather than as a number (Table 4).

11. ROM: Cervical

This test[57,78,80] evaluates the mobility of the cervical spine. An inclinometer is placed at the occiput and T-1. Sagittal plane movements (flexion/extension) are assessed by placing the inclinometer vertically perpendicular to the spine in the midline. Frontal plane motion (lateral flexion) is assessed by placing the base of the inclinometer horizontal so that the needle hangs freely. The end points of movement are recorded at both the occiput and T-1. The difference is then calculated using the equation: Occiput − T-1. If the average of three consecutive readings falls within 5° or 10% of the average, the highest of the three readings is recorded (Table 5). This procedure may be repeated a maximum of six times to try to achieve this result.[57]

Table 5. Cervical ranges of motion

Motion	Mean ± SD*	Normal range	Percent of normal
Flexion	53 ± 12.1	50°	105.6
Extension	71 ± 14.1	63°	112.6
Right lateral flexion	49 ± 7.2	45°	109.6
Left lateral flexion	50 ± 7.8	45°	112.0
Right rotation	88 ± 10.6	85°	103.3
Left rotation	90 ± 9.6	85°	105.5

*Sample includes 160 male railroad workers; average age = 35 years ± 7.5 years; height = 64.9 in ± 2.6 in; weight = 187 ± 28.6 lbs.
SD = standard deviation.
Sources: Mayer T, Tencer A, Kristoferson S, Mooney V. Use of noninvasive techniques for quantification of spinal range-of-motion in normal subjects and chronic low-back dysfunction patients. *Spine.* 1984;9:588–595. Mayer T, Gatchel RJ, Keeley J, Mayer H, Richling D. A male incumbent worker industrial database. *Spine.* 1994;19:762–764.

Supine tests

12. Modified Thomas test/hip extension test

Five steps are involved with this test.[47,81–83] The steps are as follows:

1. With the inclinometer placed 5 cm above the patella on the lateral thigh, the patient is first positioned supine with the knees straight on the bench to obtain an initial inclinometer reading, reset at zero.
2. The patient is next positioned at the end of the bench in a manner that the ischial tuberosities are supported by the end of the table's edge in a partially standing and sitting position.
3. The contralateral knee and hip are flexed to the chest to eliminate lumbar lordosis, and the patient is lowered to a supine position.
4. The testing hip is then passively flexed to a 90° angle, the inclinometer is reset to zero, and the leg is allowed to hang freely toward the floor fully relaxed.
5. The evaluator records the angle when the tested leg is fully relaxed, hip extended, and the lumbar lordosis is removed.

The normative data are 83.5° ± 1.1°, intra-assay CV is 0.7%, and inter-assay CV is 1.2%.[47]

13a. Supine vs sitting SLR/distraction (Waddell nonorganic low back pain test 3)

The reader is referred to the discussion under "8. Sitting vs Supine Straight Leg Raise/Distraction."

13b. SLR (hamstring flexibility) test

A SLR (hamstring flexibility)[46,47,61,79] test is performed with the doctor supporting the lower extremity (with crook of elbow) while holding the zeroed inclinometer mid-tibia or having it strapped to the lateral thigh (5 cm above patella), the doctor's indifferent hand stabilizes the pelvis. The leg is raised to a point of first of knee flexion (on the leg being tested) and/or the pelvis begins to rock or the opposite knee flexes. The evaluator records the hip flexion angle. Normative data range from 70° to 90°.[47]

14. Repetitive sit-up

In this test,[71–73] the patient is positioned supine with the knees flexed 90° with the ankles fixed. The patient is instructed to sit up until the thenar pad of the hand touches the patella; the patient then curls back down fully to the supine position. The number of repetitions are counted to a maximum of 50. The normative data are age, gender, and occupational specific, as depicted in Table 6.[73]

Prone tests

15. Knee flexion test/nachlas

In this test,[46,47,83,84] the doctor's position is to the side of the patient. The patient is placed in the prone position. The inclinometer is placed on the lower leg with the knee fully extended (the feet may hang over the edge to ensure full extension). With the pelvis strapped down, the knee is passively flexed (the heel is brought toward the buttocks). The angle is recorded at the moment hip flexion or hiking occurs. The normal angle equals 147.9° ± 1.6°, intra-assay CV is 0.5%, and inter-assay CV is 1.1%.[47]

16. Repetitive arch-up test

When performing the repetitive arch-up test,[71,73] the patient is placed prone with the anterior superior iliac spine (ASIS) just on the table, trunk extended off, arms at sides, and the ankles and thighs are fixed to the table by strapping.

Table 6. Repetitive sit-up test*

| | Males (n = 242) | | | | | | Females (n = 233) | | | | | |
| | Blue collar | | White collar | | All | | Blue collar | | White collar | | All | |
Age	x̄	SD	x̄	SD	x̄	SD	x̄	SD	x̄	SD	x̄	SD
35–39	29	13	35	13	32	13	24	12	30	16	27	14
40–44	22	11	34	12	27	13	18	12	19	13	19	12
45–49	19	11	33	15	24	14	17	14	22	15	19	14
50–54	17	13	36	16	23	16	9	10	20	13	11	11
35–54	23	13	35	13	27	14	17	13	24	15	19	14

x̄ = mean; SD = standard deviation.
*A maximum of 50 repetitions is allowed.
Source: Alaranta H, Hurri H, Heliovaara M, et al. Non-dynamometric trunk performance tests: reliability and normative data. *Scand J Rehab Med.* 1994;26:211–215.

The patient raises upward to the horizontal position and then down to a 45° angle. The number of repetitions is counted (maximum of 50). The normative data are age, gender, and occupational specific, as depicted in Table 7.[73]

17. Hip ROM (internal and external rotation)

To test hip ROM,[59,85] the patient is prone with the inclinometer fixed to the anterior distal third of lower leg, with the knee flexed 90°. A stabilizing strap is placed across the pelvis and internal rotation (IR) and external rotation (ER) of the hip are performed to a point of firm end feel or hip hiking. The evaluator records the angle at maximum IR and ER of the hip. The normative data established by Chesworth are 41° to 45° for internal rotation and 41° to 43° for external rotation.[85]

18. Static back endurance test

In this test,[49,71,73,82] the set-up is the same as in test 16, (ie, patient is prone with the ASISs just on the end of the table, arms at the sides, and ankles fixed). Rather than performing repetitions, the patient holds the horizontal position for as long as possible or for 240 seconds, whichever occurs first. The normative data are age, gender, and occupational specific, as depicted in Table 8.[73]

19. Grip strength dynamometry

In this test,[57,86] the patient may sit or stand. A Jamar hand dynamometer, usually in the second or third position (depending on size of hand), is used to take three readings; the three readings are averaged. The three tests, which are taken at different times during the examination, are considered reliable if there is less than 20% variation among them (this screening effort is a screen for full effort; the 20% variation "screen" can be used to evaluate for poor effort, barring pain-induced weakness is not the cause of weakness).[86] The evaluator compares normal to abnormal; no significant difference in dominant side strength is considered. If bilateral, normative data can be found in a variety of texts.[57,86]

20. Subjective outcome assessment instrumentation

Several self-administered, subjective OA instruments[4,17-24,27,40] are included in the QFCE for obvious reasons. First, they provide valuable information that has been found to be reliable regarding patient perception of condition-specific problems, general health issues and psychometrics (eg, depression). Second, they serve as valuable and sensitive ways to assess outcomes, which is a primary goal of the QFCE. Third, much has been published regarding their utility and practicality, and they complement the functional assessment the same way the history complements the physical examination. Because there are many condition-specific and general health questionnaires, it is important to stay with the same instrument used initially to collect the baseline information throughout the case management process. Information regarding these various instruments has been published elsewhere and will not be specifically discussed at this time.[4-40]

21. Post-VAS

The reader is referred to "1. Visual Analogue Scale."

Test completion

The average time for the authors to complete the QFCE is 35 minutes (excluding data analysis). No significant problems or exacerbations were experienced in performing the QFCE, and similar success with many of the same tests has been reported elsewhere.[73]

Table 7. Repetitive arch-up test*

	Males (n = 242)						Females (n = 233)					
	Blue collar		White collar		All		Blue collar		White collar		All	
Age	$\bar{x}$	SD	$\bar{x}$	SD	$\bar{x}$	SD	$\bar{x}$	SD	$\bar{x}$	SD	$\bar{x}$	SD
35–39	26	11	34	14	29	13	28	13	27	11	27	12
40–44	23	12	36	14	28	14	25	14	20	11	23	13
45–49	24	13	34	16	28	15	25	15	31	16	27	15
50–54	21	11	35	17	26	15	18	14	26	14	19	14
35–54	24	12	35	15	28	14	24	14	26	13	24	14

$\bar{x}$ = mean; SD = standard deviation.
*A maximum of 50 repetitions is allowed.
Source: Alaranta H, Hurri H, Heliovaara M, et al. Non-dynamometric trunk performance tests: reliability and normative data. *Scand J Rehab Med.* 1994;26:211–215.

Table 8. Static back endurance test*

	Males (n = 242)						Females (n = 233)					
	Blue collar		White collar		All		Blue collar		White collar		All	
Age	x̄	SD	x̄	SD	x̄	SD	x̄	SD	x̄	SD	x̄	SD
35–39	87	38	113	47	97	43	91	61	95	48	93	55
40–44	83	51	129	57	101	57	89	57	67	51	80	55
45–49	81	45	131	64	99	58	90	55	122	73	102	64
50–54	73	47	121	56	89	55	62	55	99	78	69	60
35–54	82	45	123	55	97	53	82	58	94	62	87	59

x̄ = mean; SD = standard deviation.
*The maximum amount of time allowed is 240 s.
Source: Alaranta H, Hurri H, Heliovaara M, et al. Non-dynamometric trunk performance tests: reliability and normative data. Scand J Rehab Med. 1994;26:211–215.

CONCLUSION

With the discrepancy between the inflation rate of health care (17%) and the general inflation rate (3% to 5%), the need to monitor the effectiveness of treatment becomes obvious.[3] With the objective of cost containment, there is a need for functional tests that are valid, reliable, practical, safe, and useful. The QFCE appears to fulfill these criteria as well as to facilitate the need for objective data that, when coupled with subjective OA instruments, can provide the practitioner with the necessary information to make informed and wise clinical decisions based on OA. The issue of practicality goes further as the various tests that comprise the QFCE are movements of normal daily living. As a result, the manner in which the injured person moves as well as the end point measurement result in both prescriptive and descriptive validity, respectively. The combination of low cost, movements used in activities of daily living, relatively short examination time (35 minutes), and practicality favors the use of low-tech functional capacity over high-tech instrumentation in these authors' opinion. Figs 2–4 offer examples of forms that may be used to organize data in the chart.

Because the QFCE and associated protocol require that care be taken to perform the tests exactly the same as described, a national database is being established for the purpose of determining the reliability and validity of this instrument. A call thus goes out to those who are using the QFCE to forward their results to the principal author. The protocol is available on computer disk, which will provide the summary reports, important for documentation reasons and a valuable asset for third-party payers, managed care companies as well as for easy submission of the results for the national database. Appreciation is extended in advance to those who decide to contribute.

REFERENCES

1. Relman A. Assessment and accountability: the third revolution in health care. *N Engl J Med.* 1988;319:1221–1222.
2. Donabedian A. The quality of medical care. In: Graham NO, ed. *Quality Assurance in Hospitals.* Gaithersburg, Md: Aspen Publishers; 1982.
3. Whitton M. Outcomes assessment: its relationship to chiropractic and managed health care. *J Am Chiro Assoc.* July 1994:37–40.
4. Goertz CMH. Measuring functional health status in the chiropractic office using self-report questionnaires. *Top Clin Chiro.* 1994;1:51–59.
5. Johnson D. *Dartmouth COOP Project.* Hanover, NH: Dartmouth Medical School; 1989.
6. Brazier J, Harper R, Jones SN. Validating the SF-36 health survey questionnaire: new outcome measure for primary care. *Br Med J.* 1992;305:160–164.
7. Bergner M, Bobbitt RA, Carter WB, Gilson BS. The sickness index profile: development and final revision of a health status measure. *Med Care.* 1981;9:787–809.
8. Deyo RA. Comparative validity of the sickness impact profile short scales for functional assessment in low back pain. *Spine.* 1986;11:951–954.
9. Chapman-Smith D. Measuring results—The new importance of patient questionnaires. *Chiro Report.* 1992;7:1–6.
10. Reading AE. A comparison of pain rating scales. *J Psychosom Res.* 1979;24:119–124.
11. Von Korff M, Deyo RA, Cherkin D, Barlow SF. Back pain in primary care: outcomes at 1 year. *Spine.* 1993;18:855–862.
12. Dworkin SF, Von Korff M, Whitney WC, et al. Measurement of characteristic pain intensity in field research. *Pain.* 1990;5(suppl):S290.
13. Von Korff M, Ormel J, Keefe F, Dworkin SF. Grading the severity of chronic pain. *Pain.* 1992;50:133–149.
14. Melzack P. *Pain Measurement and Assessment.* New York, NY: Raven Press; 1982.

15. Melzack R. The McGill pain questionnaire: major properties and scoring methods. *Pain.* 1975;1:277–279.
16. Melzack R. The short-form McGill pain questionnaire. *Pain.* 1987;30:191–197.
17. Fairbank J, Davies J, Couper J, O'Brien JP. The Oswestry low back pain disability questionnaire. *Physiotherapy.* 1980;66(18):271–273.
18. Hudson-Cook N, Tomes-Nicholson K. *The Revised Oswestry Low Back Pain Disability Questionnaire.* Anglo-European College of Chiropractic; 1988. Thesis. Bournemouth, England.
19. Roland M, Morris R. A study of the natural history of low back pain, part II. *Spine.* 1983;8(2):145–150.
20. Haas M, Jacobs GE, Raphail R, Petzing K. Low back pain outcome measurement assessment in chiropractic teaching clinics: responsiveness and applicability of two functional disability questionnaires. *J Manipulative Physiol Ther.* 1995;18:79–87.
21. Lawlis GF, Cuencas R, Selby D, McCoy CE. The development of the Dallas pain questionnaire for illness behavior. *Spine.* 1989;14:511–515.
22. Deyo RA, Cherkin DC, Franklin G, Nichols JC. Low back pain (forms 6.1 to 6.4). Bloomington, MN: Health Outcomes Institute; 1992.
23. Vernon H, Mior S. The neck disability index: a study of reliability and validity. *J Manipulative Physiol Ther.* 1991;14(7):409–415.
24. Jacobson GP, Ramadan NM, Aggarwal SK, Newman CW. The Henry Ford Hospital headache disability inventory (HDI). *Neurology.* 1994;44:837–842.
25. Waddell G, McCulloch JA, Kummel E, Venner RM. Nonorganic physical signs in low-back pain. *Spine.* 1980;5:117–125.
26. Korbon GA, DeGood E, Schroeder ME, et al. The development of a somatic amplification rating scale for low-back pain. *Spine.* 1987;12(8):787–791.
27. Zung WWK. A self-rating depression scale. *Arch Gen Psychiatry.* 1965;32:63–70.
28. Main CJ. 1983 modified somatic perception questionnaire. *J Psychosom Res.* 1983;27:503–514.
29. Bernstein IH, Jaremko ME, Hinkley BS. On the utility of the SCL-90-R with low-back pain patients. *Spine.* 1994;19:42–48.
30. Beck A. *Depression: Clinical, Experimental and Theoretical Aspects.* New York, NY: Harper & Row; 1967.
31. Main CJ, Wood PL, Hollis S, et al. The distress and risk assessment method: a simple patient classification to identify distress and evaluate the risk of poor outcome. *Spine.* 1992;7:42.
32. Waddell G, Newton M, Henderson I, et al. A fear-avoidance beliefs questionnaire (FABQ) and the role of fear-avoidance beliefs in chronic low back pain and disability. *Pain.* 1993;52:157–168.
33. Coulter ID, Hays RD, Danielson CD. The chiropractic satisfaction questionnaire. *Top Clin Chiro.* 1994;1:40–43.
34. Deyo RA, Diehl AK. Patient satisfaction with medical care for low back pain. *Spine.* 1986;11:28–30.
35. Cherkin D, MacCormack F. Patient evaluations of low-back pain are from family physicians and chiropractors. *West J Med.* 1989;150:351–355.
36. Ware J, Davies AR. Defining and measuring patient satisfaction with medical care. *Eval and Program Plan.* 1983;6:247–263.
37. Ware JE, Davies-Avery A, Stewart AL. The measuring and meaning of patient satisfaction. *Health Med Care Serv Rev.* 1978;1:1–15.
38. Bigos S, Battie M, Spenglere DM, et al. A prospective study of work perceptions and psychosocial factors affecting the report of back injury. *Spine.* 1991;16:1–6.
39. Cats-Baril WL, Frymoyer JW. Identifying patients at risk of becoming disabled because of low-back pain: the Vermont rehabilitation engineering center predictive model. *Spine.* 1991;16:605–607.
40. Millard RW. The functional assessment screening questionnaire: application for evaluating pain-related disability. *Arch Phys Med Rehabil.* 1989;70:303–307.
41. Mooney V. The place of active care in disability prevention. In: Liebenson CL, ed. *Rehabilitation of the Spine: A Practitioner's Manual.* Baltimore, Md: Williams & Wilkins; 1994.
42. Mooney V, Matheson LN. Objective measurement of soft tissue injury: feasibility study; Examiner's manual. Whittier, CA: Los Angeles College of Chiropractic; 1994, October, p.4.
43. Hart DL, Isernhagen SJ, Matheson LN. Guidelines for functional capacity evaluation of people with medical conditions. *J Orth Sport Phys Ther.* 1993;18:682–686.
44. Grabiner B, Liljeqvist M, Hansson T. Primary prevention of back symptoms and absence from work. *Spine.* 1993;18:587–594.
45. Newton M, Waddell G. Trunk strength testing with iso-machines, part 1: review of a decade of scientific evidence. *Spine.* 1993;18:801–811.
46. Wang S, Whitney SL, Burdett RG, et al. Lower extremity muscular flexibility in long distance runners. *J Orth Sport Phys Ther.* 1993;2:102–107.
47. Ekstrand J, Wiktorsson M, Oberg B, Gillquist J. Lower extremity goniometric measurements: a study to determine their reliability. *Arch Phys Med Rehab.* 1982;63:171–175.
48. Mayer T, Gatchel R, Kishino N, et al. Objective assessment of spine function following industrial injury: a prospective study with comparison group and one-year follow-up. *Spine.* 1985;10:482–493.
49. Biering-Sorenson F. Physical measurement as risk indicators for low back trouble over a one-year period. *Spine.* 1984;9:143–148.
50. Troup JDG, Martin JW, Lloyd DCEF. Back pain in industry: a prospective study. *Spine.* 1981;6:61–69.
51. Vernon H, Aker P, Aramenko M, et al. Evaluation of neck muscle strength with a modified sphygmomanometer dynamometer: reliability and validity. *J Manipulative Physiol Ther.* 1992;15:343–349.
52. Cassidy JD, Lopes AA, Yong-Hing K. The immediate effect of manipulation versus mobilization on pain and range of motion in the cervical spine: a randomized controlled trial. *J Manipulative Physiol Ther.* 1992;15:570–575.
53. Toppenberg RM, Bullock MI. The interrelation of spinal curves, pelvic tilt and muscle lengths in the adolescent female. *Aust J Physiother.* 1986;32:6–12.
54. Konz S. NIOSH lifting guidelines. *Am Ind Hyg Assoc J.* 1982;43:931–933.
55. Mayer T, Barnes D, Kishino N, et al. Progressive isoinertial lifting evaluation. I. A standardized protocol and normative database. *Spine.* 1988;13:993–997.
56. Matheson L. An introduction to lift capacity testing as a component of functional capacity evaluation. IRG. Whittier, CA: Los Angeles College of Chiropractic; Summer 1991.
57. American Medical Association. *Guides to the Evaluation of Permanent Impairment.* Chicago, Ill: AMA Press; 1993.
58. Nansel D, Jansen R, Cremata E, et al. Effects of cervical adjustments on lateral-flexion passive end-range asymmetry and on blood pressure, heart rate and plasma catecholamine levels. *J Manipulative Physiol Ther.* 1991;14:450–454.
59. Ellison JB, Rose SJ, Sahrmann SA. Patterns of hip rotation range of motion: a comparison between healthy subjects and patients with low back pain. *Phys Ther.* 1990; 70:537–541.

60. Reid DC, Burnham RS, Saboe LA, Kushner SF. Lower extremity flexibility patterns in classical ballet dancers and their correlation to lateral hip and knee injuries. *Am J Sports Med.* 1987;15:347–352.
61. Ekstrand J, Gillquist J. The frequency of muscle tightness and injuries in soccer players. *Am J Sports Med.* 1982;10:75–78.
62. Inamura K. Re-assessment of the method of analysis of electrogravitograph and the one foot test. *Aggressologie.* 1983;24:107–108.
63. Nelson RM. *NIOSH Low Back Atlas of Standardized Tests/Measures.* Washington, DC: US Department of Health and Human Services, National Institute for Occupational Safety and Health; 1988.
64. Hirasawa Y. Left foot to support human standing and walking. *Sci Am.* 1981;6:33–44.
65. Mayer T, Brady S, Bovasso E, et al. Noninvasive measurement of cervical tri-planar motion in normal subjects. *Spine.* 1994;18:2191–2195.
66. Youdas J, Carey J, Garret T. Reliability of measurements of cervical spine range of motion—comparison of three methods. *Phys Ther.* 1991;71:98–106.
67. Gajdosik RL, Rieck MA, Sullivan DK, et al. Comparison of four clinical tests for assessing hamstring muscle length. *J Orth Sport Phys Ther.* 1993;18:614–618.
68. Grice A. *Lumbar Exercises for Kinesiological Harmony and Stability:* Toronto, Ontario: Canadian Chiropractic Assoc; 1976.
69. Nelson RM, Nestor DE. Standardized assessment of industrial low-back injuries: development of the NIOSH low-back atlas. *Top Trauma Acute Care Rehabil.* 1988;2:16–30.
70. Moffroid MT. Distinguishable groups of musculoskeletal low back pain patients and asymptomatic control subjects based on physical measures of the NIOSH low back atlas. *Spine.* 1994;19:12;1350–1358.
71. Rissanen A, Alaranta H, Sainio P, Harkonen H. Isokinetic and non-dynamometric tests in low back pain patients related to pain and disability index. *Spine.* 1994;19:1963–1967.
72. Harding VR, Williams AC. The development of a battery of measures for assessing physical functioning of chronic pain patients. *Pain.* 1994;58:367–375.
73. Alaranta H, Hurri H, Heliovaara M, et al. Non-dynamometric trunk performance tests: reliability and normative data. *Scand J Rehab Med.* 1994;26:211–215.
74. Gatchel RJ, Mayer TG, Capra P, et al. Quantification of lumbar function, part 6: the use of psychological measures in guiding physical functional restoration. *Spine.* 1986;11:36–41.
75. Adams M, Dolan P, Marks C, Hutton C. An electroinclinometer technique for measuring lumbar curvature. *Clin Biomech.* 1986;1:130–134.
76. Fitzgerald G, Wynveen K, Rheault W, Rothschild B. Objective assessment with establishment of normal values for lumbar spinal range of motion. *Phys Ther.* 1983;63:1776–1781.
77. Keeley J, Mayer T, Cox R, et al. Quantification of lumbar function, 5: reliability of range-of-motion measures in the sagittal plane and in vivo torso rotation measurement techniques. *Spine.* 1986;11:31–35.
78. Loebl W. Measurements of spinal posture and range in spinal movements. *Ann Phys Med.* 1967;9:103–110.
79. Mayer T, Tencer A, Kristoferson S, Mooney V. Use of noninvasive techniques for quantification of spinal range-of-motion in normal subjects and chronic low-back dysfunction patients. *Spine.* 1984;9:588–595.
80. Mayer T, Gatchel RJ, Keeley J, Mayer H, Richling D. A male incumbent worker industrial database. *Spine.* 1994;19:762–764.
81. U.S. Department of Labor, Employment and Training Administration. *Dictionary of Occupational Titles.* 4th ed. Washington, DC: GPO; 1986.
82. Hyytiainen K, Salminen JJ, Suvitie T, et al. Reproducibility of nine tests to measure spinal mobility and trunk muscle strength. *Scand J Rehabil Med.* 1991;23:3–10.
83. Janda V. *Muskelfunktionsdiagnostik: muskeltest, untersuchung verkurzter muskeln, untersuchung der hypermobilitat.* Leuven, Belgium: Verlag; 1979.
84. Kendall HO, Kendall FP, Wadsworth GE. *Muscles, Testing and Function.* 2nd ed. Baltimore, Md: Williams & Wilkins; 1971.
85. Chesworth BM, Padfield BJ, Helewa A, Stitt LW. A comparison of hip mobility in patients with low back pain and matched healthy subjects. *Physio Can.* 1994;46:267–274.
86. Swanson AB, Matev IB, de Groot Swanson G. The strength of the hand. *Bull Prosthet Res.* Fall 1970:145–153.

Date	Pain			Function			
	VAS	Drawing	McGill	Health status	Neck disability	LB disability	Satisfaction
Baseline							
	___/10 now ___/10 avg. ___/10 worst	Physiologic 1. Yes 2. No		1. PF__ 6. SF__ 2. RP__ 7. RE__ 3. BP__ 8. MH__ 4. GH__ DEPRS 5. VT__ 1, 2, 3	_____%	Name: _____% _____%	
Progress							
	___/10 now ___/10 avg. ___/10 worst	Physiologic 1. Yes 2. No			_____%	Name: _____ _____%	
	___/10 now ___/10 avg. ___/10 worst	Physiologic 1. Yes 2. No			_____%	Name: _____ _____%	
	___/10 now ___/10 avg. ___/10 worst	Physiologic 1. Yes 2. No			_____%	Name: _____ _____%	
	___/10 now ___/10 avg. ___/10 worst	Physiologic 1. Yes 2. No			_____%	Name: _____ _____%	
	___/10 now ___/10 avg. ___/10 worst	Physiologic 1. Yes 2. No			_____%	Name: _____ _____%	
	___/10 now ___/10 avg. ___/10 worst	Physiologic 1. Yes 2. No			_____%	Name: _____ _____%	
	___/10 now ___/10 avg. ___/10 worst	Physiologic 1. Yes 2. No			_____%	Name: _____ _____%	
	___/10 now ___/10 avg. ___/10 worst	Physiologic 1. Yes 2. No			_____%	Name: _____ _____%	
	___/10 now ___/10 avg. ___/10 worst	Physiologic 1. Yes 2. No			_____%	Name: _____ _____%	
	___/10 now ___/10 avg. ___/10 worst	Physiologic 1. Yes 2. No			_____%	Name: _____ _____%	
Discharge							
	___/10 now ___/10 avg. ___/10 worst	Physiologic 1. Yes 2. No		1. PF__ 6. SF__ 2. RP__ 7. RE__ 3. BP__ 8. MH__ 4. GH__ DEPRS 5. VT__ 1, 2, 3	_____%	Name _____ _____%	_____%

VAS = visual analogue scale; LB = low back; avg = average; PF = physical function; RP = role physical; BP = bodily pain; GH = general health; DEPRS = depression; VT = vitality; SF = social function; RE = role emotions; MH = mental health.

Fig 2. Outcomes Assessment Record

NAME: _____ Occupation: ___WC/BC___ DATE: _____ BD: _____ AGE: _____
Dx: _____ Test #: ___1, 2, 3, 4___ Symptom Duration: _____ Prior Episodes: __YES/NO__

Test name	Normal	Patient result		Percent of normal	
1. VAS	0/10	____/10		____%	
2. Repetitive squat*	____/(max 50)	____/(45)		____%	
3. ROM/lumbar spine					
Flexion	65°	____°		____%	
Extension	30°	____°		____%	
Rt lateral flexion	25°	____°		____%	
Lt lateral flexion	25°	____°		____%	
4. Waddell #1: Pain	Negative	Positive/Negative		NA	
5. Waddell #2: Simulation	Negative	Positive/Negative		NA	
6. Gastrocnemius/ankle DF	23°	Lt: ____	Rt: ____	____%	____%
7. Soleus/ankle DF	25°	Lt: ____	Rt: ____	____%	____%
8. Sitting SLR/distraction w/test 13†	LBP: YES/NO	LBP: YES/NO		NA	
9. Waddell #4: Regional neuro	Negative	Positive/Negative		NA	
10. Waddell #5: Exaggeration	Negative	Positive/Negative		NA	
11. ROM/cervical					
Flexion	50°	____°		____%	
Extension	63°	____°		____%	
Rt lateral flexion	45°	____°		____%	
Lt lateral flexion	45°	____°		____%	
Rt rotation	85°	____°		____%	
Lt rotation	85°	____°		____%	
12. Modified Thomas					
Iliopsas	84°	Lt: ____	Rt: ____	____%	____%
13a. Waddell #3: Distraction†	Negative	Positive/Negative		NA	
13b. Straight leg raise*	70–90°	Lt: ____	Rt: ____	____%	____%
14. Repetitive sit-up*	____/(max 50)	____/(max ____)		____%	
15. Knee flexion	147° ± 1.6	Lt: ____	Rt: ____	____%	____%
16. Repetitive arch-up*	____/(max 50)	____/(max 50)		____%	
17. Hip rotation ROM					
Internal rotation ROM	41–45 (43)	Lt: ____	Rt: ____	____%	____%
External rotation ROM	41–43 (42)	Lt: ____	Rt: ____	____%	____%
18. Static back endurance*	____(max 240 s)	____ s		____%	
19. Grip strength*	Lt: ____kg Rt ____kg	Lt: ____kg	Rt: ____kg	____%	____%
20. Outcome instrument(s)					
• Oswestry LB disability questionnaire	0/50 (0%)	____%		____%	
• Neck disability index	0/50 (0%)	____%		____%	
• General health					
– SF-36, HSQ, RAND-36 (circle)	100 points (each, 8 sections)				
– Dartmouth COOP charts	9 sections (see sep. doc.)				
– Other: ____					
21. Posttest VAS	0/10	____/10		____%	

WC = white collar; BC = blue collar; BD = birth date; Dx = diagnosis; VAS = visual analogue scale; ROM = range of motion; max = maximum; Rt = right; Lt = left; DF = dorsiflexion; w/ = with; SLR = straight leg raise; LBP = low back pain; NA = not applicable; HSQ = Health Status Questionnaire 2.0.
*Normative data are determined by age, sex, and occupation.
†A positive test #13a (supine SLR) and a negative sitting/distracted SLR (test #8) = positive Waddell sign for distraction.

SIGNED _____ DATE _____

Fig 3. Quantitative Functional Capacity Results Form

NAME _____ DATE _____ DOB _____ DOI _____ TIME IN _____
Dx: _____ Prior Episodes: __YES/NO__

TEST Standing	INITIAL Date:	1ST REEXAM Date:	2ND REEXAM Date:	3RD REEXAM Date:
1. Pretest VAS	____/10	____/10	____/10	____/10
2. Repetitive squat (feet 15 cm apart) Thigh horizontal, 1 repetitive/2–3 s, note # of repetitions; max is 50	____ # of repetitions	____ # of repetitions	____ # of repetitions	____ # of repetitions
3. ROM: PAIN SCALE: LUMBAR EXTREMITY (Lt/Rt)	−1 = Decr/centralize 0 = No change +1 = Incr/peripheralize			
FLEXION (forward flexion)	FL _____ +1,0,−1	FL _____ +1,0,−1	FL _____ +1,0,−1	FL _____ +1,0,−1
EXTENSION (backward ext)	EXT _____ +1,0,−1	EXT _____ +1,0,−1	EXT _____ +1,0,−1	EXT _____ +1,0,−1
RLF (abduction)	RLF _____ +1,0,−1	RLF _____ +1,0,−1	RLF _____ +1,0,−1	RLF _____ +1,0,−1
LLF (adduction)	LLF _____ +1,0,−1	LLF _____ +1,0,−1	LLF _____ +1,0,−1	LLF _____ +1,0,−1
4. PAIN (superficial): Waddell #1	+/−	+/−	+/−	+/−
5. SIMULATION: Waddell #2				
a. Trunk rotation	+/−	+/−	+/−	+/−
b. Axial compression (5 kg)	+/−	+/−	+/−	+/−

TESTS	LT	RT	LT	RT	LT	RT	LT	RT
5. Gastrocnemius/ankle DF (knee extended)	____°	____°	____°	____°	____°	____°	____°	____°
7. Soleus/ankle DF (knee flexed)	____°	____°	____°	____°	____°	____°	____°	____°
Seated	LT	RT	LT	RT	LT	RT	LT	RT
8. Sitting SLR/DISTRACTION (Waddell #3; see test 13a) ↑ LBP: (circle)	↑ LBP: yes/no	↑ LBP: yes/no	↑ LBP: yes/no	↑ LBP: yes/no	↑ LBP: yes/no	↑ LBP: yes/no	↑ LBP: yes/no	↑ LBP: yes/no
9. Regional neuro (Waddell #4)	+/−	+/−	+/−	+/−	+/−	+/−	+/−	+/−
10. Exaggeration (Waddell #5)	+/−		+/−		+/−		+/−	
11. ROM: PAIN SCALE: CERVICAL EXTREMITY (Lt/Rt)	−1 = Decr/centralize 0 = No change +1 = Incr/peripheralize							
FLEXION (forward flexion)	FL _____ +1,0,−1		FL _____ +1,0,−1		FL _____ +1,0,−1		FL _____ +1,0,−1	
EXTENSION (backward ext)	EXT _____ +1,0,−1		EXT _____ +1,0,−1		EXT _____ +1,0,−1		EXT _____ +1,0,−1	
RLF (abduction)	RLF _____ +1,0,−1		RLF _____ +1,0,−1		RLF _____ +1,0,−1		RLF _____ +1,0,−1	
LLF (adduction)	LLF _____ +1,0,−1		LLF _____ +1,0,−1		LLF _____ +1,0,−1		LLF _____ +1,0,−1	
RT ROTATION (exterior rotation)	RR _____ +1,0,−1		RR _____ +1,0,−1		RR _____ +1,0,−1		RR _____ +1,0,−1	
LT ROTATION (interior rotation)	LR _____ +1,0,−1		LR _____ +1,0,−1		LR _____ +1,0,−1		LR _____ +1,0,−1	

PAIN SCALE

NUMERICAL SCALE	DEFINITION
+1	Increase or peripheralization of pain
0	No pain
−1	Decrease or centralization of pain

COMMENTS _____
_____ GO ON TO PAGE 2 ⇒ ⇒ ⇒

continues

NAME _____ DATE _____ DOI _____

Supine	LT	RT	LT	RT	LT	RT	LT	RT
12. Hip extension test/modified Thomas • Measure: Passive hip extension (psoas tension)	a.____°	a.____°	a.____°	a.____°	a.____°	a.____°	a.____°	a.____°
13. Hip flexion/supine SLR a. (Waddell #3: supine + vs sit − SLR) b. Measure angle at point of knee flexion	a. +/− b.____°	a. +/− b.____°	a. +/− b.____°	a. +/− b.____°	a. +/− b.____°	a. +/− b.____°	a. +/− b.____°	a. +/− b.____°
14. Repetitive sit-up test • Sit-up, knees 90°, feet anchored, 1 repetition/2–3 s, touch thenar to patella, curl back down; max of 50 repetitions	Endurance repetitions ____/50		Endurance repetitions ____/50		Endurance repetitions ____/50		Endurance repetitions ____/50	
Prone	LT	RT	LT	RT	LT	RT	LT	RT
15. Knee flexion test/modified Nachlas test	____°	____°	____°	____°	____°	____°	____°	____°
16. Repetitive arch-up test • Repetitive arch-up: Waist at table's edge, fixed at ankle, flexed 45° raises up to horizontal; 1 repetition/ 2–3 s; max of 50 repetitions	Repetitions ____/50		Repetitions ____/50		Repetitions ____/50		Repetitions ____/50	
17. Hip ROM • Internal rotation • External rotation	IR ____° ER ____°	IR ____° ER ____°	IR ____° ER ____°	IR ____° ER ____°	IR ____° ER ____°	IR ____° ER ____°	IR ____° ER ____°	IR ____° ER ____°
18. Static back endurance • Static back endurance: Patient holds trunk horizontal up to max of 240 s	Static Time ____/240 s		Static Time ____/240 s		Static Time ____/240 s		Static Time ____/240 s	
TESTS	LT	RT	LT	RT	LT	RT	LT	RT
19. Grip dynamometry Dominant: Left/Right (circle) • Use Jamar • Use position 1 or 2 • Three trials (average)	1. ____ 2. ____ 3. ____ avg ____	1. ____ 2. ____ 3. ____ avg ____	1. ____ 2. ____ 3. ____ avg ____	1. ____ 2. ____ 3. ____ avg ____	1. ____ 2. ____ 3. ____ avg ____	1. ____ 2. ____ 3. ____ avg ____	1. ____ 2. ____ 3. ____ avg ____	1. ____ 2. ____ 3. ____ avg ____
20. Outcomes instruments: a. Oswestry LB disability questionnaire b. Neck disability index c. General health SF-36, HSQ, RAND-36 COOP Other:_____	a. ____% b. ____% SF-36 ___, ___, ___, ___, ___, ___, ___ COOP ___, ___, ___, ___, ___, ___, ___ Other_____		a. ____% b. ____% SF-36 ___, ___, ___, ___, ___, ___, ___ COOP ___, ___, ___, ___, ___, ___, ___ Other_____		a. ____% b. ____% SF-36 ___, ___, ___, ___, ___, ___, ___ COOP ___, ___, ___, ___, ___, ___, ___ Other_____		a. ____% b. ____% SF-36 ___, ___, ___, ___, ___, ___, ___ COOP ___, ___, ___, ___, ___, ___, ___ Other_____	
21. Posttest VAS	____/10		____/10		____/10		____/10	

SIGNED _____ DATE _____ TIME OUT _____
SIGNED _____ DATE _____ TIME OUT _____
SIGNED _____ DATE _____ TIME OUT _____
SIGNED _____ DATE _____ TIME OUT _____

DOB = date of birth; DOI = date of injury; Dx = diagnosis; VAS = visual analogue scale; max = maximum; ROM = range of motion; LT = left; RT = right; FL = flexion; EXT = extension; RLF = right lateral flexion; LLF = left lateral flexion; RR = right rotation; LR = left rotation; DF = dorsiflexion; SLR = straight leg raise; LBP = low back pain; Decr = decrease; Incr = increase; IR = internal rotation; ER = external rotation; avg = average; HSQ = Health Status Questionnaire 2.0; COOP = Dartmouth COOP Health charts.

Fig 4. Quantitative Functional Capacity Evaluation Tests

Algorithm 1

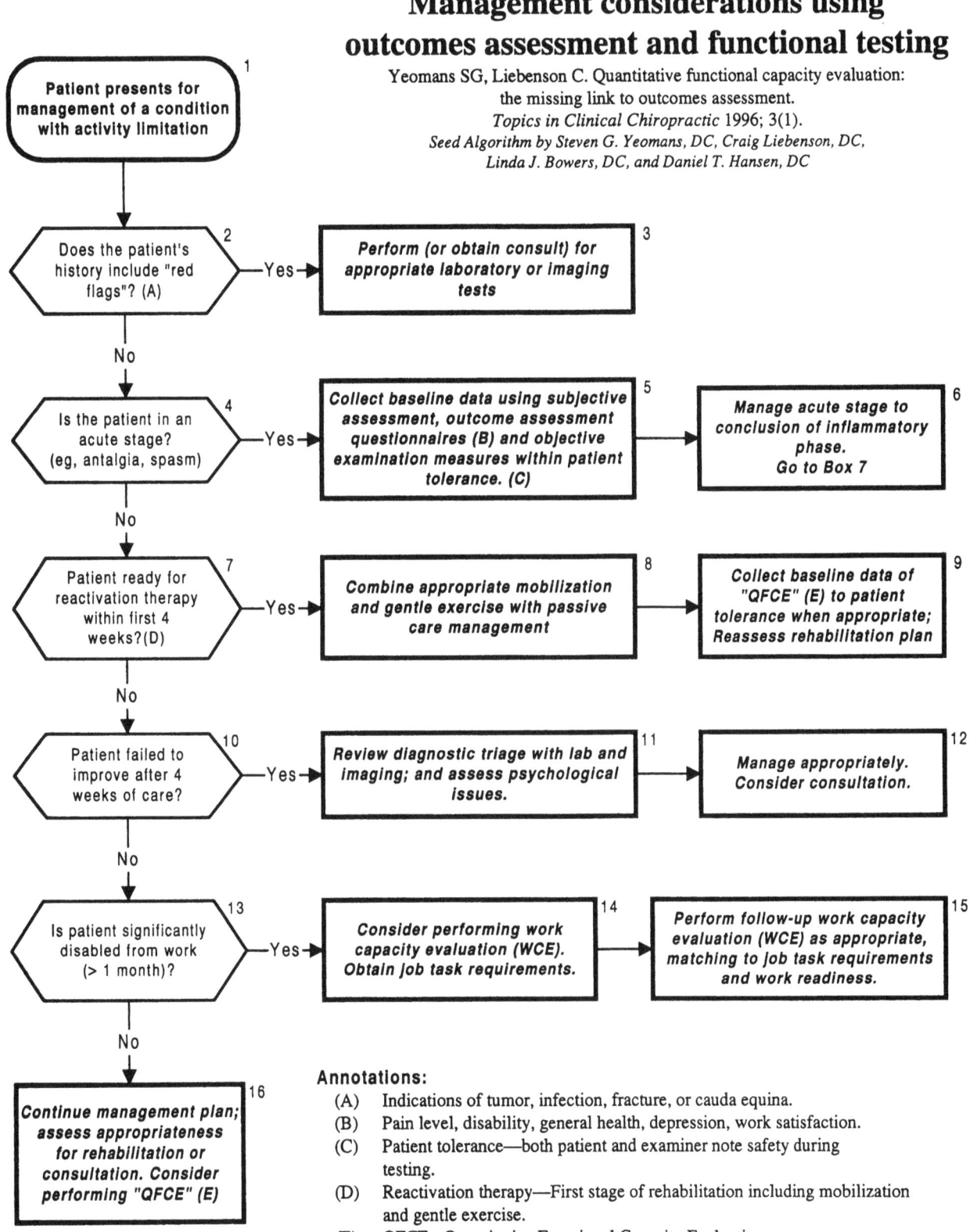

17

Opening Access to Spine Care in the Evolving Market: Integration and Communication

John J. Triano, Ralph F. Rashbaum, and Daniel T. Hansen

The past decade has seen a proliferation in public awareness of chiropractic spine care. Political pressure from professional guilds has found a synergy with the winds of social change. The timing of the current social introspection on its health care system has been coincident with the accumulation of good scientific evidence on a value of chiropractic treatment (eg, spinal high velocity, low amplitude manipulation/adjustment). The credibility of the evidence, driven in part by the nature of it being from legitimate interdisciplinary sources, supplied the critical mass necessary to transform political activism into a seed of moral and cultural authority.

There is a wave of interdisciplinary fervor progressing across the United States. We see it in the formal attention paid to the profession by federal agencies such as the Agency for Health Care Policy and Research (AHCPR) and Health Resources and Services Administration (HRSA), and scores of new complementary medicine programs within medical training. Medical facilities of all sizes are beginning to consider or are granting invitation to some of our colleagues to enter into strategic business and clinical partnerships. Does the recognition for value of our primary mode of treatment translate into an acceptance of chiropractors as the experts? The answer is "not necessarily." Response of the medical, health policy, payer, and political communities can be divided into three arms: denial, partnership, and usurpation.

Denial is reflected by the continued barriers to access created by payers and primary care providers. Too often, we still hear and feel the frustration of our patients who are told, "We don't refer to chiropractors." Medical demigods of "scientific health care" continue to use untested or ineffective methods to treat spine-related disorders rather than be swayed by the evidence. Behavior like this reflects the sovereignty of medicine past and ignores its demise.[1] Health care and health policies no longer are driven primarily by the medical industrial complex where available technology drives utilization. Technology-driven markets and technology-oriented professionals treat customer interests as secondary. Society has reduced the cultural authority of political medicine, as it has not sustained its promise for both competence and legitimacy. Health reform has failed to lower actual costs[2] and has given only lip service to increasing quality of services. Driven by customer and patient-focused ethics and unsatisfied by today's market reform, the turbulence affecting daily practice is likely not to end in the near future.

Physicians who have recognized their shifting base of support have responded in one of the remaining ways. An increasing number of legitimate health care partnerships have and are forming. These are not vacuous relationships founded purely on gimmicks to increase fees or decrease accounts receivable. They represent collegial, professional, and business relations that share individual and comanagement responsibility and rewards. These are solid and evolving relationships that use step-by-step development and validation, including use of consensus building, protocols, and quality improvement techniques. Their objective is the development of a "focused factory" or working, multidisciplinary networks providing high quality care attracting larger market share.

Finally, there is active effort to usurp manipulation as a procedure within medicine. As recently as 1994, Shekelle and associates[3] showed that 94% of all billings for manipulation were performed by chiropractors. In that same year, the AHCPR produced a monograph designed to inform family practice and internal medicine providers of the proper meth-

Adapted from *Top Clin Chiro* 1998; 5(4): 44–52
© 1998 Aspen Publishers, Inc.

ods to examine and prescribe treatment for acute, adult low back pain. Its development was motivated by the need to upgrade the ability of these providers to deal with these types of cases. In the 4 short years that have followed, the guilds for both the family practice and physical medicine and rehabilitation (PM&R) subspecialties have organized efforts to train interested members in manipulation procedures. At the 1996 PM&R conference in Chicago, the curriculum included two sessions on manipulation technique: "Foolproof Methods of Manipulation for the Novice" and "Advanced Manipulation Techniques."

The shift to a patient-centered market is not going to stop.[1] New power brokers are emerging. If we are to meet our professional potential, we must participate in the evolving power base. To achieve that, we must understand the evolving market, the basis for cultural authority and offer responsible leadership participation. We must convince the purchasers of health care as to our existing expertise and the costs of relying on unskilled and novice manipulators. We must deserve and obtain their trust. Achieving that trust offers a number of rewards as we reach our professional potential. They include an opening of the doors to patient access, increased case mix, and the privilege of appropriately serving patients who previously had been withheld from our services.

OPPORTUNITIES

There is no question that all health care providers feel the effects of the turmoil in health care today. Articles and letters in the *Dynamic Chiropractic* and its medical counterpart the *AMA News* reflect the decline of the halcyon days of fee-for-service. Except where managed care has had limited penetration, doctors from all disciplines have seen their practices decline substantially. Many have responded by diversifying into investments, nutritional pyramid marketing, and similar schemes to preserve their incomes. Some have elected to stubbornly ignore the forces of change and strike onward. Others have looked for the opportunity that historically accompanies each period of challenge. Seizing that opportunity always requires modifying how we do business. It is not, however, necessary to abandon the very elements of our practices, chiropractic or medical, which deliver clinical value.

Spine care is made even more complex by virtue of the fact that it defies the medical model of disease, and thus the comprehension of the health care system. Yet, there are elements of spine care where evidence for effective treatment exists.[4] More importantly, it is a compelling problem both in terms of suffering and costs to society. The province of spine care and who will be the leaders in it remains to be determined. It is unlikely that any one group will have the competence and legitimacy necessary to claim cultural authority over all of spine care. However, breaking down the barriers between the various providers that deal with spine care and getting them to work together brings the most resources to bear on solving the problem. The group that successfully minimizes redundancy of effort or cost while attempting to optimize outcomes of care will open access to their services.

There are several payoffs. First is the nirvana for doctors; increased access to their services, varied and complex case mix, and larger market share. Secondary benefits arise from the advantages of economies of scale that decrease the administrative costs of modern practice: credentialing, precertification, appeal process, billing fee adjustments by payer contract, and collections. This article is intended for the spectrum of health professionals who are seeking to fulfill the need for coordinated services in spine care. The article may also help health care administrators faced with increasing public dissatisfaction with the limited progress in health reform. Finally, it may help focus objectives for continuing education that may foster practical solutions and facilitate the continuity of care that our patients deserve.

TRENDS IN HEALTH INDUSTRY

Over the past 10 to 15 years, there has been a shift in how patients obtain care from a specialist. Where once barriers to see a specialist for spine-related problems were confined mostly to rigid staff model health maintenance organizations (HMOs), many other iterations of managed care adopted the same or similar barriers for patient access to specialists. The primary feature was the requirement for even the most evident complaints to be triaged through a gatekeeper. The burden was centered on one professional discipline, generally the family or general practitioner, to understand the indications and expectations for care from all other disciplines. The broader managed care phenomenon has adopted similar barriers to patient access of specialty services based on early promise of economic savings. The power of the economic argument spread to permit the patient with a spine-related complaint to be seen by nonphysician generalists (eg, physician assistants [PAs], nurse practitioners). Thus, by design, a patient with back pain was often required to see their primary care provider first. This first visit could either be with an actual generalist physician or even a physician extender (eg, PA, nurse practitioner).

The commensurate training of the generalist was attempted through devices like the development of the AHCPR guidelines for management of acute adult low back pain. Appropriately, the patients are not entirely satisfied with this arrangement.[5] Between the use of economic incentives to minimize specialist referrals and the attempt of some primary care providers (PCPs) to manage cases beyond their expertise, there is little evidence for either improved quality or savings in health care delivery to the spine. After delays and failed care, many patients eventually ended up in the care of specialists anyway, but now with the added problem of chronicity of their symptoms, or they sought care from alternative health care providers.[6]

These observations and subsequent studies showing continued preference and increased satisfaction with specialist care, have curtailed the insistence on PCP triage. Health care plans now design competitive products that allow patients better access to specialists and complementary providers, such as in preferred provider organizations (PPOs) and point-of-service arrangements.[7]

The administrative turmoil has fostered scientific paradox. We have entered a phase of nihilism that has affected the determination of appropriate care for patients with back pain. A 7-year series of studies looked at the epidemiology, diagnosis, and treatment of back pain through projects championed by Deyo and others.[8] Their scientific conclusions have been extrapolated to imply that the treatment of spine pain may be hopeless. Those proponents hold that back pain is so endemic as to be "normal." Similarly, because most episodes are essentially self-limiting, the diagnosis is trivialized to that of being disc or nondisc in origin. Concern for reducing patient suffering has been subordinated to living with the natural history. Thus minimized as a problem for which little can be done, we see now a new turf war heralded by the battle cry for primary care providers to "reclaim back pain" as a rightful component of their domain.[9] Somehow, the irony of the 4 short years between the development of the AHCPR guidelines targeted on PCP ineptitude in spine care management, and today's medical chauvinism has yet to strike home. Interestingly, over the past 15 years, the use rate for chiropractic services appears to have doubled, with the great majority of the chiropractic patients receiving care for musculoskeletal conditions.[10]

It can be argued that primary care providers could certainly serve a function in the management of back and neck pain, if indeed they are comfortable doing so. Cherkin has studied this issue for almost 10 years.[5,11] Patients sense this and have historically reported greater satisfaction when they felt that their physician was confident with their back problem. The work of T.S. Carey and others (personal communication, February 1996) expanded on this phenomenon by exposing general practitioners to the rudiments of spinal manipulation. The result was a greater comfort in physician attitude toward treating back pain patients. With their greater understanding, they also demonstrated an increased tendency to refer to chiropractors for spinal manipulation.

THE RESOURCES OF THE MODERN HEALTH INDUSTRY

The medical industrial complex has taken on new leadership partners. The old system was technology driven in which the availability of technical know-how drove provider utilization patterns. Under the evolving health care system, employer and payer purchasers have taken on a new profile that not only influences utilization patterns but also the development or suppression of new knowledge, often based on economic criteria.

The health industry itself includes first professional-licensed providers (MD, DO, DC); allied providers (eg, RNs, PAs); ancillary therapists (eg, physical therapists [PTs], occupational therapists [OTs]); clinical support staff (medical assistants, including chiropractic assistants, therapy assistants, and technologists); and administrative support staff. Obviously there are subcategories traditionally based on specialty and subspecialty training. Their service is also subdivided into primary, secondary, and tertiary settings depending on the clinical focus and disorder progression. Sites oriented to secondary and tertiary care include hospitals, urgent care centers, and specialty diagnostic centers and clinics. The new entries affecting day-to-day case management include all of the elements of health care financing including insurance, case management, health administration, and regulation.

The concept of who is the principal customer has also changed. The chiropractic and Hippocratic oaths are now straining to accommodate often-conflicting priorities of patients, employers in business and industry, and government programs. The doctor, facing a patient encounter many times each day, must balance the opposing demands by determining the "issues that matter"—the outcomes of care (Table 1).

The opportunity of today's practice arises from fulfilling the needs and expectations of the customer base. On an individual basis, it means developing a strategic business plan that matches solutions to customer demands without losing site of the important outcomes. Triano and Hansen[12] have shown that the extent to which a doctor or health care system can demonstrate achievement of these outcomes, they will be rewarded by increased market share. In that study, the providers enjoyed twice as many referrals.

Cost-effectiveness is a reality that cannot be ignored. It requires a clearly defined goal of treatment agreed upon by patient, provider, and payer, and a means of achieving it as rapidly as possible. These are the elements of value. Unfortunately, until recently most of the emphasis has been driven

---

Table 1. Outcomes: the issues that count in modern spine care

- ***Diagnostic***—proper pain generator identification, complicating factors
- ***Treatment***—clinical progress and response to care
- ***Economic***—[value = quality/cost]; early return to preinjury status
- ***Social***—patient satisfaction with care

by economists, entrepreneurs, or health system predators with costs being the focus. As the patient base has felt the effects and begun to voice dissatisfaction, the time is ripe for cross-trained health care providers to merge clinical wisdom with skills in business, economics, market trends, finance, and public health issues. For spine problems, the "focused factory"[13] of integrating multidisciplinary teams offers a natural opportunity to best address both the needs of the customers and the access to the providers.[14]

COMMUNITY PERSPECTIVES

The heightened awareness in the health care community that the patient or customer has expectations and preferences that impact physician choice, clinical efficiency, sensitivity for cost of care, and patient quality of life causes a focus of involvement at the community level. How is it we know about these expectations in the community with the respective customers? A Texas Back Institute team of investigators developed a community-based survey process, utilizing survey instruments, focus groups, and consensus exercises to ascertain trends and relationships of expectations of the health care episode.[15] The community-based customers included patients, physicians (primary care physicians, orthopaedic surgeons, chiropractors, and physiatrists), payers (insurance, HMOs, and PPOs), and employers (local and national corporations). The purpose of this exercise was to determine what the customer expectations or needs are during an episode of back pain. The episode of back pain was described for four distinct phases ranging from the preepisode asymptomatic state, through the interval of symptom development and first consultation with a provider, to the interval of treatment encounters and end point of care, and even issues beyond the end point of care. Vignette-based survey instruments and focus groups were performed for each of the four customer groups reflecting changing expectations during the four phases of the episode of care. The four clinical vignettes were carefully designed to represent the four stages of spinal health. Specific questions that served as focal points of discussion were separately validated. Key words or phrases were identified and collapsed in the subsequent group exercises. Where there was agreement, the key words or phrases were distinguished as patient focus vs system focus depending on the perceived benefit or actual involvement of the patient. The relative proportion of patient-focus responses to system-focus responses were then charted for each constituency group. As can be seen in Fig 1, a greater homogeneity of focus was observed among patients, employers, and primary

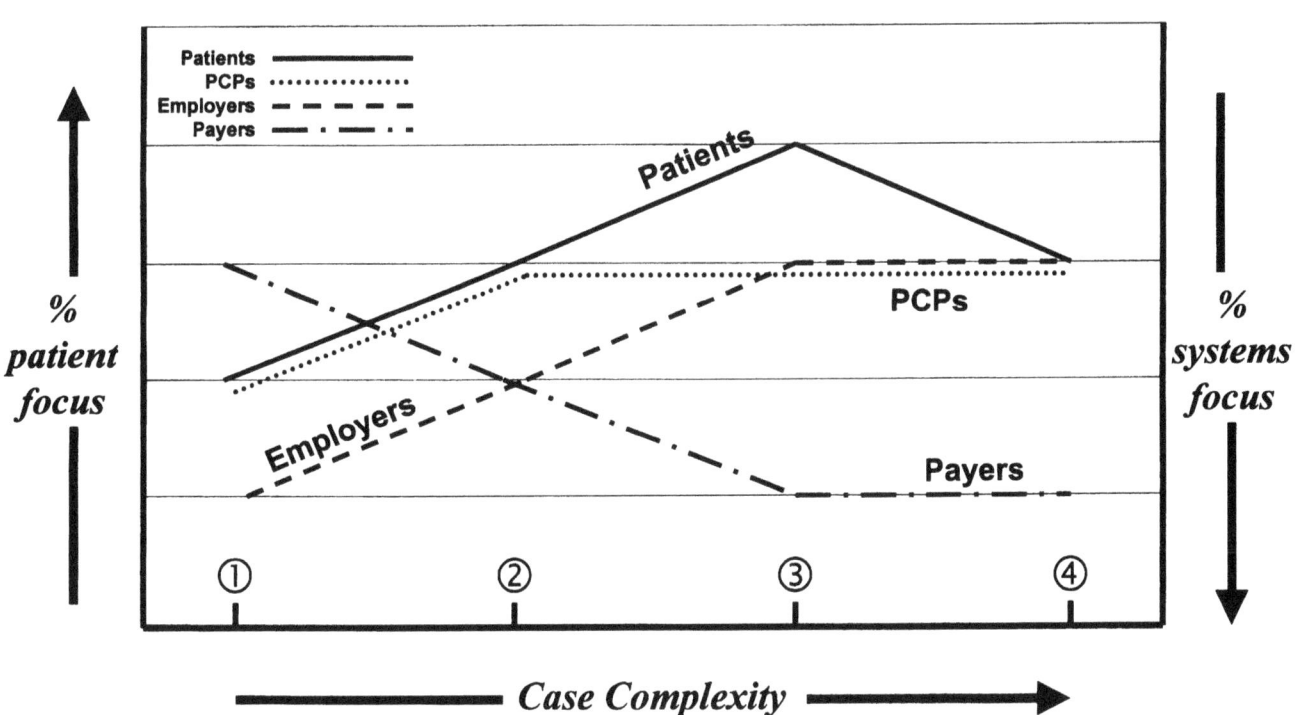

Fig 1. Customer expectations: Survey and focus groups. PCP, primary care providers. (1) Preepisode/asymptomatic state. (2) Interval of symptom development to consultation with provider. (3) Interval of treatment encounters ranging to the endpoint of care. (4) Later interval beyond the endpoint of care.

care providers. This relationship was not expected; but, it does reflect a set of expectations arising from the community for the Texas Back Institute to respond.

And interestingly, there were a number of expectations and attitudes where there was strong agreement, and conversely strong disagreement (Table 2). Those where there was strong agreement across the four groups had emphasis on education and cooperative efforts involving payers and business. Additionally, for those cases where the management and treatment was protracted or complicated, the use of patient liaisons or case managers was an area of identified need. The constituent groups could not agree, however, on use of provider resources. There was strong sentiment by patients that they would prefer specialists over primary care providers for the back problems, and expressed stronger disagreement about being seen by a physician extender (PA or nurse practitioner).

This exercise provided the Texas Back Institute with valuable input from the community that has since facilitated its strategies to integrate its delivery services to the various markets served in the state of Texas.

FOCUSED SPINE CARE MARKETS

The concept of focused-factories in health care is relatively new.[14] They were an evolution from the scramble associated with attempts to price health care under capitation as "carve outs" for certain procedures or specific diseases.[16] Diabetes and end-stage renal diseases are examples where this approach has resulted in reasonable value in care for these patients. Focused factories and provider networks for specific disorders offer a comprehensive set of health services that take advantage of economies of scale and depth in expertise for treating a narrow range of problems. The focused factory is a single site "one-stop shop" where all services likely to be needed are available. The provider network consists of a multidisciplinary group that works closely together with common consensus on appropriate care. In so doing, they can meet both the clinical needs of the patient with increased efficiencies. For instance, by nature of having a common medical record, redundancy of diagnostic procedures can be avoided. It is not uncommon for diagnostic imaging obtained by one provider or at an emergency department to be unavailable to the doctor who ultimately becomes the manager of the case. With the common medical record, those results are immediately available and management decisions can address need for advanced imaging or a modification in the treatment plan without delay or added cost.

Injury care represents a significant portion of neuromusculoskeletal (NMS) practice. Disorders range from the uncomplicated strain or sprain to the more complicated fractures, total joint failure, or central or peripheral nerve syndromes. The services offered by NMS providers often overlap with each group (DC, orthopedist, PM&R, PT, OT) having a primary area of expertise. They use similar evaluations and the same array of diagnostic technologies for differential diagnosis. With these facts, there is logic in bringing all of these resources together into one complementary group with a common mission—the prevention and treatment of neuromusculoskeletal disorders. Value of services in spine care develops as four nonpartisan principles are realistically applied to patient care.

1. Initial assessment, regardless of provider type, identifies the need for urgent or emergent care (progressive neurologic deficit, fracture, infection, cancer, or systemic disease).
2. If need for urgent or emergent care is absent, focus the treatment plan on evidence that there is an optimum approach that should be followed initially.
3. If evidence for a preferred treatment method is absent, identify any contraindication to the approach primarily used by the provider performing the assessment. If none, initiate a trial of therapy.
4. Review results of the initial therapy plan within a short interval (2 weeks). If progressing to resolution, proceed. If not responding as expected, modify the treatment plan or refer to an alternative methodology.

Injury care

Injured workers and motor vehicle accident victims are good examples of a focused population. The commonality of mecha-

Table 2. Customer expectations in spine care

Strong agreement	Strong disagreement
• Prevention education in formal (K–12) education settings	• Provider resources
• Community-based outreach partnerships (business and payers)	Specialists > PCPs
• Use of EAP services	Use of physician extenders
• Use of case managers (liaisons)	• "Optimum benefit" as a basis to stop care
• Patients learn to manage long-term effects	• Need for long-term follow-up

nisms of injury and the knowledge of typical course and outcome permits predictions that generally apply. Management, in a sense, can be done by exception. Evidence-based protocols can be applied that give guidance from triage to rehabilitation. Progress can be monitored with valid outcome measures to anticipate the need for changing the treatment plans early when progress begins to lag. The effect is to address the expectations of the patients and payers with focus to reduce work-time loss, enhancing functional status upon return to work. All, hopefully, accomplished at a minimum for both direct and indirect health costs. While there is ample evidence of significant regional variations in practice,[17,18] it is clear that chiropractic practice can be cost- and time effective.[17,19,20] Appropriately coupled as a part of the health care team, there is every reason to believe that such efficiency can be leveraged even for chronic, severe, and complex cases.

Limitations in achieving such ends are strengthened by perceptions that an alarming number of health care providers have entered into questionable, if not illegal, practices purely for financial gain.[21] Injury care is particularly susceptible to misleading billing schemes including upcoding, multiple fee schedules, and misrepresentation of provider type performing services. In response, public and private sector health care organizations have integrated many aspects of managed care into their delivery and reimbursement mechanisms (eg, preauthorization, provider credentialing, concurrent peer or utilization review, retrospective review)[22] and antifraud investigation functions.

Complicated cases

Clinical outcomes depend on a balance between the constellation of factors that affect patient status (Table 3), and the effectiveness of treatment administered. Depending on the individual case complexity, that effectiveness may rely on the dexterity with which the managing physician coordinates multiple providers and services. The effects of age, pathology, comorbid disease, postsurgical anatomy, and psychosocial factors most often define complexity. The greater the complexity, the more resources may be necessary to bring the patient's problem under control.

For example, segmental instability, failed back syndrome, pseudoarthrosis, degenerative scoliosis, and severe osteopenia are all physical features of pathology or postsurgical anatomy. Each requires modification and adaptation of manipulation techniques to accommodate the more fragile tissues. Similarly, patients with diabetes, peripheral vascular disease, or neuropathy may not be able to tolerate adjunctive thermal therapies. Those with gastric sensitivity may not be able to have a referral for antiinflammatory medications.

A case in point is a 58-year-old female originally diagnosed with painful discs from two-level lumbar degenerative disc disease. She was treated unsuccessfully by anterior, interbody fusion. Following her surgical recovery, her pain was unchanged at a VAS level of 8.5/10. A chronic gastrointestinal ulcer condition prevented use of antiinflammatory medication. Her chiropractic provider requested a provocative diagnostic injection of the sacroiliac joint. The patient responded with 100% relief of pain for 4 hours. Interferential therapy at 4,000 Hz was used for pain management and a second application of 80–120 Hz reduced local spasm. Manipulation of the sacroiliac was implemented using continuous passive motion and modified diversified procedures to account for the recent surgery. Resistive exercises and stretching were used daily at home. After 4 weeks, a 30% reduction of pain was noted, motion was returned to normal but endurance for upright activity remained limited at 30 minutes. At that point, manipulation under joint anesthesia (MUJA) techniques were applied where the patient underwent sacroiliac injection followed within 1 to 4 hours by manipulation in the chiropractor's clinic. Together, the combined skills and knowledge of the chiropractor and pain management specialist unraveled complexity poorly amenable by either technique alone.

Table 3. Factors affecting clinical outcomes

Patient clinical status	Treatment methods	Complementary services
• Age and sex	• Manipulation	• Advanced diagnostics
• Comorbid illness	• Mobilization	• Medication
• Primary diagnosis	• Modalities	• Psychologic counseling
• Condition severity	• Muscle energy technique	• Physical therapy
• Clinical stability	• Exercise	• Occupational therapy
• Financial status		• Injection techniques for muscle, joint, and disc
• Work or life habits		
• Cultural, ethnic attributes		
• Psychosocial functioning		

INTEGRATION OF THE CHIROPRACTOR INTO THE MULTIDISCIPLINARY SETTING

The integrated delivery system focusing on specific disease entities is an emerging practice style that offers many attractive features to payers and patients.[16,23] There is growing sentiment that the fragmented system where a PCP at one site attempts to manage care of specialists scattered in other sites is inefficient and as costly as health care before reform. Not only does it disrupt continuity of care, introducing expensive delays in appropriate treatment, but it also requires the new case management industry to make multiple contacts and office visits at higher administrative expense to the benefits plan. A multidisciplinary "one-stop shop" for spine care, for example, affords several advantages. First, treatment administered under one roof and managed by a single primary contact provider centralizes communications and medical records. It minimizes the number of case manager contacts and travel costs. Early detection of patients failing to respond to therapy can be made with rapid transition to alternate approaches.

For the practitioner, there are equally compelling advantages. Each provider sees a significant increase in value of practice support by participating in economies of scale. That is, he gets more support for the money. Teams of staff can be afforded that focus on modern health administrative services from credentialing providers, billing and collections, patient precertification to practice marketing. Administrators can administrate and doctors can focus their attention on the delivery of care. Payer groups, increasingly, are inclined to credential entire groups of providers as a unit as they tend to result in greater subscriber satisfaction with continuity of care and availability of specialists.

Optimum skill sets of integrated providers

As a new practice style, the information and skill sets that a successful participant possesses are more extensive than required for private or single specialty group practice. Substantive familiarity with procedures likely to be encountered by patients seeing other members of the multidisciplinary practice is vital. Each doctor in the group will be the attending physician and be expected to coordinate services necessary for individual cases. As such, he or she will request consultation with members of other disciplines. The doctor's credibility in the eyes of the patient will depend on the ability to make appropriate referrals, counsel on realistic expectations, and evaluate the outcome of the test or treatment procedure that was requested.

For the case of the 58-year-old female described above, in addition to the usual diagnostic and manipulative skills expected of chiropractors, they must be facile with a number of other elements (Table 4).

Triage, consultation, referral, comanagement, networking

One particular challenge found in this multidisciplinary facility was the varying levels of understanding (and comfort) of physicians, surgeons, therapists, and scheduling staff as to why a patient would see a chiropractor, and what would the chiropractor do? In the spirit of reducing the variation in understanding, and to facilitate the appropriate routing of patients to the chiropractic providers, a job aid was developed and improved using formal consensus methods involving the appropriate end users. (The result of that process is found in Fig 1.) This job aid, used as an internal document, defines those indications for chiropractic access, assessment, and management decisions. This job aid actually has three dimensions.

- The first is reading across the page (left to right) distinguishing those reasons or circumstances that a patient

Table 4. Extended information necessary for the chiropractor to adequately perform as the managing professional for the failed back, postfusion, sacroiliac patient*

- General indications for instrumented anterior interbody fusion
- Expected pathoanatomic weaknesses introduced by surgery
- Expected postsurgical course
- Ability to diagnose postfusion nonunion/pseudoarthrosis
- Familiarity with early and late phase complications
- Indications for and value of provocative sacroiliac injections
- Familiarity with procedure technique sufficient for a general description to the patient
- Ability to evaluate the short- and long-term effects
- Awareness of general contraindications for the procedure
- Awareness of alternate medical approaches and primary contraindications
- Detailed knowledge of modifications to standard manipulation procedures to accommodate postfusion pathoanatomy
- Knowledge of expected joint anesthesia effects to judge appropriate application and results of manipulation
- Detailed knowledge of adjunctive therapies useful for pain management augmenting stability of manipulation results
- Rehabilitation methods, limitations, and contraindications

*As described in the text.

would be directed to a chiropractor at Texas Back Institute; and when with a chiropractor, a list of services provided by the chiropractic staff.
- The second dimension is the vertical component (reading from top-down) segregating the issues of access or triage from assessment and diagnostic workup, to management and treatment issues.
- The third dimension is reflective of the legend designating that the services would be performed by the chiropractor as the primary provider managing the case, vs those circumstances where it is advisable for collaborative care with another specialist physician.
- And finally, the contraindications are also listed according to their need for team management or as an absolute contraindication to manipulation therapies.

This job aid has been quite useful as an internal instrument, enhancing communication among providers and staff, but also an aid in training new staff. Value has also been realized when it is used in communications with external customers, such as case managers, primary care networks, and payers.

Within a multidisciplinary culture, whether it is an established community clinic or regional clinic system, or an informal collection of collegial professional relationships in a community, expectations mature in these groups with respect to what are the best resources for specialized testing and treatment procedures. A chiropractor who works closely with an orthopaedic group or neurology group will quickly learn the "favored" resources for obtaining special imaging studies, injection procedures, neurodiagnostic studies, minimally invasive surgical procedures, and chronic pain management sequences. In the realm of spine care, there are many diagnostic and therapeutic procedures that are commonly performed. And in a community or regional health market, there can be several physicians and even physician types that can be available to perform these services. Convenient location, accessibility, and availability for your patients are important issues to be considered when choosing a provider or facility to refer your patient to. But, more importantly is the aspect of quality work. That "community" of spine specialists you will likely want to deal with are those who are intolerant of poor quality studies, poor reports, patient complaints, and just bad medicine. Fig 1 identifies the most appropriate specialist for the various spine-related procedures. This job aid also identifies what the procedure consists of, and what you as a referring provider should expect. The traffic (and communication) goes both ways. Thus, you will also see how a chiropractor may appear on this same job aid if the user were some other physician type. Fig 2 provides a triage form that facilitates referral to chiropractors at the Texas Back Institute.

COMMUNICATION: PROFESSIONALISM AND COURTESIES

Trust is earned with time and familiarity. It grows naturally from the combination of observed professionalism, collegial interaction, and the demonstration of high-quality care. Patients referred who are treated well and have good outcomes are impressed with both their doctors. No physician, regardless of discipline, is willing to continue to send patients to or comanage patients with a provider who has poor outcomes. Similarly, there will be hesitation if standard conduct of good professionalism and etiquette are ignored. Health plan administrators and case managers are no different in their response to interactions with the treating or referring physician.

Such interactions are founded on mutual respect. Respect is demonstrated through more than courteous verbal and written exchange. It is the fundamental ingredient of all interactions from contractual relationships to marketing and patient management. Whether by network participation or focused factory, the administrative services (credentialing, precertification, billing, collections, marketing), financial risks, and benefits should be on par basis among the participants. The simplest way to achieve this is to focus on the common denominator of practice—the patient—through the development of consensus-based treatment protocols and pathways. Arrangements that are based on the strata of disciplines (DC vs MD vs DO) ultimately retain more of the friction of turf conflict. Those that are based on patient care minimize and expend that friction during the healthy discussions over appropriate triage and care. Consensus takes time invested in regular, substantive, and focused interactions between all of the providers who are a part of the team. The exercise of developing the protocols exposes the evidence supporting referral, the ambiguities remaining and the clinical logic that permeates the group. As patient comanagement progresses, our experience shows an expanding understanding of how cross referrals (DC–MD, MD–DC, MD–complementary, DC–complementary) can speed patient recovery and strengthen the cohesion of the group.

What does it take to open access to care in the evolving market? In our experience, it is the development of collaborative relationships that strategically focus on customer expectations, offering greater value of service.

REFERENCES

1. Enzmann DR. *Surviving in Health Care.* Mosby; St. Louis, MO: 1997.
2. Wechsler J. Small business executives back consumer protections. *Manag Healthcare.* 1988; August: 7.
3. Shekelle PG, Adams A, Chassin MR, Hurwitz EL, Brook RH. Spinal manipulation for low back pain. *Ann Intern Med.* 1992;117(7):590–598.
4. Bigos S, Bowyer O, Braen G, et al. *Acute Low Back Problems in Adults. Clinical Practice Guidelines No. 14.* Rockville, MD: AHCPR; 1994. AHCPR Publication No. 95-0642.
5. Bush T, Cherkin D, Barlow W. The impact of physician attitudes on patient satisfaction with care of low back pain. *Arch Fam Med.* 1993;2(3):301–305.
6. Eisenberg DM, Kessler RC, Foster C, Norlock FE, Calkins DR, Delbanco TL. Unconventional medicine in the United States: prevalence, costs, and patterns of use. *N Engl J Med.* 1993;328:246–252.
7. Barnett PB. Clinical communication and managed care. *Med Group Manage J.* 1998;45(4):60–66.
8. Deyo RA. Tsui-Wu JY. Descriptive epidemiology of low back pain and its related medical care in the United States. *Spine.* 1987;12:264–268.
9. Deyo RA. Plenary Presentation. Institute for Healthcare Improvement Congress on Low Back Pain; St. Louis, Missouri; February 18, 1998.
10. Hurwitz EL, Coulter ID, Adams AH, Genovese BJ, Shekelle PG. Use of chiropractic services from 1985 through 1991 in the United States and Canada. *Am J Public Health.* 1998;88(5):771–776.
11. Cherkin D, Deyo RA, Berg AO. Evaluation of physician education intervention to improve primary care for low back pain: impact on patients. *Spine.* 1991;16:1,173–1,178.
12. Triano JJ, Hansen DT. Chiropractic and quality care, are they exclusive? *QME Quarterly.* (In press).
13. Hagland M. Focused factories: Giving consumers what they want. *Healthcare Forum J.* 1997;Sep/Oct:23–26.
14. Coile RC. Chiropractic treatment: An "alternative medicine" becomes mainstream health care. *Health Trends.* 1995;7(9):1–8.
15. Hansen DT, Triano JJ, Raines L. Assessment of Customer Expectations During Episodes of Back Pain. Presented at the Congress on Back Pain, Institute for Healthcare Improvement; St Louis, Missouri; February 18, 1998.
16. Pristave RJ, Becker S, McCarthy LI. Development of provider networks for specific diseases. *Health Care Innovations.* 1995;Sept/Oct:9–37.
17. Jarvis JB, Phillips RB, Morris EK. Cost per case comparison of back injury claims of chiropractic versus medical management with identical diagnostic codes. *J Occ Med.* 1991;33:847–852.
18. Carey TS, Garrett J, Jackman A, McLaughlin C. The outcomes and costs of care for acute low back pain among patients seen by primary care practitioners, chiropractors, and orthopedic surgeons. *N Engl J Med.* 1995;333:913–917.
19. Mosley CD, Cohen IG, Arnold RM. Cost-effectiveness of chiropractic in a managed care setting. *Am J Manag Care.* 1996;2(3):280–284.
20. Triano JJ, Hondras M, McGregor M. Differences in treatment history with manipulation for acute, subacute, chronic and recurrent spine pain. *J Manipulative Physiol Ther.* 1992;15(1):24–30.
21. Dahan DH. MD/DC clinic advertisement. *Dynamic Chirop.* 1998;16(19):29.
22. McElheran LJ, Sollecito PC. Delivering quality chiropractic care in a managed care setting. *Top Clin Chirop.* 1994;1(4):30–40.
23. Triano JJ, McGregor M, Skogsbergh DR. Use of chiropractic manipulation in lumbar rehabilitation. *J Rehabil Res Dev.* 1997;34(4):394–404.

	PROCEDURE	INDICATIONS PURPOSE OF PROCEDURE	COMMUNITY RESOURCES Appropriately performed by:
DIAGNOSTICS	**Clinical Laboratory**	Differential diagnosis Confirmation of "Red Flags"	Clinical laboratory Primary care center Internal medicine specialist
	Diagnostic Imaging Plain film, MRI/CT, bone scan, discogram, myelogram	Differential diagnosis Confirmation of "Red Flags" Confirm anatomy Confirm pathology Rule out contradictions for SMT	Chiropractic office (plain films) Imaging center Radiologist Neuroradiologist
	Neurophysiologic Testing Nerve conduction velocities (NCV) Electromyelogram (EMG) Somatosensory evoked potentials (SSEP)	Differential diagnosis Muscle & nerve function	Neurologist Physical medicine & rehab (PM&R)
	Diagnostic Injections SI, facet joint inj, epidural steroid (ESI) selective nerve root block (SNRB) muscle inj (myofascial)	Location of pain generator Tolerance to injections	Dolorologist, anesthesiologist PM&R, ortho/neurosurgeons Neuroradiologists
	Functional Assessment Biomechanical assessment Functional capacity evaluation Worksite evaluation	Assessment of structural stability Assessment of functional stability Ability to perform physical demands of job Assess "fit" of employee to job/tasks	Occupational medicine specialists Occupational therapists Chiropractors PM&R Physical therapists
	Behavioral Assessment	Assessment of high risk/labile patients Screening for chronic pain/disability syndrome	Psychologist
THERAPEUTICS	**Medical Management**	Management of pain, inflamation, muscle spasm, infection, depression, narcotics.	Medical practitioner, surgeon, osteopath, physician's assistant, nurse practitioner
	Therapeutic Injections SI, facet joint inj, epidural steroid (ESI) selective nerve root block (SNRB) muscle inj (myofascial), costovertebral, rhizotomy	Management of joint or nerve pain, muscle spasm, trigger points.	Dolorologist, anesthesiologist PM&R, ortho/neurosurgeons Neuroradiologists
	Mechanical/Manual therapy Mobilization, manipulation, muscle techniques	Management of joint dysfunctions, faulty body mechanics, muscle dysfunction, trigger points.	Chiropractors, osteopaths PM&R Physical & occupational therapists
	Physiological Therapeutics Hot/cold therapies, sound, light, traction, laser, etc.	Tissue healing, pain management, inflammation	Physical therapists Chiropractors
	Spine Surgery Non-fusions, fusions, deformity repair, infection repair, fracture/dislocation repair	Nerve entrapment release, discectomy, instrumented or non-instrumented fusions, scoliosis repair, spinal cord implants	Fellowship trained spine surgeons (ortho or neuro)
	Rehabilitation Therapeutic exercise, conditioning, job retraining (work hardening), back school	Therapeutic stretch and exercise, aerobic conditioning, coordination, work readiness, education	PM&R Physical therapists Chiropractors
	Behavioral Medicine	Chronic pain or disability syndromes, psychoses, depression, somatization, non-compliant, suicidal	Psychologists Psychiatrists
	Chronic Pain Management	Chronic pain or disability syndromes, nociceptive pain, non-responsive to previous pain management, addiction management, non-compliant	Multidisciplinary team - including spine surgeon, PM&R, psychologist, PT/OT, chiro and social service (rehab counselor)

Fig 1. Job aid: diagnostic and treatment implications by provider type.

What Leads a Patient to a Chiropractor
Circumstances, patient complaints or patient symptoms that lead to seeking chiropractic consultation or appointment:

Services the Chiropractor Provides
Administrative, clinical and consultative procedures and services provided by chiropractic providers:

ACCESS / TRIAGE DECISIONS

☐ Direct referral from MD/DO/DC	☐ **No Red Flags** (B) and:	☐ 1st physician-available triage	☐ Physical examination
☐ Direct referral from PT/OT/LMT	♦ Headache	☐ Conservative care consultation	☐ Ortho / neuro examination
☐ Physician requests DC or manip.	♦ Neck pain	☐ Pre-/post surgical consultation	☐ Non-invasive imaging
☐ Pt. requests DC or manip/adj.	♦ Mid-back (thoracic) pain	☐ MVA / work injury work-up	☐ Biomechanical assessment
☐ Patient request no surg or meds	♦ Low back / pelvis pain	☐ Impairment rating	☐ Scoliosis evaluation
☐ Non-critical trauma (A)	♦ Extremity symptoms		
☐ Favorable response to prev manip			

ASSESSMENT DECISIONS

☐ Painful spine motion	☐ Painful incr stiffness in local jnt	☐ Biomechanical assessment	☐ Physical examination
☐ Focal tenderness over joint	☐ Normal or stable motor function	☐ Scoliosis evaluation	☐ Ortho / neuro examination
☐ Focal muscle hypertonicity	☐ Normal/stable sensory function	☐ Health risk assessment	☐ Non-invasive imaging
☐ Focal muscle tenderness		☐ Ergonomic assessment	

MANAGEMENT DECISIONS

☐ Acute LBP w/in 1st mo of sympts	☐ Cumulative trauma disorders	☐ Tolerance to manual methods	■ Manipulation, post-injection
☐ Acute soft tissue injury	☐ Uncomplicated DJD / DDD	☐ Passive care: manipulation	■ Post-surgical mgmt (mechanical)
☐ Subacute neck pain - manip.	☐ Referred UE/LE spine rel sympt	☐ Passive care: cont. passive mob	■ Failed surgery management
☐ Pain/spasm assoc w/acute radic	☐ Extremity pain/dysfunction	☐ Passive care: muscle/trig point	■ Chronic pain management
☐ Recurrent back/neck pain	☐ Non-progr spondylo(w&w/o slip)	☐ Active care: therapeutic stretch	■ Chronic pain behav/emo overlay
☐ Chronic neck pain	■ Patient refusal of surgery	☐ Active care: therapeutic exercise	■ Pain management (w/meds)
☐ Chr back pain w/ or w/o leg pain	■ Complicated multi-joint disorders	☐ Pt education: biomechanics	■ Supportive care, disability syndr
☐ Chronically limited ROM	■ Suspected or known instability	☐ Scoliosis management/bracing	■ Supportive care, compl rehab
☐ Tension, other non-migraine HA	■ Consult: non-surgical options		

CONTRAINDICATIONS TO MANIPULATIVE THERAPIES

Legend: ■ Relative contraindication: team manage ■ Absolute contraindication

■ Undiagnosed neuro deficits	■ Suspected / known acute fx (C)	■ Area w/ malignancy	■ Clin evidence of vert-basilar synd
■ Congen / acquired deformities	■ Region w/ acute episode of RA	■ Area w/ bone/joint infection	■ Advanced osteoporosis
■ Hx circ. (CVA/TIA) deficits (C)	■ Acute myelopathy/ cauda equina	■ Progressive neuro deficits	
■ Benign bone tumors	■ Spondy w/ progressive slippage		

Annotations:
(A) Non-critical spinal trauma: lack of any spinal fracture or hard neurological signs.
(B) Red Flags: History or exam findings indicative of infection, fracture, cancer or progressive neurological deficits
(C) Contraindicated until complication or risk of complication has been ruled out by appropriate diagnostic testing.

Legend: ☐ Primary Management ■ Collaborative Care

Fig 2. Chiropractic management: indications/contraindications.

Index

A

Access to spine care, 182–192
  community perspectives, 185–186
  complicated cases, 187
  customer expectations, 185–186
  focused markets, 186–187
  injury care, 186–187
  opportunities, 183
  outcomes factors, 187
Accountability, technology assessment, history, 158–159
Algorithm by consensus, xviii
Articular dysfunction, outcomes measurement, 38
Autonomic function, 41

B

Back pain
  clinical algorithm
    diagnostic imaging, 125
    initial screening, 67
    mechanical low back pain, 68–69
  diagnostic imaging
    analysis, 120–122
    appropriateness, 119–120
    goals, 119–120
    seed algorithm, 122–123
  orthopedic testing, 59–66
    data collection, 60
    data interpretation, 60
    determining sources, 60–61
    evaluation of mechanical back pain, 61
    muscle pain, 64
    referred leg pain, 63–64
    rheumatic conditions, 64–65
    ruling out tumors, infections and visceral referral, 61
    sciatic leg pain, 61–63
    somatization disorder, 65
Bayesian analysis
  action threshold, 33
  decision analysis, 33–35
  defined, 33
  exclusion threshold, 33
  prior probability, 33–34
Blinding, technology assessment, 42
Bloodborne pathogen
  Occupational Safety and Health Administration, 20
  protection, 20

C

Care pathway, xv, xvii
Case series, technology assessment, 9
Case study, technology assessment, 10
Cervical disorder, etiologies, 71
Cervical range of motion, quantitative functional capacity evaluation, 171
Cervical spine
  clinical algorithm
    assessment, 87
    diagnostic imaging, 104–105
  diagnostic imaging, 96–101
    computed tomography, 99–100
    computed tomography myelography, 100
    conventional tomography, 101
    delayed instability, 98
    diagnostic goals, 96
    indications for imaging, 97
    indications for pillar views, 98
    initial diagnostic work-up, 96
    magnetic resonance imaging, 100–101
    myelography, 101
    patient selection, 97
    plain film radiography, 97
    prognostic significance, 98–99
    radiographic interpretation, 97–98
    subacute instability, 98
  mechanical assessment, 70–85
    active ranges of motion, 76–78
    acute or severe cervical condition, 75
    cervical active excursion ranges, 77
    cervical examination, 74–81
    chief complaint, 72
    common cervical mechanical conditions, 80–81
    common cervical regional muscular patterns, 75
    computed tomography, 83
    differential diagnosis of abnormal muscular findings, 77

expanded current and past medical histories, 72–73
functional strength testing, 79
history of present condition, 72
magnetic resonance imaging, 84
mechanical etiology, 72
mechanical provocation testing, 78, 82
monitoring strategies for functional restoration, 74
muscular function testing, 78, 79
neurologic examination, 78–81
nonmechanical pathology, 72
objectifying subjective information, 73–74
observation, 75
palpation, 75–76
passive ranges of motion, 78
patterns from muscular and joint structures, 73–74
radiographic imaging, 81–82
special studies, 81–84
structures of mechanical importance per quadrant, 76
videofluoroscopy, 84
vital signs, 74–75
work-up approach, 70–81
whiplash-induced injury, 96–101
computed tomography, 99–100
computed tomography myelography, 100
conventional tomography, 101
delayed instability, 98
diagnostic goals, 96
indications for flexion-extension lateral views, 98
indications for imaging, 97
indications for pillar views, 98
initial diagnostic work-up, 96
magnetic resonance imaging, 100
myelography, 101
patient selection, 97
plain film radiography, 97
prognostic significance, 98–99
radiographic interpretation, 97–98
subacute instability, 98
Cervical spine myelopathy, mechanical factors, 71
Chemical hazard, protection, 25
Child abuse, reporting, 25–26
Chiropractic
changing face of clinical practice, 59–60
contemporary management scenario, 38
evaluation of manpower resources, 9
integrated model, 39–41
integration of chiropractor into multidisciplinary setting, 188
management contraindications, 192
management indications, 192
systematic approach, 39–41
Chiropractic subluxation, technology assessment, 37–43
Clinical algorithm, xv, 29
action box, xx, xxi
back pain
diagnostic imaging, 125
initial screening, 67
mechanical low back pain, 68–69
caveat, xv
cervical spine
assessment, 87
diagnostic imaging, 104–105
clinical state box, xx, xxi
critiquing, xxiii
decision box, xx, xxi
defined, xvii
develoment, xviii, xxvi
diagnostic sequences, xx
endpoints of therapeutic cycles, xx
end-users, xx
evidence-based medicine
assessment of quality of evidence, 16
sequence for evidence-based assessment, 17
history, xvi
implementation, xviii
improving, xxiii
link box, xx, xxi
neck pain, diagnostic imaging, 125
quantitative functional capacity evaluation, 181
relevance, xv
terminology, xvi
testing, xxiii
titling, xx, xxiii
use of annotations, xx, xxiii
whiplash-induced injury, diagnostic imaging, 104–105
writing, xix
Clinical Efficacy and Assessment Project, 7
Clinical guideline, xvii
Clinical Laboratory Improvement Act, 18–20
Comanagement, 188–189
Communicable disease, reporting, 21–22
Communication, 189
Consensus development, technology assessment, 10
Consultation, 188–189
Cost-effectiveness analysis, 5–6
Council on Health Care Technology, 7
Courtesies, 189

D

Decision analysis, 28–36
Bayesian analysis, 33–35
caveats, 35–36
defined, 28
Decision making
diagnostic test, 31–32
expert algorithms, 29
hypothetico-deductive decision making, 29–30
integration of approaches, 30
mental processing error, 30–31
disease misclassification, 30
information gathering errors, 30
information integration errors, 30
overview, 29–33
pattern recognition, 29
physician behaviors, 29–30
reducing errors in practice, 31
Diagnostic and Therapeutic Technology Assessment, 7
Diagnostic imaging
back pain
analysis, 120–122
appropriateness, 119–120
goals, 119–120
seed algorithm, 122–123
cervical spine, 96–101
computed tomography, 99–100
computed tomography myelography, 100
conventional tomography, 101
delayed instability, 98
diagnostic goals, 96
indications for flexion-extension lateral views, 98
indications for imaging, 97
indications for pillar views, 98

initial diagnostic work-up, 96
magnetic resonance imaging, 100–101
myelography, 101
patient selection, 97
plain film radiography, 97
prognostic significance, 98–99
radiographic interpretation, 97–98
subacute instability, 98
neck pain
analysis, 120–122
appropriateness, 119–120
goals, 119–120
seed algorithm, 122–123
Diagnostic test
decision making, 31–32
design considerations for studying, 42
interpretation, 32
predictive value, 31–32
Diagnostic ultrasound
musculoskeletal system, 126
spine, 126–129
consensus statements, 128
controversies, 127–128
evaluation, 126–129
technology assessment, 126–129
Documentation, 142
Dynamic spinal loading, 40

E

Electromyography, 40
Evidence-based medicine, clinical algorithm
assessment of quality of evidence, 16
sequence for evidence-based assessment, 17
Exaggeration/overreaction, quantitative functional capacity evaluation, 171
Expert panel, 149–155
clinical decision making, 153
first round "modified-Delphi" methodology, 150
indications list development, 149–150
literature review, 149–150
method, 149–150
mobilization of cervical spine, 150–155
patient preferences, 155
research on appropriateness method, 150

second round "nominal group" methodology, 150
spinal manipulation, 150–155
utility of appropriateness ratings by non-physicians, 154–155
value of appropriateness studies to chiropractic profession, 153–154

F

Functional testing, quantitative functional capacity evaluation, 181

G

Gastrocnemius/ankle dorsiflexion test, quantitative functional capacity evaluation, 170
Grip strength dynamometry, quantitative functional capacity evaluation, 173
Gross range of motion, 39–40

H

Hamstring flexibility test, quantitative functional capacity evaluation, 172
Handwashing
guidelines, 24
procedure, 24
Health care delivery
resources, 184
trends, 183–184
Hip range of motion, quantitative functional capacity evaluation, 173
Hypothetico-deductive decision making, decision making, 29–30

I

Imaging
lumbar spine, 106–117
arthritides, 109, 111, 112
computed tomography, 107
congenital abnormalities, 108–109, 110
indications, 107
infectious disease, 110–111
magnetic resonance imaging, 107–108

myelography, 107
neoplasms, 111–115, 116, 117
plain film radiography, 106
radionuclide imaging, 108
trauma, 109–110, 113, 114, 115
radiology guidelines, 136–137
case study, 137–139
Infection control
office procedures, 24–25
supplies, 24
Intersegmental range of motion, 40

J

Job aid, diagnostic and treatment implications by provider type, 191

K

Knee flexion test/nachlas, quantitative functional capacity evaluation, 172

L

Laboratory testing, office-based, regulation, 18–20
Lumbar spine, imaging, 106–117
arthritides, 109, 111, 112
computed tomography, 107
congenital abnormalities, 108–109, 110
indications, 107
infectious disease, 110–111
magnetic resonance imaging, 107–108
myelography, 107
neoplasms, 111–115, 116, 117
plain film radiography, 106
radionuclide imaging, 108
trauma, 109–110, 113, 114, 115

M

Managed care organization, technology assessment, 161–162
Mechanical assessment, cervical spine, 70–85
active ranges of motion, 76–78
acute or severe cervical condition, 75

cervical active excursion ranges, 77
cervical examination, 74–81
chief complaint, 72
common cervical mechanical conditions, 80–81
common cervical regional muscular patterns, 75
computed tomography, 83
differential diagnosis of abnormal muscular findings, 77
expanded current and past medical histories, 72–73
functional strength testing, 79
history of present condition, 72
magnetic resonance imaging, 84
mechanical etiology, 72
mechanical provocation testing, 78, 82
monitoring strategies for functional restoration, 74
muscular function testing, 78, 79
neurologic examination, 78–81
nonmechanical pathology, 72
objectifying subjective information, 73–74
observation, 75
palpation, 75–76
passive ranges of motion, 78
patterns from muscular and joint structures, 73–74
radiographic imaging, 81–82
special studies, 81–84
structures of mechanical importance per quadrant, 76
videofluoroscopy, 84
vital signs, 74–75
work-up approach, 70–81
Medical waste
  disposal, 23
  excluded from regulations, 23
  office guidelines, 23–24
  processing, 22–24
  production, 22–23
  storage, 23
  transport, 23
  transport container criteria, 23
  treatment, 23
  types regulated, 22
Mental processing error, decision making, 30–31
  disease misclassification, 30
  errors of information integration, 30
  information gathering errors, 30

Meta-analysis, technology assessment, 10
Modified Thomas test/hip extension test, quantitative functional capacity evaluation, 172
Musculoskeletal system, diagnostic ultrasound, 126

N

National Institutes of Health
  Office of Medical Applications of Research, 7
  Technology Assessment Conferences and Workshops, 7
Neck pain, diagnostic imaging analysis, 120–122
  appropriateness, 119–120
  clinical algorithm, 125
  goals, 119–120
  seed algorithm, 122–123
Networking, 188–189

O

Occupational health regulations, 18–27
Occupational Safety and Health Administration, bloodborne pathogen, 20
Office of Health Technology Assessment, 7
Opinion survey, technology assessment, 10
Orthopedic testing, back pain, 59–66
  data collection, 60
  data interpretation, 60
  determining sources, 60–61
  evaluation of mechanical back pain, 61
  muscle pain, 64
  referred leg pain, 63–64
  rheumatic conditions, 64–65
  ruling out tumors, infections and visceral referral, 61
  sciatic leg pain, 61–63
  somatization disorder, 65
Outcomes, 184
Outcomes assessment
  articular dysfunction, 38
  assessment options, 166

quantitative functional capacity evaluation, 181
state of the art, 165–168
Outcomes assessment record, 177

P

Pain, 39
Pain provocation test, 39
Palpatory tenderness, 39
Pattern recognition, decision making, 29
Performance analysis, technology assessment, 9
Physical function, 39
Physical performance measure, 41
Physiologic measure, 41
Plain film radiography, diagnostic criteria, 132
Practice parameter, xvii
Praxis, 31
Professionalism, 189
Prone test, quantitative functional capacity evaluation, 172–173
Public health offices, state and national directory, 50–52
Public health regulations, 18–27
Public health resources, internet, 53–55

Q

Quality assurance
  radiography
    maintenance schedule, 144
    technical strategies, 135–136
  radiology, 142–145
    analysis, 142–143
    control apparatus, 143–145
    darkroom, 142–143
    documentation, 142
    generator, 143–145
    imaging receptors, 143
    maintenance, 142–143
    processor, 142–143
    radiographic exposure log, 142
    radiographic techniques, 145
Quantitative functional capacity evaluation, 165–174
  cervical range of motion, 171
  clinical algorithm, 181
  completion, 173

criteria, 167
exaggeration/overreaction, 171
functional testing, 181
gastrocnemius/ankle dorsiflexion test, 170
grip strength dynamometry, 173
hamstring flexibility test, 172
hip range of motion, 173
initial and final test, 168
knee flexion test/nachlas, 172
modified Thomas test/hip extension test, 172
outcomes assessment, 181
prone test, 172–173
regional neurology, 171
repetitive arch-up test, 172–173
repetitive sit-up, 172
repetitive squat, 168, 169
sitting test, 170–171
sitting vs. supine straight leg raise/distraction, 170–171
soleus/ankle dorsiflexion test, 170
standing test, 168
static back endurance test, 173
subjective outcome assessment instrumentation, 173
supine test, 172
supine vs. sitting SLR/distraction, 172
tests, 180
trunk rotation, 170
visual analogue scale, 168
Quantitative functional capacity results form, 178–179

R

Radiology
imaging guidelines, 136–137
case study, 137–139
influencing clinical behaviors, 136
minimizing radiation exposure, 135–140
optimizing clinical use, 131–140
patient protection, 135–136
quality assurance, 142–145
analysis, 142–143
control apparatus, 143–145
darkroom, 142–143
documentation, 142
generator, 143–145
imaging receptors, 143
maintenance, 142–143
maintenance schedule, 144
processor, 142–143
radiographic exposure log, 142
radiographic techniques, 145
technical strategies, 135–136
retakes, 135
subluxation, 88–93
appropriateness of radiography, 89–90
clinical decision making impact, 91–92
functional lesion, 89
functional lesion hypothesis, 91
future trends, 93
historical significance, 88–89
malposition hypothesis, 90–91
malposition lesion, 89
performance characteristics of appropriate test, 89
rationale for ordering radiographs, 88, 89
videofluoroscopy, 91
usefulness, 131
value as diagnostic tool, 132
reality check, 134–135
value for biomechanical assessment, 132–134
reality check, 134–135
reliability, 133–134
validity, 133
value for monitoring therapeutic progress, 134
RAND Panel for Appropriateness of Manipulation and Mobilization of the Cervical Spine, 149–155
clinical decision making, 153
first round "modified-Delphi" methodology, 150
indications list development, 149–150
literature review, 149–150
method, 149–150
mobilization of cervical spine, 150–155
patient preferences, 155
research on appropriateness method, 150
second round "nominal group" methodology, 150
spinal manipulation, 150–155
utility of appropriateness ratings by non-physicians, 154–155
value of appropriateness studies to chiropractic profession, 153–154
Randomized controlled clinical trial, technology assessment, 9
Reactive leg length discrepancy, 40–41
Referral, 188–189
Referred leg pain, 63–64
Regional neurology, quantitative functional capacity evaluation, 171
Repetitive arch-up test, quantitative functional capacity evaluation, 172–173
Repetitive sit-up, quantitative functional capacity evaluation, 172
Repetitive squat, quantitative functional capacity evaluation, 168, 169
Reproducibility, technology assessment, 42

S

Sample selection, technology assessment, 42
Sciatic leg pain, 61–63
Seed algorithm, xvii
development, xviii
graphic programs, xxii
testing, xxi
Seed guideline, xvii
development, xviii
graphic programs, xxii
testing, xxi
Seed pathway, xvii
development, xviii
graphic programs, xxii
testing, xxi
Sensitivity, technology assessment, 42
Sitting test, quantitative functional capacity evaluation, 170–171
Sitting vs. supine straight leg raise/distraction, quantitative functional capacity evaluation, 170–171
Soleus/ankle dorsiflexion test, quantitative functional capacity evaluation, 170
Specificity, technology assessment, 42
Spine, diagnostic ultrasound, 126–129
consensus statements, 128
controversies, 127–128
evaluation, 126–129
Standards of care, xvii

Standing test, quantitative functional capacity evaluation, 168
Static back endurance test, quantitative functional capacity evaluation, 173
Static postural assessment, 40
Static postural misalignment, 40
Subjective outcome assessment instrumentation, quantitative functional capacity evaluation, 173
Subluxation
  assessment methods
    reliability, 41
    usefulness, 43
  defined, 38
  measurement problems, 38
  radiography, 88–93
    appropriateness of radiography, 89–90
    clinical decision making impact, 91–92
    functional lesion, 89
    functional lesion hypothesis, 91
    future trends, 93
    historical significance, 88–89
    malposition hypothesis, 90–91
    malposition lesion, 89
    performance characteristics of appropriate test, 89
    rationale for ordering radiographs, 88, 89
    videofluoroscopy, 91
Supine test, quantitative functional capacity evaluation, 172
Supine vs. sitting SLR/distraction, quantitative functional capacity evaluation, 172

T

Technology, defined, 5
Technology assessment, 3–13

accountability, history, 158–159
attributes of practitioner knowledge of, 13
blinding, 42
case series, 9
case study, 10
chiropractic subluxation, 37–43
chiropractic techniques and procedures, 157–162
  chiropractic colleges, 159–160
  history, 158–159
  intercollegiate technology assessment, 160–161
consensus development, 10
consistency of application, 42
contemporary situation, 3–4
  provider-centered issues, 4–5
defined, 5
description, 5
diagnostic ultrasound, 126–129
four screen model, 11
guideline processes, 9–10
historical aspects, 7–9
inappropriate use, 10–13
managed care organization, 161–162
meta-analysis, 10
misconceptions and faulty assumptions, 11
opinion survey, 10
organizations involved, 7
performance analysis, 9
randomized controlled clinical trial, 9
reproducibility, 42
resource development in chiropractic, 7–9
resource list, 45–49
roles, 12
sample selection, 42
sensitivity, 42
social and non-technical aspects, 6, 7
specificity, 42

technique entrepreneurs, 161
uses, 6
Tissue compliance, 40
Triage, 188–189
Trunk rotation, quantitative functional capacity evaluation, 170
Tuberculosis, protection, 20–21

V

Vertebral subluxation, undefined, 37–38
Visual analogue scale, quantitative functional capacity evaluation, 168

W

Whiplash-induced injury
  cervical spine, 96–101
    computed tomography, 99–100
    computed tomography myelography, 100
    conventional tomography, 101
    delayed instability, 98
    diagnostic goals, 96
    indications for flexion-extension lateral views, 98
    indications for imaging, 97
    indications for pillar views, 98
    initial diagnostic work-up, 96
    magnetic resonance imaging, 100
    myelography, 101
    patient selection, 97
    plain film radiography, 97
    prognostic significance, 98–99
    radiographic interpretation, 97–98
    subacute instability, 98
  clinical algorithm, diagnostic imaging, 104–105

www.ingramcontent.com/pod-product-compliance
Ingram Content Group UK Ltd.
Pitfield, Milton Keynes, MK11 3LW, UK
UKHW051117200426
11947UKWH00038B/1825